For Betsy,

my co-author

Sandy

INTRODUCTORY HEARING SCIENCE

Physical and Psychological Concepts

SANFORD E. GERBER, Ph.D.

Associate Professor of Audiology
Speech and Hearing Center
University of California, Santa Barbara;
Research Associate
Ear Institute at
St. Francis Hospital
Santa Barbara, California

W. B. SAUNDERS COMPANY 1974
Philadelphia • London • Toronto

W. B. Saunders Company: West Washington Square
Philadelphia, Pa. 19105

12 Dyott Street
London, WC1A 1DB

833 Oxford Street
Toronto, Ontario M8Z 5T9, Canada

Library of Congress Cataloging in Publication Data

Gerber, Sanford E

Introductory hearing science.

1. Audiology.   I. Title. [DNLM: 1. Hearing.   2. Psychoacoustics.   WV270 G362i]

RF294.G25   617.8′9   73–89177

ISBN 0–7216–4104–0

Introductory Hearing Science   ISBN 0-7216-4104-0

Print No.   9   8   7   6   5   4   3   2   1

INTRODUCTORY HEARING SCIENCE

Physical and Psychological Concepts

SANFORD E. GERBER, Ph.D.

Associate Professor of Audiology
Speech and Hearing Center
University of California, Santa Barbara;
Research Associate
Ear Institute at
St. Francis Hospital
Santa Barbara, California

W. B. SAUNDERS COMPANY 1974
Philadelphia • London • Toronto

W. B. Saunders Company: West Washington Square
                         Philadelphia, Pa. 19105

                         12 Dyott Street
                         London, WC1A 1DB

                         833 Oxford Street
                         Toronto, Ontario M8Z 5T9, Canada

Library of Congress Cataloging in Publication Data

Gerber, Sanford E

Introductory hearing science.

1. Audiology.   I. Title. [DNLM: 1. Hearing.   2. Psychoacoustics.   WV270 G362i]

RF294.G25   617.8'9   73–89177

ISBN 0–7216–4104–0

Introductory Hearing Science   ISBN 0-7216-4104-0

Print No.   9   8   7   6   5   4   3   2   1

CONTRIBUTORS

BENJAMIN B. BAUER, E.E.
Vice President and Director, Acoustics Research Department, CBS Laboratories, Stamford, Connecticut.

JOSEPH RAYMOND DI BARTOLOMEO, M.D., F.A.C.S.
Research Associate, Speech and Hearing Center, University of California, Santa Barbara. Chairman, Department of Otolaryngology, Santa Barbara Medical Clinic. Chairman, Department of Otolaryngology, St. Francis Hospital. Director, Ear Institute, Santa Barbara.

DONALD G. DOEHRING, Ph.D.
Professor of Human Communication Disorders, Psychology, and Otolaryngology, McGill University, Montreal, Quebec, Canada.

SANFORD E. GERBER, Ph.D.
Associate Professor of Audiology, Speech and Hearing Center, University of California, Santa Barbara. Research Associate, Ear Institute, Santa Barbara, California.

MARK PEREGRINE HAGGARD, M.A., Ph.D.
Professor and Chairman, Department of Psychology, Queens University, Belfast, Northern Ireland.

DONALD F. KREBS, Ph.D.
Director, San Diego Speech and Hearing Center (A Division of Children's Health Center). Consultant in Audiology, U.S. Naval Hospital, San Diego, California.

HARRY LEVITT, Ph.D.
Professor of Speech and Hearing Sciences, City University of New York Graduate School. Consultant to Lexington School for the Deaf.

J. KENNETH MANHART, P.E.
Principal Acoustical Engineer, Industrial Acoustics Company, Inc., New York, New York.

ROBERT EUGENE SANDLIN, Ph.D.
Lecturer, San Diego State University. Consultant, U.S. Naval Hospital, San Diego. Director of Professional Services, San Diego Speech and Hearing Center, San Diego, California.

BARRY VOROBA, Ph.D.
Instructor, Audiology and Speech Pathology, Brooklyn College, City University of New York, Brooklyn, New York.

HISASHI WAKITA, Ph.D.
Research Engineer at the Speech Communications Research Laboratory, Inc., Santa Barbara, California.

FOREWORD

Despite the tremendous progress that has been made over the past 20 years in the field of hearing, no new introductory textbook has been produced. Those who have been searching for a book pertaining to fundamentals of hearing science will find Dr. Gerber's *Introductory Hearing Science* to be a work which has long been needed in this field. The text is a careful presentation of basic principles elucidated by numerous graphs and illustrations.

In this book Dr. Gerber and his collaborators, who represent distinct areas of competence and are specialists in their own right, offer the undergraduate student their broad experience as scientists, clinicians, and dedicated teachers. They represent different institutions and environments which are not restricted to the university setting.

As an otorhinolaryngologist I feel that this book fills the longstanding need for a "basic book" on the subject of hearing. It certainly satisfies my requirements and exceeds my expectations.

BASHARAT JAZBI, M.D., D.L.O.

PREFACE

It is now more than 35 years since the publication of *Hearing* by Stevens and Davis, and over 20 years since the appearance of Hirsh's *The Measurement of Hearing*. In the last few years there has been a substantial publication effort for books about audiometry, but there have been no books on basic auditory science. We intend this book to fill part of the need for an introductory book.

As a university teacher of audiology, I have been disturbed by the apparent fact that my students have so little information about the physical and psychological processes inherent in audition when they begin my classes. Published materials fall into three classes: too hard, too easy, too old. We use the two classic volumes mentioned above, but their very age indicates that some of the things we teach at present cannot be found there. There are no new books introductory to the study of audiology. This may be due in part to the absence of any one person completely qualified to write such a book. With that in mind, I attempted to assemble a panel of experts and asked each of them to contribute to this volume.

Audiology is a science and is subject to the methods of science and its techniques of measurement. The book is divided into four parts after the Introduction. Part One consists of only one chapter, which deals with the structure and function of the auditory organ. Part Two deals with the physics of sound and with electroacoustic devices to draw the direct relevance of physics to the study of audition and to consider the specifics of acoustics required for the study of auditory processes and the applied physics of sound in electroacoustic transducers, audiometers, and hearing aids. Having completed the study of physical acoustics and electroacoustics in Part Two, we turn our attention in Part Three to psychological acoustics: absolute and relative thresholds, pitch, loudness, temporal phenomena in hearing, and binaural hearing. The study of the physics and psychology of hearing is eventually directed toward the study of hearing for speech. Therefore, Part Four of the book is devoted to this important topic. It deals with the acoustic properties of speech and speech sounds, and concludes with a chapter on speech perception.

My contributing authors and I have entered into this book project in the hope that it could serve as an introductory text for the undergraduate student of audiology and speech pathology or experimental psychology. In fact, we are hopeful that the book will be of interest and utility to students of other disciplines as well. For example, students of music, of communications engineering, and of otolaryngology ought to find it useful to acquire a basic understanding of psychoacoustics and the acoustics of speech.

I am grateful to many people for their efforts in this project. The confidence of the W. B. Saunders Company for taking on the project is central to our appreciation. One of those very undergraduates to whom the book is addressed, Miss Elizabeth Skarakis, did all the bibliographic checking and correcting; she accomplished a monumental task with efficiency and good humor. Ann Bredhof and Jan de Grandchamp did a lot of the typing, fitting it into their other chores. And, especially, my wife Louise, who takes pride in all of my accomplishments, is responsible for the work coming to fruition.

SANFORD E. GERBER

CONTENTS

Chapter Twelve

INTRODUCTION: METHODS AND MEASUREMENTS

Audiology is the science of hearing in all its aspects. In this book, one attempts to learn some basic scientific facts about hearing. Audiology is one of those words combined from Greek and Latin: the Greek *logos* in the sense of discourse or reckoning, and the Latin *audire,* meaning to hear. Therefore, "audiology" literally means to discourse about hearing. And the *science* of hearing, audiology, is to discourse about hearing in a systematic way.

METHOD

The question, "How do we know what we know?" is essential to any scientific endeavor. So, what is scientific method? Or, better for our purposes, what is *psychophysical* method?

In 1965, Mueller reminded us that most people have some notion of *threshold:* we believe that some sounds are loud enough to be heard and others are not; some lights are bright enough to be seen and others are not; some stimuli are above threshold and others are not. But how would we go about learning this given a real person? We can ask him; but the problem is, how do we ask him? What do we ask him to *do*? To what do we ask him to respond, and in what way do we present the stimuli to which we want responses? His responses to audible stimuli constitute the subject matter of this book.

An excellent discussion of psychophysical method was that given by the late distinguished psychologist S. S. Stevens in 1951, and the reader is urged to look there to find the rest of the meat to go on these bones. Stevens listed seven of the methods by which we may elicit psychological responses to physical events; the relation between the physical and psychological worlds is described by the word *psychophysics*. The table

1

Some Methods of Psychophysics

METHOD	BRIEF CHARACTERIZATION	USUAL STATISTICAL INDEX	PROBLEMS TO WHICH MOST APPLICABLE
1. Adjustment (average error)	Observer adjusts stimulus until it is subjectively equal to or in some desired relation to a criterion.	Average of settings (average error of settings measures precision).	Absolute threshold Equality Equal intervals Equal ratios
2. Minimal change (limits)	Experimenter varies stimulus upward and/or downward. Observer signals its apparent relation to a criterion.	Average value of stimulus at transition point of observer's judgment.	All thresholds Equality
3. Paired comparison	Stimuli are presented in pairs. Each stimulus is paired with each other stimulus. The observer indicates which of each pair is greater in respect to a given attribute.	Proportion of judgments calling one stimulus greater than another. (These proportions are sometimes translated into scale values via the assumption of a normal distribution of judgments.)	Order Equal intervals (under 'distribution' assumption)

4. Constant stimuli	Several comparison stimuli are paired at random with a fixed standard. Observer says whether each comparison is greater or less than the standard. (A special case of paired comparisons.)	Size of difference limen equals stimulus distance between 50 and 75 per cent points on psychometric function.	All thresholds Equality Equal intervals Equal ratios
5. Quantal	Various fixed increments are added to a standard, with no time interval between. Each increment is added several times in succession. Observer indicates apparent presence or absence of the increment.	Size of sensory quantum equals distance between intercepts of rectilinear psychometric function.	Differential thresholds
6. Order of merit	Group of stimuli, presented simultaneously, are set in apparent rank order by the observer.	Average or median rank assigned by observers.	Order
7. Rating scale (single stimuli)	Each of a set of stimuli is given an "absolute" rating in terms of some attribute. Rating may be numerical or descriptive.	Average or median rating assigned by observers.	Order Equal intervals Stimulus rating

shown lists Stevens' seven psychophysical methods. First is the method of *adjustment* (or average error) which is useful for measuring absolute thresholds, equality, equal intervals, or equal ratios (cf. Chapter 5). Second is the method of *limits* (or minimal change), the one usually applied in clinical audiometry as it is useful for the measurement of any threshold. Third is the method of *paired comparison* by which a subject may be asked to judge which of two tones is louder, or which of two lights is brighter, or which of two substances is sweeter. The method of paired comparison is applicable to any problem in which the stimuli are to be ordered or arranged according to equal intervals. The fourth method, *constant stimuli,* is the case wherein several different stimuli are to be compared with a fixed reference. The method of constant stimuli is the one used to make judgments of equal loudness (cf. Chapter 7). In Stevens' fifth method, the *quantal* method, fixed increments are added to some standard stimulus, and the subject is asked only to judge if he perceives the increments, as for example in the measurement of differential thresholds (cf. Chapter 5). The sixth is the *order of merit* method whereby the experimenter asks the observer to place stimuli in some kind of rank order. Last is the *rating scale* method (or method of single stimuli) by which observers are asked to make absolute judgments. These are frequently numerical judgments—for example, of the kind where listeners may be asked to assign a number to each of a series of tones to describe their loudnesses. Certainly, there are more than seven psychophysical methods, but these are the ones traditionally employed. Chapter 5 discusses these methods more fully.

MEASUREMENT

What sorts of scales may be rendered by psychophysical methods? Again, the student is referred to Stevens (1951) for a lengthier discussion. The point is that we need somehow to describe the results of psychophysical experiments and must perforce develop appropriate scales. Four scales are commonly used in psychophysics: nominal, ordinal, interval, and ratio.

SCALES

The *nominal* scale is one in which numbers are used as names, but are not used to describe relative or absolute merit or size. For example, one should not suggest that because he wears number 18, Roman Gabriel is twice as good a quarterback as Sonny Jurgensen who wears number 9. The numbers indicate only that he is another person.

On the other hand, the numbers in an *ordinal* scale do indicate a kind of rank order if not an actual size. We know that Second Street is usually the block after First Street, but it is not necessarily bigger or better than

First Street. The numbers indicate only the order of occurrence. Hence, these ordinal numbers are not only names, but also help us to know where to expect them.

To know the size of a difference requires an *interval* scale. On an interval scale, the numbers do indicate relative distances, relative sizes, or relative merits. On an interval scale, the distance from First Street to Second Street must be equal to the distance from Second Street to Third Street; quarterback number 18 really is twice as good as quarterback number 9; and I do weigh twice as much as someone who scales half the number of pounds. Probably, the interval scale is the one which most pervades our daily lives.

The *ratio* scale describes not only the sizes of things being scaled but also their sizes relative to other similar things. Scales of pitch (Chapter 6) and of loudness (Chapter 7) are ratio scales. On a ratio scale, the distance from First Street to Second Street is more than the distance from Second Street to Third Street (2:1 as compared with 3:2). Ratio scales are critical to our understanding of auditory processes. In Chapter 2 you are introduced to the notion of the "decibel" which is a numeric device to describe ratios.

STATISTICS

Given the methods of gaining information, and given the kinds of numbers which may be applied to data derived by these methods, we are still required to find the means to make reasonable generalizations about what we have learned. These means are usually called "statistics." We measure ultimately by statistical procedures. When we say that one stimulus value is greater than another to observers, we imply that we have some assurance that this is true. Furthermore, we imply that we know how often it is true and when it can be expected to be true in the future. We say that some differences are "significant" and others are not. So, statistics are implicit throughout the following material, and are often explicit.

CONCLUSION

It is evident that the book which follows is quantitative in nature. Audiology is a quantitative science, and, finally, a clinical science. For the clinician it is mandatory to know how much hearing has been lost, how much regained, how useful is a hearing aid, how beneficial a therapy. So, audiology eventually becomes audiometry, that is, the measurement of hearing. Measurement means assigning numerals to things according to rules. "Having determined the rules for assignment, we must now proceed to determine what are the observable events in hearing" (Hirsh, 1952). These observable events are the subject matter of this book.

REFERENCES

Hirsh, I. J. (1952): *The Measurement of Hearing*. New York, McGraw-Hill Book Co.
Mueller, C. G. (1965): *Sensory Psychology*. Englewood Cliffs, N.J., Prentice-Hall.
Stevens, S. S. (1951): Mathematics, measurement, and psychophysics. In S. S. Stevens
(ed.): *Handbook of Experimental Psychology*. New York, John Wiley & Sons.

Part One

ANATOMY AND PHYSIOLOGY OF THE EAR

Before we can intelligently discuss the several physical and psychological phenomena involved in audition, we must have some picture of the place in which these originate. The first chapter reviews the anatomy (structure) and the physiology (operation) of the peripheral auditory system. Of course, the student of audiology is required to have a more detailed and thorough understanding of aural anatomy and physiology than we have presented, and he will acquire this important knowledge during his studies. These topics are important for our present purpose also, and the single chapter of Part One reviews these for us. In Chapter 1, we explain that the ear operates as a series of transducers,* amplifying, altering, and modifying the incoming sound wave. We demonstrate the series of physical changes which an audible stimulus undergoes from acoustic to mechanical to hydraulic forms and emphasize the basic fact of biological early warning provided by this system.

---

*See Chapter 3 for an explanation of this word.

Chapter One

ANATOMY AND PHYSIOLOGY OF THE EAR

Joseph R. Di Bartolomeo

For all forms of animal life, the ear serves as one of the most important sensory organs. In lower animals, the purpose of hearing is mainly protective while in higher animals, it provides for both the reception of sound and spatial orientation. While one ear alone permits the reception of sound, the presence of two enables one to localize the direction of sound (cf. Chapter 9). In man, the hearing organ is not only protective, but also enables him to satisfy one of his most basic needs—his determination to exchange thoughts and to communicate. In serving man this way, the ear has been recognized as his most important sensory organ.

Anatomically, the ear is one of the most complex structures within the human body. It is housed within the temporal bone, the hardest bone of the body, to allow for adequate protection of the delicate ear structures. The central core of the temporal bone is hollowed out with channels and cavities to provide for the basic apparatus of the ear. Within one of these chambers, we find the smallest bones and the smallest muscles of the body. Other critical structures, such as the facial nerve, lie interlaced among these structures of the ear. The facial nerve innervates the muscles that give us facial expression. Another nerve which courses through the ear, the chorda tympani, provides the fibers for the sensation of taste of the anterior two-thirds of the tongue and for stimulation of saliva-producing glands. Finally, the temporal bone is the main corridor through which pass the major blood vessels of the brain; the internal carotid artery and internal jugular vein.

EMBRYOLOGY

In man, the ear is the first organ of special sense to become differentiated. Many of its elements are actually derived from the branchial apparatus which serves the respiratory function in aquatic and amphibious creatures (Fig. 1–1). During the early stages of fetal development, six visceral arches appear on the lateral aspect of the head as ridges separated from each other by a series of furrows. Just above the groove between the first (mandibular) and second (hyoid) branchial arches is the primordium of the ear which begins as a placodal thickening. The placode becomes dimpled to form an auditory pit which further invaginates to become the definitive *otocyst*. The auricle and external auditory canal develop from the first branchial groove between the first and second branchial arches. The middle ear cavity and Eustachian tube arise from the inner depression between the first and second arches called the first pharyngeal pouch. The first branchial arch gives rise to the malleus and incus, while the stapes develops from the second branchial arch. Unlike the outer and middle ear structures which develop from mesenchyme (i.e., the primordium for connective tissue structures), the inner ear is derived from ectoderm in the region of the hindbrain.

It is amazing that the inner ear has reached its full adult size and form by the end of the fourth fetal month. By the sixth week of embryonic life,

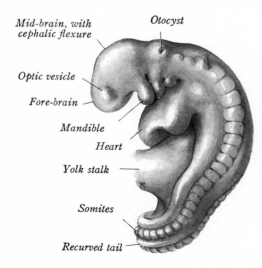

Mid-brain, with
cephalic flexure

Otocyst

Optic vesicle

Fore-brain

Mandible

Heart

Yolk stalk

Somites

Recurved tail

Figure 1–1 Human embryo of 26 days, showing first and second branchial grooves and the otic pit preliminary to formation of otocyst. (From Arey, L. B.: Developmental Anatomy, 7th ed. Philadelphia, W. B. Saunders Co., 1965.)

the semicircular canals are well formed. At approximately the ninth fetal week, the ossicles have achieved a miniature size of the general configuration characteristic of their appearance in the adult. However, they will increase their overall dimension approximately three times over the next three months. The ultimate size of the stapes is attained by the end of the seventh fetal month. During the last month of fetal life, full pneumatization of both tympanum and epitympanum is virtually attained, but the actual tympanic space continues to enlarge after birth. Since the cochlear end organ is the last of the labyrinthine structures to develop, it is more subject to developmental anomalies than the vestibular system.

At first, the mastoid antrum is present only as a single air cell. After birth, the antrum enlarges backward and downward within the mastoid process and becomes recognizable at the end of the second year. In the newborn infant, the external auditory canal is approximately two-thirds its adult size. Also, the auricle is not fully developed until the fifth or sixth year of life. Even before man is born, the ear is the first organ of special sense to be differentiated. In fact, responses to sound can be demonstrated in a fetus of 26 weeks (Johannson, Wedenberg, and Westin, 1964).

GROSS STRUCTURES

The ear may be anatomically divided into three separate parts: the external ear, the middle ear, and the inner ear (Fig. 1–2).

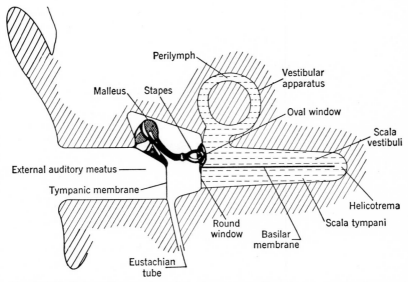

Figure 1–2 Schematic drawing of the human ear. Sound waves enter the external meatus, and move the tympanic membrane which sets the three ossicles in motion. When the stapes footplate moves inward, the perilymph inside the cochlea flows in the direction of the helicotrema and makes the round-window membrane bulge outward. All these movements can be observed with the aid of a microscope. (From Stevens, S. S. (ed.): Handbook of Experimental Psychology. New York, John Wiley and Sons, Inc., 1951, p. 1076.)

THE EXTERNAL EAR

The external ear consists of an auricle and an external auditory canal. The auricle (or pinna) is a corrugated flap of skin-covered cartilage which projects from the side of the head. It has an inferior pendulous portion which is free of cartilage, called the lobule. At the lowermost portion of its attachment to the head, the auricle has a scooped-out area called the *concha* which leads to the opening of the external auditory canal. The cartilage of the auricle continues inward to become the supporting structure for the outer third of the ear canal. The inner two-thirds of the ear canal is formed by the bone of the temporal bone. Anterior to the opening of the external auditory canal is a small, flat projection of skin called the *tragus*. The skin at the entrance of the ear canal contains both sebaceous glands and hair follicles. While fine hair may line the cartilaginous portion of the ear canal, large terminal hairs are usually present on the tragus. These occur especially in males and represent a secondary sexual characteristic. The bony portion of the ear canal ends blindly at the tympanic membrane. The external canal contains the glands which produce *cerumen*, commonly known as earwax. This material usually consists of white, watery droplets when produced, which, over a period of time, become darkened, thickened, sticky, and semi-solid.

There are two constrictions which occur within the external auditory canal. One is at the junction of the cartilaginous and bony portions, and the second is deeper to it at a region called the *isthmus* of the ear canal. The isthmus is the narrowest portion of the ear canal.

THE MIDDLE EAR

The *tympanic membrane* separates the external auditory canal from the middle ear. The middle ear cavity is approximately the size of a large pea and resembles a small room with six sides. The lateral wall is partly made up of the tympanic membrane (Fig. 1–3). This is a pearly gray, pie-shaped structure of approximately nine millimeters in diameter and slightly higher than it is wide. Its thickness is about 0.01 millimeter although composed of four layers. The superficial layer is continuous with the lining of the external auditory canal and is composed of skin. The inner surface is a mucous membrane which is continuous with the lining of the middle ear. Between these two surfaces is a double-thick middle layer of supporting connective tissue. Superiorly, there is a wedge-shaped area which is lacking the supporting layer, called the pars flaccida. The lateral surface of the eardrum membrane is seen as a concave structure with a central prominence called the *umbo*. This name is derived from the Latin meaning "the knob on the center of a warrior's shield." In the superior quadrant of the middle ear cavity we find one of the ossicles, the malleus, embedded within the layers of the tympanic membrane in a position similar to the spoke of a wheel.

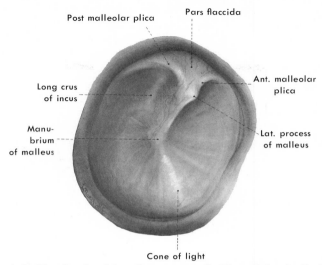

Post malleolar plica

Pars flaccida

Long crus
of incus

Ant. malleolar
plica

Manu-
brium
of malleus

Lat. process
of malleus

Cone of light

Figure 1-3 The drumhead (membrana tympani). (From Boies, L. R., Hilger, J. A., and Priest, R. E.: Fundamentals of Otolaryngology, 4th ed. Philadelphia, W. B. Saunders Co., 1964, p. 8.)

In total, the ossicles are three in number and form a chain from the tympanic membrane to the oval window (Fig. 1–4). The chain traverses the middle ear cavity suspended by ligaments and connected as joints. Since the ossicles resemble the blacksmith's forge, they are popularly known as the hammer, the anvil, and the stirrup. The hammer, or *malleus*, is the longest of the ossicles and is attached to the tympanic membrane. The anvil, or *incus*, resembles a bicuspid tooth and forms the link between the malleus and the stirrup. The stirrup, or *stapes*, is the smallest bone of the body. The flat portion of the stapes (the footplate) is embedded within the *oval window* (fenestra ovalis) in the medial wall of the middle ear cavity. In this way, a direct connection is provided between the middle ear and the inner ear.

Along the medial wall of the middle ear, several structures can be identified (Fig. 1–5). Superiorly, we see the bulge of the horizontal semicircular canal of the inner ear. Below this, we find the facial nerve and still lower is the oval window. Beneath this is the promontory which is actually a bulge in the medial wall caused by the inner ear. The lowermost structure is a central depression which is a small pocket called the *round window* (fenestra rotunda) which also leads to the inner ear. The facial nerve passes through the middle ear to supply the muscles of the face. One of its branches, the chorda tympani, passes between the malleus and incus to supply taste to the anterior two-thirds of the tongue and stimulatory fibers to the salivary glands. The anterior side of the middle ear contains the opening of a tube which extends from the middle ear to the back of the nose. This structure is the *eustachian tube*, named after

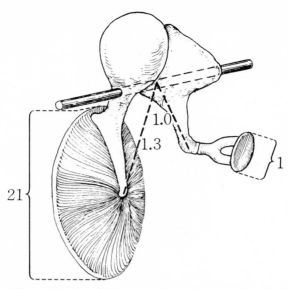

Figure 1–4 The areal ratio of the tympanic membrane and oval window, and the lever ratio of the ossicular chain. (From Paparella, M. M., and Shumrick, D. A. (eds.): Textbook of Otolaryngology, Vol. I. Philadelphia, W. B. Saunders Co., 1973, p. 268.)

Bartolomeo Eustachio (1520–1574), who at one time held the chair of anatomy at the University of Rome. In 1562, he wrote what is probably the earliest work dealing exclusively with the ear, "Epistola de Auditis Organis." The eustachian tube is approximately 1½ inches long in the adult. The opening of the eustachian tube into the middle ear is surrounded by bone for one-third its length. The remaining two-thirds is cartilage and opens into the nasopharynx. In the posterior wall of the middle ear space we see a passage, called the aditus ad antrum, leading backward to the mastoid antrum. Two small muscles, the *stapedius* and the *tensor tympani*, can be seen within the middle ear space. The stapedius muscle, which is the smallest muscle in the body, acts as a check rein on the stapes. The tensor tympani is attached to the malleus where its function is evident from its name.

THE INNER EAR

The inner ear lies in the petrous portion of the temporal bone. Here we find the sensory end organ receptors for hearing (the *cochlea*) and equilibrium (the *labyrinth*). The inner ear may be compared to a tortuous series of passageways which are double-chambered. The outer chamber, the wall, is completely bony and called therefore the *bony labyrinth* (Fig. 1–6). The inner chamber contains the sensory organs for hearing and for

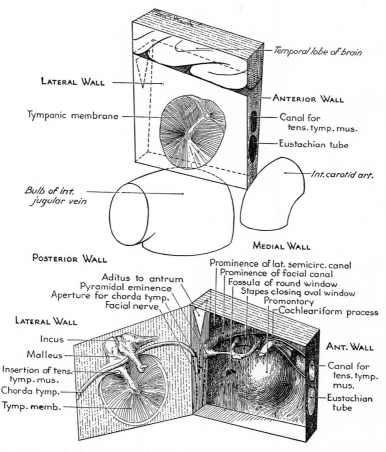

Figure 1-5 A diagrammatic scheme of the shape and relationships of the middle ear structures. (From Boies, L. R., Hilger, J. A., and Priest, R. E.: Fundamentals of Otolaryngology, 4th ed. Philadelphia, W. B. Saunders Co., 1964, p. 9.)

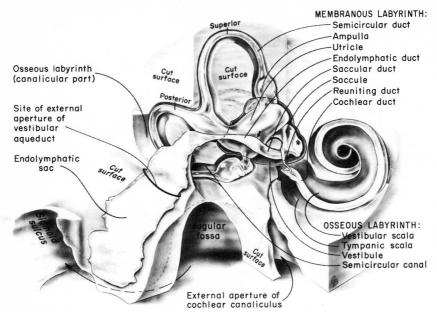

Figure 1–6 Membranous and osseous labyrinth. Reconstruction prepared by the Born method. Adult, 69 years of age. (Wisconsin Collection.) This demonstrates especially the relations between the membranous and bony labyrinths, but in particular, the form, size, and relations of the endolymphatic sac. The saccus extends for a considerable distance beyond the external aperture of the vestibular aqueduct into the posterior cranial fossa. In the latter position it occupies a foveate impression on the posterior surface of the petrous pyramid where it may be prolonged inferiorly to the level of the sulcus for the sigmoid venus sinus. The unlabeled arrow points to the utriculo-endolymphatic duct; the asterisk is on the saccule. (From Paparella, M. M., and Shumrick, D. A. (eds.): Textbook of Otolaryngology, Vol. I. Philadelphia, W. B. Saunders Co., 1973, p. 93.)

balance and is called the *membranous labyrinth* (Fig. 1–7). The space between the membranous labyrinth and the bony labyrinth is filled with a supporting fluid called *perilymph*. The membranous labyrinth itself is a passageway which contains a fluid within its inner lumen called *endolymph*. These two passageways begin at the *vestibule.*

Just beyond the oval window niche is found the vestibule of the inner ear. This is similar to an antechamber or central foyer joining two passageways leading to the labyrinth posteriorly and the cochlea anteriorly. The cochlea is a tube which is curled upon itself two and a half times and so resembles a snail (Fig. 1–6). From the vestibule, the labyrinth is a passageway that extends posteriorly and itself soon divides into three circular or ring-shaped passages called the *semicircular canals*. Both the labyrinthine and cochlear structures are surrounded by a bony capsule called the *otic capsule* which contains the perilymph as a fluid cushion. Furthermore, the labyrinth and the cochlea themselves are hollowed out to contain the inner fluid, endolymph. The endolymph, then, is continuous

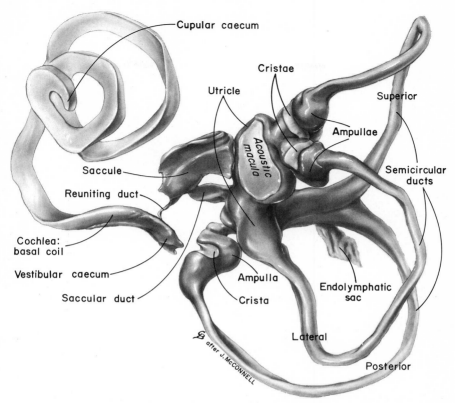

Figure 1-7 Membranous labyrinth. (From Paparella, M. M., and Shumrick, D. A. (eds.): Textbook of Otolaryngology, Vol. I. W. B. Saunders Co., 1973, p. 95.)

throughout the cochlea and membranous labyrinth. In the semicircular canals, the endolymph bathes the small sensory organs for balance known as the *crista*; while in the cochlea, the endolymph is in contact with the terminal hair cells of the sensory organ for hearing, the *organ of Corti* (Fig. 1–8), named for Alphonse Corti who described it in 1851. For a detailed discussion of the inner ear, the reader is referred to an appropriate text such as *Otolaryngology*, edited by Paparella and Shumrick.

PHYSIOLOGY OF THE EAR

Lower forms of animals, such as fish, are able to perceive vibratory phenomena transmitted directly from the aquatic (fluid) environment to the fluids of the inner ear. The vibrations set up in the surrounding water can directly affect the fluid of the inner ear. However, the lifespan of higher vertebrates is usually spent on land in an airfilled milieu. Thus, in

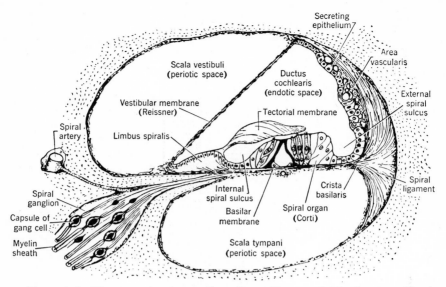

Figure 1–8 Diagrammatic cross section of a cochlear canal. The ductus cochlearis (or scala media) contains the organ of Corti with its hair cells, the ultimate end organs of hearing. (From Stevens, S. S. (ed.): Handbook of Experimental Psychology. New York, John Wiley and Sons, Inc., 1951, p. 1117.)

the natural environment of man, air molecules provide the medium for the transmission of sound. Since the organ of Corti of man rests within a fluid medium, a mechanism is required to transduce the energy of sound from a gaseous to a fluid medium. The middle ear provides a system to match the impedances for sound transmission from air to fluid; otherwise, 99 per cent of sound energy (30 dB) will be lost (Fig. 1–9). In this way, the qualities of sound transmission in air (high amplitude with low pressure) are converted to those of a fluid medium (low amplitude, high pressure). The factors of mass, stiffness, and friction diminish the efficiency of sound transport in the normal ear. Anatomically, the *mass* of the sound conductive system is represented by the tympanic membrane, the ossicular chain, and the intralabyrinthine fluids. It is the pressure gradient on both sides of the tympanic membrane, the tension of the tympanic membrane, the tone of the middle ear muscles, and the ligaments and articulations which account for the *stiffness* of the sound conducting mechanism. The *frictional* resistance is brought about by the action of the middle ear muscles.

THE EXTERNAL EAR

In lower animals, the auricle is able to be directed for better collection of sound. However, in man this ability is of little purpose. The hairs

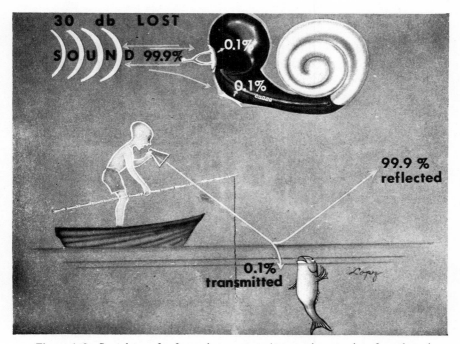

Figure 1-9   Sound transfer from air to water. At any air-water interface there is a 30-decibel loss of sound energy. This is just as true in the ear as in the sea. (From DeWeese, D. D., and Saunders, W. H.: Textbook of Otolaryngology, 2nd ed. St. Louis, Mo., C. V. Mosby Co., 1964, p. 317.)

at the entrance of the ear canal trap dust, insects, and other small particles. The wax produced possesses bactericidal qualities to guard against infection from microorganisms. The skin of the ear canal and the drum membrane has a pattern of migration which allows the ear canal to be self-cleansing. The pattern of migration is centrifugal, beginning at the umbo and extending to the opening of the canal. The overall rate of growth is equivalent to that of a fingernail, completely being replaced every three months. By having the tympanic membrane concave and cone-shaped (cf. Figs. 1-3 and 1-4), similar to a loudspeaker, it affords less distortion and broader frequency characteristics than a flat disc.

THE MIDDLE EAR

The tympanic membrane with its embedded malleus and the ossicular chain together provide a *transformer mechanism* for matching the impedance of air to that of the inner ear fluids. The ossicular chain is a lever system with a mechanical advantage of approximately 1.3:1. A second factor, the aerial ratio of the tympanic membrane to the oval window membrane, is probably even more important. The effective aerial ratio is recognized at 14:1. The aerial ratio between these two membranes increases the force of the vibrations at the oval window significantly. Thus, the transformer ratio (product of the ossicular chain lever ratio and the aerial ratio) between the tympanic membrane and the oval window membrane is approximately 18.3:1 (Paparella ànd Shumrick, 1973). The eustachian tube aids in the equalization of pressure on both sides of the tympanic membrane. Normally, the eustachian tube is closed, but it is opened by the action of the tensor and levator muscles of the palate. The opening is usually patent for about one-fifth to one-tenth of a second during the acts of swallowing, yawning, or chewing. As the stapes footplate is depressed into the oval window niche, it initiates the vibration through the inner ear fluids.

THE INNER EAR

The cochlea is a 32-millimeter-long passageway divided into an upper level (*scala vestibuli*) and a lower level (*scala tympani*) by the cochlear duct (Fig. 1–8). The scala vestibuli and the scala tympani both contain perilymph and may be compared to a U-shaped tube filled with fluid and having a diaphragm at each end: at one end is the oval window and at the other is the round window. Since fluid always maintains a fixed volume, inward displacement of the oval window causes an outward displacement at the round window.

Separating these two scalae is the *cochlear duct* which contains the organ of Corti, the sensory end organ for hearing (Fig. 1–8). The cochlear duct is a wedge-shaped compartment separated from the scala vestibuli above by *Reissner's* membrane and from the scala tympani below by the *basilar* membrane which acts as a resonating membrane within a resonating tube. The sensory end organ, the organ of Corti, lies upon the basilar membrane and contains approximately 23,000 hair cells on its free surface. The vibration of the stapes at the oval window is transmitted to the perilymph of the scala vestibuli. The vibrations are further transmitted through Reissner's membrane to the endolymph and still further through the basilar membrane to the scala tympani where they pass downward, causing a displacement of the round window. It has been demonstrated that the hair cells are arranged in rows along the two and a half turns of the cochlea (Fig. 1–10). The range of sound reception along the cochlea enables man to perceive sounds from below 100 to above 20,000 Hz. The receptors for the higher frequencies are located at the basal turn of the cochlea, while those for the low-frequency sounds are located at the apical turn. In this way, the response of the cochlea is similar to the scale of a piano. In the cochlea, two essential phenomena take place, namely *transmission* and *transduction*. Transmission accounts for the transfer of acoustic energy from the oval window to the hair cells, while transduction is a process by which the sound energy pattern is converted at the organ of Corti into electrical action potentials in the auditory nerve endings.

Figure 1–10 Innvervation of the organ of Corti (cat). Auditory nerve fibers (AN), with their cell bodies in the ganglion of Corti (GC), end in the organ of Corti (OC). Internal hair cells (IHC) receive radial fibers (RF) and collaterals from internal spiral fibers (ISF). External hair cells (EHC) receive collaterals mainly from external spiral fibers (ESF). An external hair cell is innervated by many fibers; an internal hair cell by a few. The function of the internal spiral and centrifugal (CF) fibers is unknown. (From Stevens, S. S. (ed.): Handbook of Experimental Psychology. New York, John Wiley and Sons, Inc., 1951, p. 1119.)

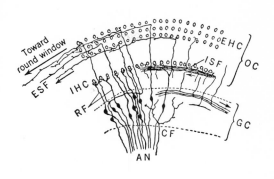

SUMMARY

Various forms of energy are converted to serve the function of hearing in man. The energy of the transmission of sound through the movement of air molecules must be converted at the tympanic membrane into mechanical energy to cause displacement of the footplate of the stapes. Inward displacement of the footplate of the stapes initiates the vibration of inner ear fluid, or hydraulic energy, which distorts the hair cells. Displacement of the hair cells relative to their cell bodies produces cochlear microphonics. This is probably the final mechanical event preceding neuronal stimulation. From this point on, the electrical energy continues as an impulse along the cochlear nerve ascending along various pathways.

At birth, it is the organ of hearing that provides us with our first awareness of the world around us. Thereafter, the ear continues to remain the ever faithful servant of man, while awake or asleep, even to the instant he draws his final breath.

REFERENCES

Johannson, B., Wedenberg, E., and Westin, B. (1964): Measurement of tone responses by the human foetus, *Acta Oto-laryngologica* 57:188–192.

Paparella, M. M., and Shumrick, D. A. (eds.) (1973): *Otolaryngology*. Vol. 1, Philadelphia, W. B. Saunders Co.

Part Two

INTRODUCTION TO
AUDITORY PHYSICS

Audiology is the science of hearing, *audiometry* is the study of the measurement of hearing, and *psychoacoustics* is the study of the links between the perceptual world and that part of the physical world which comes under the heading of *acoustics*. In order to understand psychoacoustics, it is imperative that we understand the nature of the stimulus and its receiver. Thus, we must study anatomy and acoustics, as well as electroacoustics in order to familiarize ourselves with the instruments for the generation, transmission, and reception of sound stimuli.

Does it follow, therefore, that audiologists need be biologists or physicists? No, but it does follow that we must appreciate the sciences with which we must interact since, after all, we cannot adequately describe what we hear without acquiring some understanding of the physics of the environment and the structure of the sensor. In the succeeding chapters of this second part, we consider physical acoustics and electroacoustics. Physical acoustics is that branch of physics which treats of sound in all its aspects, which deals directly with the properties of sound waves and the phenomena which affect them. Electroacoustics, though, is that branch of engineering concerned with devices which deal with acoustic phenomena; for example, microphones, loudspeakers, audiometers, and hearing aids. In the chapters of this section, we get ever closer to the daily concerns of audiometrists and clinical audiologists as we progress from anatomy, to the physics of sound, to hearing aids.

The law of the conservation of energy is central in physics and biophysics. It states that energy cannot be consumed; it cannot be used up, for the quantity of energy is constant. However, the form in which energy is found at a given moment can be altered, that is, energy can be *transduced*; it can be changed from one form to another. The study of electroacoustics, then, deals with the ways in which electrical energy and acoustic energy may be transduced into one another. An electroacoustic transducer is one which converts acoustic energy into electrical energy (e.g., a microphone) or, vice versa, converts electrical energy into acoustic energy (e.g., a loudspeaker).

A collection of electroacoustic transducers assembled expressly for the measurement of hearing constitutes an audiometer. Similarly, a hearing aid is an assemblage of electroacoustic transducers for the enhancement of hearing. The audiometer is central to the audiologist's diagnostic function, and the hearing aid is principal in his rehabilitative function.

To this extent, then, we must all be biological and physical scientists. We must be facile and conversant with the biology, physics, and electronics of our trade.

Chapter Two

ACOUSTICS FOR THE STUDY OF HEARING

J. Kenneth Manhart

The profession of audiology is so intimately associated with the study of sound—its generation, transmission, and measurement—that it is necessary for the audiologist to have a working, though not necessarily detailed, comprehension of the physical behavior of sound waves. Furthermore, in order to be able to report, communicate, and educate, it is essential that he acquire proficiency in working with the terms and units that are used to define or measure the properties of sound. His ability to function effectively in his profession requires knowledge of the performance and limitations of the audio equipment he uses, and an appreciation of the methods used for the measurement, control, specification, and interpretation of physical quantities that are related to sound.

ACOUSTIC WAVES

The type of acoustic or sound waves of interest here are those that are propagated in air. It is well to remember, however, that in the hearing process, sound energy does exist in acoustical, mechanical, hydraulic, and electrical forms. For example, hearing involves an airborne sound wave received by the outer ear as acoustic energy which is converted by the ossicles of the middle ear into mechanical energy, transformed to hydraulic energy in the endolymph (fluid) of the inner ear, to electro-chemical (or neural) energy which is deciphered by the brain and interpreted as sound. To accomplish the hearing process, both the frequencies and amplitude (or intensity) of the components of the sound must be within the limits of the response of the ear. These limits are called "hearing range." Sound energy certainly does occur at frequencies too low (infrasonic) or too high (ultrasonic) for the ear to respond. High-intensity sound can also exist as shock waves, a sudden release of energy as occurs in explosions, rifle fire, or sonic booms. For the most part, studies of these phenomena are for acoustical disciplines other than audiology.

WHAT IS SOUND?

In the general sense, sound is a pressure wave which consists of pulsations or vibrations of molecules of an elastic medium (gas, liquid, or solid). In this chapter, the word "sound" denotes a physical disturbance of air particles caused by vibrating objects, e.g., vocal cords, the diaphragm of an earphone or loudspeaker, bells, etc. Sound can also be generated by high-speed or unsteady air flow such as occurs in the exhaust of jet engines, sirens, and fans. In these cases it is the high-energy level of the turbulence which causes the pressure disturbance or vibrating air particles resulting in aerodynamic sound.

Sound waves differ from vibratory motion of other kinds in two important respects:

1. Sound waves in free air are three-dimensional, i.e., they propagate or spread out in all directions once they are generated, though not necessarily with equal efficiency in all directions (cf. Directivity, page 45). The popular example of wave motion that uses the notion of a stone cast into a body of quiescent water and the ripples spread outward in two dimensions (on the surface only) is not really representative of a sound wave. The differences are major: the waves of sound spread in three dimensions in ever-enlarging spheres in the elastic medium that is in contact with the vibrating source of sound.

2. Sound in air is propagated as a longitudinal wave; that is, the motion of air molecules lies in the direction of propagation. In the example of the water ripples above, the vibrations of the water molecules are at right angles to the direction of propagation of the wave.

For the case of the sound wave, the movement of each air molecule is purely local, making small to-and-fro motions similar to the vibrating surface causing the displacement. The motion is transmitted to adjacent air molecules where the action is repeated. The to-and-fro molecular motion must be clearly distinguished from the velocity of the wave travelling through the medium. The molecule does not travel along with the sound wave. The long coil springs used as toys (such as the "Slinky") by children demonstrate wave propagation of this type exceptionally well. The individual wire coil merely moves back and forth; the wave travels down the length of the spring.

FREQUENCY

The most common approach to study a complex vibratory phenomenon is to view it as an assembly of its basic parts or the simplest regular vibrations which are called *sinusoidal* vibrations. For example, any material is composed of elements called molecules which are unique and distinct from one another.

We must first understand the most fundamental vibratory motion, i.e., a sinusoidal wave motion. Such a waveform, as shown in Figure 2–1, might be caused by the diaphragm of a loudspeaker; the forward motion compresses the air, the rearward motion reduces the pressure. This motion results in the vibration of air particles; the amplitude of vibration is measured in terms of air pressure. The to-and-fro motion of the air molecules creates a series of compressions (increased pressure) and rarefaction (reduced pressure) of the normal or steady-state value of atmospheric pressure. Therefore, the waveform shows how the air pressure changes with time when it is measured at a given point. This sequence of one compression followed by one rarefaction is known as one cycle, and the number of times the sequence is repeated (the number of cycles) in one second is called the *frequency*. Until the last few years, frequency was noted as cycles per second, designated cps or c/s. By international agree-

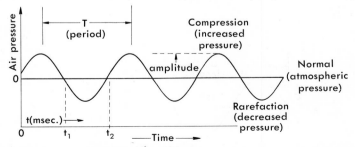

Figure 2–1 Sinusoidal wave: the waveform shows how the air pressure changes with time when it is measured at a given point.

ment, frequency units are now denoted as Hertz (Hz), named after the great German scientist who pioneered in studies of electromagnetic waves. Accordingly, the abbreviation Hz is used throughout this book to denote frequency; a frequency, $f = 256$ Hz, means that 256 cycles as described above occur each second. The nominal frequency range of normal young adult hearing is from 20 to about 20,000 Hz. Musicians often refer to frequency as "pitch" because low-frequency sound is low-pitched and high frequency is high-pitched (cf. Chapter 6).

A pressure wave having the amplitude vs. time characteristics shown in Figure 2–1 would be a pure tone, i.e., only one frequency is involved. Pure tones do not occur often in nature but may be approximated by a siren or whistle. Most sounds are made up of combinations of tones of different frequencies which may have different amplitudes and which may or may not be harmonically related. Additional discussion of this point is found on page 35 under Spectra.

As you can see in Figure 2–1, the changes of air pressure repeat regularly in the same fashion; thus, the wave is *periodic*. The reciprocal of frequency f is the period T in seconds, or

$$f(\text{Hz}) = \frac{1}{T(\text{sec})}$$

showing that frequency has the units of 1/seconds; T represents the time in seconds required to complete one cycle; thus, e.g., the period of a 500 Hz wave is 1/500 or 0.002 second.

WAVELENGTH AND SPEED OF SOUND

Let us consider a propagating sinusoidal sound wave in terms of the changes of air pressure at a distance along some straight line from a given point at a given time. In this case, the sinusoidal wave is as shown in Figure 2–2. This is different from Figure 2–1 because the horizontal scale is in distance, not time. The length which is equivalent to a period T in Figure 2–1 is now called a *wavelength*, λ (lambda). The wavelength of sound is the distance between corresponding points on two successive waveforms.

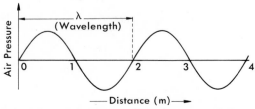

Figure 2–2 Sinusoidal wave: the waveform shows how the air pressure changes with distance from a given point at a given time.

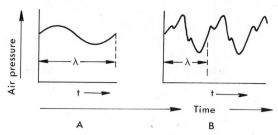

Figure 2–3 Wavelengths for different forms of sound waves; a, sinusoid; b, composite waveform.

Figure 2–3 shows the wavelengths for different forms of sound waves. Since we are looking at the wave propagating through the air, we know the wavelength of sound is related to the frequency of the wave. The speed of sound relates the frequency f to the wavelength λ by

$$\lambda(\text{m}) = \frac{c\,(\text{m/sec})}{f\left(\frac{1}{\text{sec}}\right)} = cT(\text{m}).$$

The frequency in this case shows how many waveform repetitions take place while the sound propagates in a second, and is given by

$$f(\text{Hz}) = \frac{c\,(\text{m/sec})}{\lambda(\text{m})}$$

where c is sound velocity in meters/second. For a given gas, the speed of sound is almost completely dependent upon the absolute temperature of the gas. In the English and metric systems of units, this resolves—for sea-level pressure—to

$$c = 49.03\ \sqrt{R}\ (\text{English})\ \text{ft/sec, or}$$
$$c = 20.05\ \sqrt{T}\ (\text{metric})\ \text{m/sec}$$

where R = absolute temperature in degrees Rankine, i.e., 459.7° plus the temperature in degrees Fahrenheit,

and T = absolute temperature in degrees Kelvin, i.e., 273.2° plus the temperature in degrees Centigrade.

As an example, for a temperature of 68° F (20° C):

English	*Metric*
$c = 49.03\ \sqrt{459.7 + 68}$	$c = 20.05\ \sqrt{273.2 + 20}$
$c = 1125\ \text{ft/sec}$	$c = 343\ \text{m/sec}$

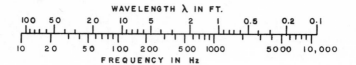

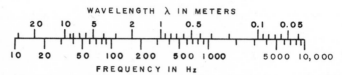

Figure 2–4   The relation between frequency and wavelength in meters and in feet. (From Harris: Handbook of Noise Control. Copyright © 1957 by McGraw-Hill, Inc. Used by permission of McGraw-Hill Book Company.)

For most uses, the accuracy to be achieved by using these equations is not necessary, and the relation shown in Figure 2–4 is adequate. Note, however, that if the gas or medium of propagation is other than air, the speed of sound will change. For example, the speed of sound in hydrogen at 0° C (32° F) is 1270 m/sec or 4165 ft/sec, which is about four times its speed in air. This means that the wavelength λ will be different for a given frequency in different gases; e.g., the wavelength λ is

$$\begin{array}{cc} \textit{In Air} & \textit{In Hydrogen} \\ \lambda = \dfrac{c}{f} = \dfrac{1087 \text{ ft/sec}}{1000 \times 1/\text{sec}} = 1.087 \text{ ft.} & \dfrac{4165 \text{ ft/sec}}{1000 \times 1/\text{sec}} = 4.165 \text{ ft.} \end{array}$$

For other gases, the speed of sound may be obtained from appropriate references such as the *Handbook of Chemistry and Physics*.

PHASE ANGLE

We have yet another way of representing a sinusoidal wave. Let us consider a bead moving with a constant speed along a wire hoop with a radius of, say, 1.0 m. The location of the bead can be expressed in terms of its angle and the vertical distance from the baseline as shown in Figure 2–5. As you can see from the figure, one cycle of motion of the bead concludes when it comes back where it started, i.e., when the angle becomes 360°. The same pattern is repeated as the bead keeps moving around the wire hoop.

Sometimes we need to describe the relative locations of two sinusoidal waves with identical frequencies. The term "phase difference" is often used to do this. An example is shown in Figure 2–6: the phase

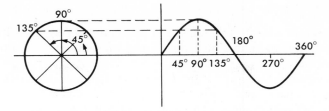

Figure 2-5 Phase angle representation of a sinusoidal wave; one cycle of motion of the bead in the hoop concludes when it comes back to where it started.

difference between the two waves A and B is 90°; wave B lags 90° from wave A, or wave A leads 90° from wave B.

Thus far, you have learned three ways of representing the sinusoidal wave: time vs. amplitude, distance vs. amplitude, and phase angle vs. amplitude. In the acoustics of hearing and of speech, these three representations are often used and you must be familiar with them.

COMPLEX WAVES

In the previous section, we became familiar with some of the basic characteristics of sinusoidal waves. As mentioned before, the sinusoidal wave plays an important role in understanding acoustic aspects of speech events since it is the fundamental mode of any vibration. For the same reason, it is the type of waveform used for the calibration of most audiometric equipment.

To look deeper into the motion of vibrating systems (e.g., a cymbal, a string, a column of air, etc.), we note that the natural modes of oscillation depend upon the physical properties of the system (i.e., the diameter and thickness of a cymbal, the length of an air column, etc.) and the manner in which a vibrating system is excited (a bowed violin string sounds different from a plucked string). These may be thought of as a combination — in suitable proportions — of several modes oscillating together. Hence, the most general motion of a vibrating surface is composed of the sum of a sinusoidal oscillation of the fundamental frequency f_0, another at the second harmonic frequency $(2f_0)$, another at the third $(3f_0)$, etc. The fundamental mode repeats itself in $T_0 = \dfrac{1}{f_0}$ seconds, the second har-

Figure 2-6 Phase difference between two sinusoidal waves.

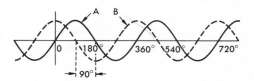

monic mode repeats itself in $T_1 = \dfrac{1}{2f_0}$, or $T_0 = 2T_1$, that is, the second harmonic has twice the frequency and one-half the period of the fundamental, the third harmonic has three times the frequency and one-third the period, etc.

The harmonic structure of the wave is very significant in determining the *timbre* or character of a sound. It is this timbre which allows one to distinguish between middle C on a piano and middle C on a violin. If a pure-tone audiometer becomes maladjusted, it can generate a spectrum having energy at various overtones, and the danger would be that one could not tell if the patient responded to the fundamental frequency (in this case, the one set by the tester) or to one or more of the overtones.

While it may not be obvious from the above discussion, it can be shown that any sound waveform can be made up of fundamentals and harmonics with suitable control of frequency amplitude and phase. The mathematical function that describes this is called the Fourier series which shows that any continuous waveform can be separated into a set of sinusoidal waves. The amplitude and frequency of each wave and the relative phase differences do the trick. Simple examples are given in Figure 2–7. In Figure 2–7(a) the frequency of wave B (the second harmonic) is twice that of A and the amplitude of wave B is half that of A. Wave C is the result of waves A and B added together; conversely, wave C can be decomposed into two harmonically related sinusoidal waves A and B. Figure 2–7(b) shows a different combination of two waves A and B. Although wave B is still the second harmonic of wave A, the result is a different complex wave C. In this case, wave B is shifted 90° against wave B in 7(a). You can observe how different resultant waveforms are obtained by changing the phase of one or both of the fundamental two waves. If wave B has the same amplitude as wave A, and has the same phase as wave B in 7(a), then yet another complex wave C is obtained as shown in 7(c).

As we saw in the examples, any waveform which looks very complicated can be composed from a sufficient number of sinusoidal waves by adjusting the amplitude and phase of each wave in an appropriate manner. Other waveforms which often occur in acoustic studies are shown in Figure 2–8.

Conversely, we may wish to decompose a complex wave into its harmonic sinusoidal structure rather than synthesize it. The same Fourier analysis (or wave analysis) may be used to accomplish this decomposition of a speech wave. It can be stated that any continuous waveform can be decomposed into a number of sinusoidal waves, although for very complex waveforms, the number of frequencies required may approach infinity. What, then, is the advantage of decomposing the complex wave into sinusoidal waves? We will find an answer for this question in the section on Spectra and also in Chapter 11.

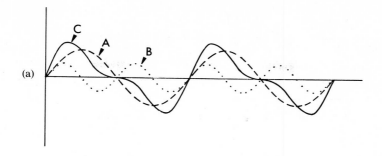

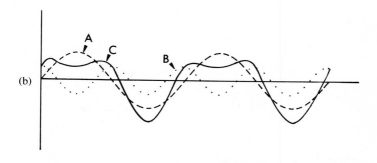

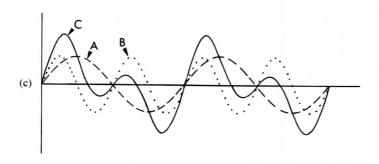

Figure 2–7 Complex waves: wave C is the sum of waves A and B.

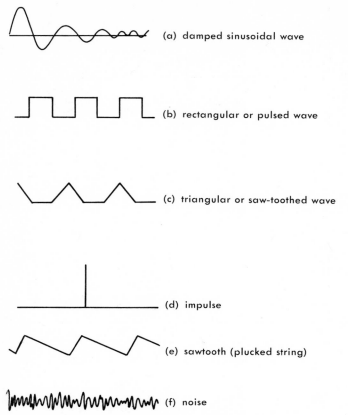

Figure 2-8   Various common types of waveforms.

AMPLITUDE OF SOUND WAVE

In the previous definition of sound, the physical description of a sound wave was given. We noted that pressure varied from point to point above and below atmospheric pressure. The instantaneous variations of pressure constitute the sound wave, and they are extremely small in comparison with the atmospheric pressure itself. For example, the undisturbed atmosphere at sea level has a static pressure of 14.7 lbs/in², which is equivalent to 1.0132×10^5 (about 100,000) Newtons/m². A sound wave having a level of 80 decibels has a pressure fluctuation of ±0.2 Newton/m². Consequently, to indicate only the sound wave, Figure 2-1 is often shown as having the atmospheric pressure designated as zero, and the more meaningful positive and negative fluctuations referred to zero, as shown in Figure 2-9.

How does one go about getting a meaningful measure of the amplitude of a sound wave? If one were to measure the mean pressure of the

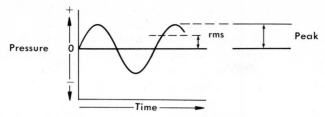

Figure 2–9   Pressure wave with positive and negative fluctuations referred to zero.

wave in Figure 2–9 over one cycle, he would find the value to be zero because there would be equal amounts of positive and negative pressures. Similar problems would result for other periodic waveforms. Therefore, the mean value of a sound wave is not a useful measure.

The wave also has a peak value which is the maximum absolute value of the instantaneous sound pressure that occurs during the cycle, i.e., during the period T. This has only indirect meaning because in the case of random acoustic energy, the peak may go (theoretically) to infinity, and the value obtained by measurement may depend strongly on the characteristics of the measuring instrument.

The measure most commonly used is the root-mean-square (or rms) value of the wave. This value has a direct relationship to the energy content of the sound wave and is noted as p_{rms}. The rms pressure is obtained by squaring the instantaneous values of the sound pressure for each point along the wave, adding the squared values, averaging them over the time of the sample, and taking the square root of the sum. This approach avoids the zero mean value by virtue of the squaring process for the negative pressures (squaring a negative number results in a positive number). For a pure sinusoidal wave only, the relation between the peak and rms values are

$$p_{rms} = \frac{1}{\sqrt{2}}\, p_{peak} = 0.707\, p_{peak}.$$

SPECTRA

The simplest form of a sound wave is a sinusoid, but, as was stated above, most sounds (including speech) have a much more complex waveshape. It also has been said that any continuous waveform having finite energy can be formed by a suitable combination of sinusoidal waveforms. This concept may be a bit difficult to grasp, but it is true, and the reader who is so inclined is referred to the detailed mathematical explanation which is found in discussions of the Fourier transform (e.g., Beranek).

This distribution of sound energy with frequency is known as a sound *spectrum*. The method used to identify the frequency components of a noise, a musical tone, or other sound, is a *spectral* or frequency analysis. By this method, the frequency or frequency band and the amplitude of each are determined. The analyses may result in a line spectrum, a continuous spectrum, or a band spectrum. Let us look at each of these terms.

LINE SPECTRUM

The example of a sinusoidal sound wave, being the simplest, is examined first. Figure 2–10(a) shows a single frequency displayed as pressure vs. time and pressure vs. frequency graphs. Note that there is only one line on the frequency graph; it is positioned along the abscissa (the horizontal or frequency axis) at the value of the frequency which, in this example, may be 500 Hz. A pure-tone audiometer would generate such a single frequency, usually at intervals from 125 to 8000 Hz. This display of the frequency/amplitude distribution is known as a *line*

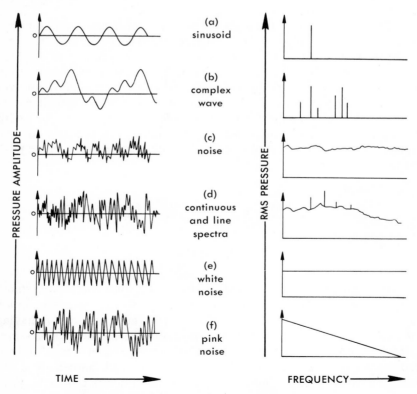

Figure 2–10 Various waveforms and their line spectra.

spectrum which consists of one or more vertical lines along the frequency scale.

Figure 2–10(b) shows the case of a slightly more complex waveform, i.e., one comprised of several sinusoidal waves. The basic waveform (or *fundamental* frequency) repeats itself with period T seconds. The amplitude and frequency distribution of sound is shown by the frequency graph. The frequency is represented by the position along the abscissa, and the amplitude of the sound at each frequency is shown by the height of the line above the abscissa. When the lines are integral multiples of the fundamental (i.e., one, two, three, etc. times the lowest frequency), these multiples are called *overtones* or *harmonics* (a musician would call them "partials"). For example, 600 Hz is the fourth harmonic of 150 Hz, since $4 \times 150 = 600$ (150 is the fundamental).

CONTINUOUS SPECTRUM

In the two cases just discussed, sound energy existed only at discrete frequencies with no energy between frequencies. A continuous spectrum, Figure 2–10(c), implies a continuous distribution of sound energy over a band of frequencies; that is, some sound energy exists at each frequency within the band. Sounds of this kind are usually random, such as the roar from a waterfall or a jet airplane engine, implying the existence of energy at an infinite number of waves with different amplitudes. These are known as *aperiodic* sounds, which is to say, non-periodic or not having a repetitive waveform. If the acoustic energy is distributed so that each cycle per second has equal energy, it is designated as *white noise* by analogy to white light. If each cycle has slightly less energy than the preceding cycle, so that there is an equal amount of energy for each octave band (doubling of frequency), it is known as *pink noise.*.

Upon occasion, as shown in Figure 2–10(d), we observe a continuous spectrum combined with a line spectrum. A noisy fan having a characteristic whine or the five o'clock whistle in a noisy factory are examples. Sometimes we wish to examine only the part of a continuous spectrum which contains the conspicuous line. For that we can look at only a *band* of frequency extending from f_1 to f_2.

SCALES

So far we have been talking about the pressure amplitude — meaning the strength — of a sound wave. Where do we place numbers along this scale? In Figure 2–1 we observed a time scale using the units of seconds and a frequency scale using the units of Hertz. Perhaps you noticed that those two scales are different types; the time scale is linear, whereas the numbers on the frequency scale increase by a factor of 10 for each equal

TABLE 2-1

NUMBER	USING THE NUMBER OF ZEROS OR EXPONENTS	NUMBER OF ZEROS
1	$10^0 = 1$	0
10	$10^1 = 10$	1
100	$10^2 = 10 \times 10$	2
1000	$10^3 = 10 \times 10 \times 10$	3
10000	$10^4 = 10 \times 10 \times 10 \times 10$	4
100000	$10^5 = 10 \times 10 \times 10 \times 10 \times 10$	5
1000000	$10^6 = 10 \times 10 \times 10 \times 10 \times 10 \times 10$	6

increment along the abscissa, i.e., 1, 10, 100, 1000, etc. The latter scale uses logarithmic increase which is also used for the pressure amplitude scale.

The normal ear provides an increase of sensory response with an increase of sound pressure. However, the range between the smallest and the largest sound pressures that the ear can sense as sound is approximately a million to one. It is tempting to use the words softest and loudest sound pressures to show the wide range, but it is necessary to be careful with these terms. The sound pressure itself is not soft or loud; it is the ear and the brain that make these judgments (cf. Chapter 9). Note, too, that the ear has no great difficulty responding to a range of sound pressures over one million to one, but what is needed is a convenient and meaningful way of placing this great range on a piece of paper and to accurately remember numbers which have many zeros. For convenience, then, we use a scale that is based on a scale of tens, using the number of zeros and not the actual number. The relations shown in Table 2-1 demonstrate that we are really familiar with this method of presentation. From Table 2-1, it can be seen that 150 in the "Number" column lies between 2 and 3 in the "Number of Zeros" column; similarly, 75,000 lies somewhere between 4 and 5. The right-hand column, "Using the Number of Zeros or Exponents," shows a form of the logarithmic scale to the base 10.* If we use the "Number of Zeros" column, and, for example, assign the number one to some reference sound pressure, then the expression "level" is related to a ratio of the two numbers, one of which is the reference quantity.

THE DECIBEL

A level, in decibels, is the logarithmic *ratio* of two quantities, one of which is a reference quantity. The other term is at some "level" above or below (generally above) the reference quantity. The expression is gen-

---

*Base 10 is used for the frequency scale presentation.

erally used in two ways: to designate a level of sound power, or to designate a level of sound pressure which is a derivative of sound power. Using the notation of power, the level is defined as

$$\text{Sound Power Level (PWL)} = 10 \log \frac{W_1}{W_0} \text{ dB, re } W_0$$

where W_1 is the sound power in watts and W_0 is the reference sound power, or 10^{-12} watt. Thus, if we had a sound source radiating one watt of sound power, the sound power level would be

$$\text{PWL} = 10 \log \frac{1}{10^{-12}} = 10 \log 10^{12} = 12 \times 10 \log_{10} = 120 \text{ dB}.$$

If the sound power doubles, the increase is 3 dB, i.e.,

$$\text{PWL} = 10 \log \frac{2}{1} = 10 (\log 2 - \log 1) = 10 (.3 - 0) = 3 \text{ dB}.$$

SOUND PRESSURE LEVEL

The ear and most sound measuring and generating instruments (microphones, earphones, loudspeakers, etc.) are devices that respond to or generate sound pressures. True, a sound source may radiate a number of acoustic watts of sound power, but the sensing or the measurement of the sound is done via sound pressure measurements. However, the decibel is a term that is also applicable to sound pressure because, as with the case of sound power, we require a scale that is associated with the ratio of two numbers. In this chapter, the assumption is made (but it is not always true) that the sound power (W) is proportional (but not equal to) the square of the sound pressure, or W is proportional to p^2.

The reference pressure used most commonly for noise measurements in air is $p_0 = 2 \times 10^{-4}$ microbar (μ bar).* This level is used to designate zero on the scale of sound pressures (hence the subscript 0). It was selected because that pressure represents approximately the threshold of hearing for normal ears at 1000 Hz when measured under quiet laboratory conditions. Recall that the term sound pressure level is used for convenience; what is really meant is the sound pressure level squared. Thus, the sound pressure level, corresponding to a pressure p_1, is

---

*In the foreseeable future, most acoustical laboratories will have adopted a different sound pressure reference. This reference level in the SI (international) systems of units employs the Newton per square meter (N/m^2) instead of the microbar (μbar) or the dyne per square centimeter (d/cm^2). Thus, the international reference is 2×10^{-5} N/m^2 which renders dB less than a reference level of 2×10^{-4} μbar. We have continued to use the older traditional system in the succeeding chapters.

$$\text{Sound pressure level} = 10 \log_{10} \frac{p_1^2}{p_0^2} \text{ dB re } 2 \times 10^{-4} \text{ } \mu\text{bar.}$$

The above equation is usually written as

$$\text{Sound pressure level} = 20 \log_{10} \frac{p_1}{p_0} \text{ dB re } 2 \times 10^{-4} \text{ } \mu\text{bar.}$$

The transition is made using some rules of logarithms. A similar, but more obvious, example is given below. Given that the logarithm of 100 is 2 (cf. Table 2–1), then

$$\log_{10} 100 = \log_{10} 10^2 = 2 \log_{10} 10 = 2(1) = 2$$

and $\qquad \log_{10} 1000 = \log 10^3 = 3 \log_{10} 10 = 3(1) = 3$

$$\text{because } \log_{10} 10 = 1.$$

A comparison of sound power level and sound pressure level is made in the following expressions:

Sound Power Level	Sound Pressure Level
$10 \log_{10} \dfrac{W_1}{W_0}$	$20 \log_{10} \dfrac{p_1}{p_0}$
dB re 10^{-12} watt	dB re 2×10^{-5} N/m².

These relations of the quantities of sound power level and sound pressure level are not always simple. Sound power level is related to the total sound power (in watts) radiated by the source, whereas sound pressure level is a measure of the pressure at a given point. Referring to the example given earlier, sound power level is related to the amount of energy generated when a stone strikes the surface of a pond of water, sound pressure level is related to the amplitude of the waves that radiate from the disturbance, and the greater the distance from the source, the smaller the wave amplitude.

Whenever the term "decibel" is used, it is essential to cite the reference level so that a reader will know whether the units are in terms of power or rms pressure. The preferred method of presentation is the kind used above, e.g., 86 dB re 2×10^{-5} N/m² or 108 dB re 10^{-12} watt. For sound power, the level is referred as dB re 10^{-12} watts. For sound pressure, the level is referred as dB re 2×10^{-5} N/m². Note that doubling the power level results in a 3 dB increase, but doubling the sound pressure level results in a 6 dB increase. A word of caution: in media other than air, the reference level may be different, e.g., 0.1 N/m² for underwater acoustics.

Example: What is the SPL re 2×10^{-5} N/m² for a wide-band noise having an rms pressure of 1 N/m²? A few extra steps are included to assist you in following the procedure.

$$\text{SPL} = 20 \log_{10} \left[\frac{1}{2 \times 10^{-5}} \right] = 20 \left[\log_{10} \frac{10^5}{2} \right] = 20 \left[\log_{10} \frac{10 \times 10^4}{2} \right]$$

$$= 20 \left[\log_{10} 5 + \log_{10} 10^4 \right] = 20 \left[.7 + 4 \right] = 94 \text{ dB re } 2 \times 10^5 \text{ N/m}^2.$$

Conversely, we are often concerned with establishing the pressure associated with a given SPL. To determine this value, it is necessary to rearrange the equation to be able to calculate the rms pressure.

Example: A SPL of 90 dB is measured in the canal of the ear. What is the actual rms pressure at the point of measurement? To work this problem, you will have to acquaint yourself with antilogarithms.

$$SPL = 20 \log \frac{p_1}{p_0} \text{ ; rearranging } p_1 = p_0 \text{ antilog } \frac{SPL}{20} = p_0 \text{ antilog } \frac{90}{20}$$

where p_0 is the reference level of 2×10^{-5} N/m^2

$$p_1 = 2 \times 10^{-5} \text{ antilog } 4.5 \text{ N/m}^2$$

$$p_2 = 2 \times 10^{-5} (31630) = 2 \times 10^{-5} \times 3.16 \times 10^4 = .634 \text{ N/m}^2.$$

ADDITION OF SOUND PRESSURE LEVELS

Frequently, it becomes necessary to add two or more sound pressure levels not at the same frequency that are measured individually at one point. The correct result is not obtained by the addition of the individual SPLs, but is proportional to the addition of the sound pressures. Recall again that we are really working with the root-mean-square values of sound pressure, and the pressure resulting from the addition of *n* different noises is:

$$p^2 = p_1^2 + p_2^2 + p_3^2 + \cdots p_n^2$$

where $p_1, p_2, p_3 \ldots p_n$ are the rms magnitudes of the individual pressures.

Fortune is kind in that one is not required to go through this procedure for a straightforward addition of SPLs. The computation has been reduced to a chart which may be used to solve most problems of this type; the chart is shown in Figure 2–11. The procedure consists of taking two SPLs, noting the difference in the levels ($SPL_1 - SPL_2$), going to the table and observing the SPL difference which is then added to the higher of the two SPLs. This operation is repeated (adding the sum to the next SPL) until all of the SPLs have been summed. For example, let us determine the resulting SPL at a given location for two noise sources. Operating independently, they generate 84 dB (SPL_2) and 89 dB (SPL_1), re 2×10^{-5} N/m^2 respectively at the point of observation. The difference $SPL_1 - SPL_2$ is 5 dB. According to Figure 2–11, the number to be added to the higher SPL is 1.2 dB, resulting in 90.2 dB re 2×10^{-5} N/m^2.

As a second example, let us add six numbers, representing the SPLs of six adjacent octave bands, and determine the overall level that would result.

Octave Band Center Frequency	(Hz)	125	250	500	1000	2000	4000
SPL (dB)		56	59	61	67	74	60

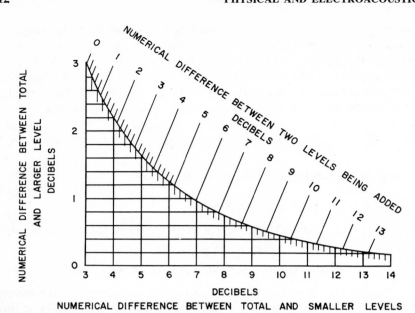

Figure 2–11   Addition of sound pressure levels. (From Peterson, A. D. G., and Gross, E.: Handbook of Noise Measurement. General Radio Company, 1963.)

After performing this calculation a few times, one usually ends up pairing those bands having SPLs closest to one another. This procedure is tabulated below:

$L_1 - L_2$	74 − 67;	61 − 60;	59 − 56
Difference, dB	7	1	3
Correction,* dB	.8	2.5	1.8
$L_1 +$ Correction	74.8	63.5	60.8
Difference			2.7
Correction		------1.9	
$L_2 +$ Correction	74.8	65.4	
Difference		9.4	
Correction*	.5—		
Overall SPL	75.3 dB re 2×10^{-5} N/m^2		

*corrections from Figure 2–11.

When the SPL in one band is much larger than in the next highest band, the increase to the higher SPL is small.

The above examples are given for broadband noise sources. For the case where the two sources are at the same frequency, addition becomes more complicated because the relative phases must be considered. Where two sources have the same frequency, the same amplitude, and the same phase, the sum of the two pressures is twice that of either of the original waves ($p_2 = p_1 + p_1 = 2p_1$), so

$$\text{SPL} = 20 \log \frac{2p_1}{p_1} = 20 \log 2 = 20 \, (.3) = 6 \text{ dB.}$$

For additional discussion of this point, the reader is referred to Beranek (1971).

PROPAGATION OF SOUND

If a sound wave propagates in one direction only (as in a duct or a tube infinitely long), it is said to be a "free progressive wave," which is referred to more commonly as a *plane* wave. The term "plane" refers to flatness or uniformity of the wave front. In such a wave, for a constant level sound source, the sound pressure amplitude would be the same everywhere along the direction of propagation and remains constant except for the losses due to the absorption of sound in air. This type of wavefront does not occur often except at great distances from a sound source in open air, about which more is said later.

INVERSE SQUARE LAW

A much more common type of wave approximates a free progressive spherical wave. Such a wave assumes a non-directional noise source (i.e., radiating sound equally in all directions) in free air without any reflecting surfaces near the source or receiver or in the line between the two. The wavefront of such a wave has a spherical shape as it radiates outward with time at a nominal speed of about 1100 feet per second in air. For this type of wave, the area of the bubble-shaped wavefront increases in size as the distance from the sound source increases. On the surface of such a spherical wave, the total sound energy remains constant. Therefore, as the wavefront area increases, the sound energy per unit area is gradually diminished, resulting in a reduction of sound pressure amplitude (p) inversely with distance (r) from the sound source:

$$p = \frac{A}{r} \cos \; k(r - ct)$$

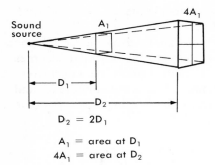

Figure 2–12 The inverse square law.

$D_2 = 2D_1$

A_1 = area at D_1

$4A_1$ = area at D_2

where $k(r - ct)$ is an argument of the trigonometric function which indicates the wave is travelling in the $+$ direction. This can be observed by setting $(r - ct) = 0$; therefore, $r = ct$ and r increases with t, the time of propagation of the wave; c is constant.

The intensity I of the sound wave decreases as the square of the distance from the sound source:

$$I = \frac{W}{4\pi r^2}$$

where I = intensity of the sound wave in watts/m², W = sound power of the source in watts, and $4\pi r^2$ = area of a sphere having a radius r meters. This relation has led to the expression "inverse square law" for intensity. Recall also the SPL involves a p^2 term (and thus an r^2 term), so it can be shown that the SPL drops off 6 dB for each doubling of the distance or 20 dB for each increase of 10 in distance. Figure 2–12 shows this effect. The procedure for determining the SPL at a distance D_2 from a source on a line with a distance D_1, when the SPL at D_1 is known ($D_2 > D_1$), is

$$SPL_{D_2} = SPL_{D_1} - 20 \log \frac{D_2}{D_1} \text{ dB.}$$

Special rooms have been built to create a *free-field* condition where the walls, floor, and ceiling are sound-absorptive such that almost no sound energy is reflected from the surface. Such enclosures are called *anechoic,* meaning echo-free.

NEAR-FIELD AND FAR-FIELD

Let us look more closely at the way that sound pressure levels decrease with distance from the source. It has been found to be convenient to divide the sound field into two regions known as the "near-field" and the "far-field." While texts in the physics of sound offer mathematical explanations describing the different properties of the two, a precise definition is really quite complicated because the limit of the near-field is a function of frequency. The sound field behaves differently in these two regions; i.e., the inverse square law is applicable only in the far-field. In the near-field, the sound pressure level may decrease at a greater or lesser amount than the 6 dB with distance doubling because the acoustic intensity is not related directly to the mean square pressure. Frequently, it is necessary to establish the limits experimentally. This is done by identifying the closest point to the source that, if the distance to the source were doubled, would result in a 6 dB reduction of SPL.

A reasonable guide to defining these regions may be in terms of the wavelength of the frequencies of interest. When the distance from the receiver to the source is greater than 10 times the wavelength of the lowest frequency of interest or three times the largest linear dimension of the noise source, whichever is larger, the receiver is probably in the far-field. Looking at the source from any point in the far-field, the source should appear small, so that the sound appears to originate from one point. This leads to the expression "point source."

In addition to the reduction of SPL in the near-field and far-field, losses also occur due to air absorption. These losses are a function of air temperature and humidity and are generally negligible at distances less than 100 feet.

DIRECTIVITY

We have assumed so far that, in a free field, sound is radiated uniformly in all directions from the source, a condition that is not generally true. Most sound sources radiate sound more efficiently in some directions than in others; this effect is known as *directivity*. The degree of directivity is generally related to the geometry of the source; for example, the directivity pattern of a trumpet lies along a line forward from the bell; while a cymbal radiates more efficiently in two directions, those which are normal (perpendicular) to the upper and lower surfaces, and very little to the side which is in the plane of the cymbal. A jet airplane engine provides an excellent example of a directive source: as it approaches, you hear the whine associated with the fan in the inlet; as it passes overhead, the jet roar becomes much more noticeable. As the airplane recedes, the sound level decreases as the effects of distance (inverse square loss) and air attenuation (air absorption) reduce the level of the sound.

A plot of directivity is known as a *directivity pattern* such as that shown in Figure 2–13. It is generally assumed that the directivity pattern does not change shape with distance from the source. The directivity pattern relates the sound power generated by the source to the sound pressure level at a given distance and direction. Frequently, a series of radiation patterns will be given for a single sound source, each pattern for a particular frequency band. In the example shown in Figure 2–13, the SPL at D_1 is 113 dB, at D_2 is 107 dB, at D_3 is 101 dB, etc.; the distance from D_2 to D_3 is double that from D_1 to D_2.

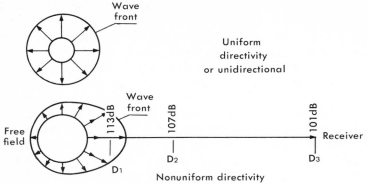

Figure 2–13 A directivity pattern does not change shape with distance from the source.

REFLECTION

In the section on the inverse square law, a free field was assumed, which means the absence of any reflecting surface. Obviously, this is not the case when a noise source is near the ground, for the surface of the earth acts as a reflector. The presence of a surface causes a major change of the sound field. In the free field, the sound wave arriving at the position of a receiver travelled on a straight line between the source and the receiver. Sound radiated in other directions never reached the receiver.

With a reflective surface near a continuously sounding noise source, there are two ways that sound energy can reach the position of the receiver: the direct path and the path along the reflected ray as shown in Figure 2–14. It should be clear that, in the example of the reflected wave, there is more sound energy at the receiver position than there was for the case of the free field (Fig. 2–13), and the sound level is slightly greater. For the case where the sound source is abrupt, such as a clap or a yell, and if the distance along the two paths is great, one will hear the noise followed by an echo which is, in this case, the reflected sound.

The effectiveness of a single hard flat surface such as a wall or a partition to reflect sound energy is related to the length and width of the surface and the relation of these dimensions to the wavelength of sound. If the dimensions of the reflecting surface are several wavelengths, the reflection will be almost complete. On the other hand, if the frequency is low, the wavelength may be greater than either the length or width of the surface and the reflection would be very incomplete. For this latter example, where the wavelength of the sound is larger than the size of the wall, the sound pressure will bend around the wall. This effect is known as *diffraction* and was possibly demonstrated to you the last time you saw a parade with a marching band. When the band was playing around the corner of a building, you heard the drums and the bass horns because the low-frequency sound was diffracted around the corner. When the

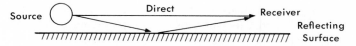

Figure 2–14 With a reflective surface near a continuously sounding noise source, there are two ways that sound energy can reach the receiver.

band turned the corner toward you, you heard the trumpets and the brass, the high frequencies which did not diffract around such a large surface, now being propagated on a straight line to your ears. If more than one reflecting surface exists, then additional reflections will occur with a consequent increase of sound energy which will be greater than that of the direct sound alone.

REVERBERATION

When the number of reflecting surfaces provides a complete enclosure, the effect of the multiple reflections is to cause reverberation. Imagine an enclosure having hard concrete walls, ceiling, and floor. With a sound source operating continuously, the enclosure becomes filled with direct and reflected sound waves, making conversation extremely difficult. Generally, one does not hear the individual reflections like echoes because of the large number and rapidity of reflections.

If the sound source were suddenly stopped, the sound level would decay or gradually diminish. The sound you hear after the source is stopped is the reflected sound which continues until all of the wave energy is absorbed by striking the walls (nothing is 100 per cent reflective) and in the air. This prolongation of sound is termed *reverberation*. The time required for the sound field to decay to inaudibility is called *reverberation time*.

ABSORPTION OF SOUND

When a sound wave is incident on a surface, some sound energy is reflected and some is absorbed. The fraction of sound energy that is absorbed by the surface is designated as the *sound absorption coefficient* (α). The absorption coefficients vary with frequency and with the angle at which the wave strikes the surface, and range from 0.01 to 1.00 (one per cent to 100 per cent). These values are usually presented as absorption coefficients at the center frequencies of selected octave bands and are specified as normal or random incidence absorption coefficients. If the sound wave strikes the absorptive surface at a 90 degree angle, the result is a normal incidence coefficient; if a reverberant field exists and waves strike the surface at all angles, the result is a random incidence coefficient. This latter is the unit generally used for determining and reporting absorption coefficients.

The amount of absorption is dependent upon the material, with lightweight fluffy materials such as fiberglass being among the most efficient absorbers. Dense materials such as steel or concrete have absorption coefficients in the range of .01 to .02. Carpeting, drapes, and overstuffed furniture usually provide some useful sound absorption in the mid and high frequencies. In addition to materials, people themselves absorb sound. The values are usually given in terms of square foot units of absorption called *Sabines*. The same unit results if one takes the absorption coefficient of a material and multiplies it by the number of square feet of that material in a room.

Sound absorbent materials are used primarily to reduce reflections from a surface. Their application to the walls of a room will reduce reverberation and echoes, but will not do much to stop the transmission of sound through a wall. Their use will prevent the build-up of sound due to the reflection from hard (non-absorptive) surfaces. The reader is referred to the *Bulletin of the Acoustical Materials Association* for additional discussion of sound absorption and tables of absorption coefficients.

SOUND TRANSMISSION LOSS

The quantity used to rate the ability of a wall to insulate against the transmission of airborne sound is called the *transmission loss* (T.L.). It is defined as the difference between the incident and transmitted sound intensity levels (note: or the sound pressure squared levels). The unit of T.L. is the decibel without reference to 2×10^{-5} N/m^2.

As a sound wave strikes a wall, some of the energy is transferred to the wall, setting it into vibration. The heavier and the better damped the wall, the less will be the vibration amplitude and the better the sound insulation it will provide.

T.L. is a function of both frequency (it generally increases with frequency) and the angle at which the incident sound wave strikes the panel. Multiple walls provide greater transmission loss than a single wall of the same weight.

At a given frequency, the transmission loss of a wall increases with the mass, i.e., if the mass is doubled, the T.L. increases theoretically about 6 dB (in reality, it is closer to 4.5 dB). This effect is called "mass law" and is useful as a guide. The empirical formulas relating T.L. to mass are

$$\text{T.L.} = 23 + 14.5 \log_{10} m, \quad \text{where } m \text{ is in lbs/ft}^2, \text{ or}$$

$$\text{T.L.} = 13 + 14.5 \log_{10} m, \quad \text{where } m \text{ is in kg/m}^2.$$

Any small openings such as cracks or holes through the wall can reduce its potential ability to reduce noise quite drastically.

Noise Reduction (N.R.) and T.L. are terms that are frequently confused with one another. N.R. is generally what is really measured in the field, i.e., determined by measuring the SPLs on each side of a wall and taking the difference:

$$N.R. = SPL_1 - SPL_2.$$

N.R. is also a smaller number than the T.L.:

$$N.R. = T.L. - K,$$

where K is a function of the total sound absorption in the receiving room.

The transmission loss for a given panel is fixed and changes only if the properties of the panel are changed, such as its mass, stiffness, etc. Noise reduction on the other hand is a variable. It depends upon the T.L. and other factors such as the amount of sound absorption in the receiving room and any other sound paths between the microphones on each side of the wall.

To achieve high T.L., an impervious and massive wall is required between a noise source and a receiver. T.L. and absorption are two separate functions. Both serve to reduce noise but in different ways. T.L. requires mass, and lightweight materials are generally ineffective methods to achieve T.L. Absorption requires porous or fibrous materials which are usually inefficient as a barrier to sound. Recall the example of the baby: the diapers solve the problem of absorption, the rubber pants solve the problem of transmission loss. One does not provide the function of the other—ask any mother.

REFERENCES

Beranek, L. L. (ed.) (1971): *Noise and Vibration Control.* New York, McGraw-Hill Book Co.
Harris, C. (ed.) (1957): *Handbook of Noise Control.* New York, McGraw-Hill Book Co.
Peterson, A. P. G., and Gross, E. E., Jr. (1963): *Handbook of Noise Measurement.* 6th Ed. West Concord, Mass., General Radio Co.

Chapter Three

ELECTROACOUSTIC TRANSDUCERS

Benjamin B. Bauer

INTRODUCTION

The most widely used mode of aural communication takes place when we interact directly with other people — as when we engage in conversation with someone or deliver a lecture to a small group. However, sometimes we find that, even under these favorable circumstances, aids to human voice and hearing are needed. For this purpose, we employ a variety of simple devices. Consider:

1. A megaphone horn is often used by an athletic coach to better project his voice to the players.
2. A stethoscope tube with diaphragm at one end and ear couplers at the other is used by a doctor to listen to faint chest sounds.

50

3. A person cups a hand around his ear in a noisy location to exclude
   unwanted sounds and to reinforce desired sounds.

These are examples of purely acoustical aids to communication based, in
the order listed, on the acoustical properties of horns, the sound transmission characteristics of tubes, and the diffraction and resonance behavior
of open cups.

A more powerful class of aids to aural communication is based upon
the technology of energy conversion and electronic signal amplification.
In these devices, sounds are first converted to equivalent electrical signals
(i.e., transduced from one form of energy to another) whereby they can be
transmitted over wires, amplified, recorded, broadcast over great distances, etc., and thereafter transduced back into the original sounds. Examples abound in modern life: telephone, radio, phonograph, tape recorder, public address system, audiometer, hearing aid—all depend on
transducers for their operation.

In this chapter, we study electroacoustic transducers (i.e., transducers which convert acoustic into electric energy, or vice versa): their
operating principles, the basic elements of their design and structure, their
application to devices we use in our daily life such as microphones,
earphones, and loudspeakers, and their proper utilization and calibration.
These applications touch upon many of the various activities engaged in
by audiologists.

GENERAL DESCRIPTION

Electroacoustic transduction, in almost every case, is carried out in
two steps as exemplified in Figure 3–1 which depicts a so-called "moving-
coil" transducer. First, the sound waves impinge upon an extended

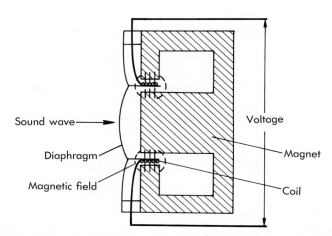

Figure 3–1 Stylized representation of a moving-coil electroacoustic transducer.

member, called a diaphragm (or, depending upon its shape, sometimes called a piston, a cone, or a ribbon), causing it to vibrate in response to the alternating sound pressure falling on one or both of its surfaces. The vibrations of the diaphragm, in turn, actuate some type of mechanism capable of transforming the vibratory motions into electrical signals, in this example, a tubular coil of wire cemented to the diaphragm at one end and at the other end immersed in a magnetic field. In the reverse operating mode, vibratory electrical signals are applied to a transducer which transforms electrical impulses into mechanical forces (the coil of wire described above may be used for this purpose) which, in turn, cause the diaphragm to vibrate, producing audible sound.

In the above example, the diaphragm can be thought of as a mechanoacoustic transducer, and the coil of wire in the magnetic field as an electromechanical transducer. Coupled together, they produce an electroacoustic transducer. Often, the term "transducer" is extended to mean not just the electroacoustic transducer per se, but also the total transducing mechanism including even an external case or cabinet and its immediate accessories—in other words, the complete device which performs the transducing function.

Most of the transducers studied here are reversible; that is to say, they are capable of transducing energy backward and forward, from one form to another, as in the above example of a coil of wire immersed in a magnetic field. Some transducers, however, are irreversible. An example of an irreversible electroacoustic transducer is a doorbell or chime which generates a sound with the application of a pulse of current but does not produce equivalent current with the application of a sound wave. Another example is a carbon-granules transducer used in an ordinary telephone handset which generates electrical signals when its diaphragm is actuated by sound waves, but which does not produce sounds when vibratory electrical signals are applied to its terminals.

CLASSIFICATION OF TRANSDUCERS

We classify transducers according to (1) the type of device in which they are employed; (2) the electromechanical principle used; and (3) their performance characteristics, such as fidelity of sound reproduction, response to sounds in various directions, electrical parameters, etc. The significance of these terms is discussed in the following sections.

TRANSDUCING DEVICES

MICROPHONES

Transducers especially intended for receiving sounds of human voice, music, etc., and converting them into corresponding electric signals

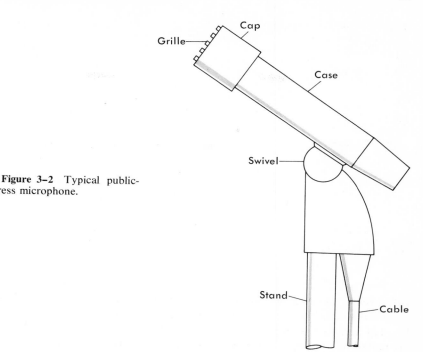

Figure 3-2 Typical public-address microphone.

are called microphones. Microphones of highest quality, capable of capturing sounds with great fidelity over the whole range of human hearing for the purpose of making disc or tape records, are designated as recording microphones. Those of somewhat less fidelity, but robustly built to withstand rough handling, accidental dropping, etc., and often adjusted especially to favor the transmission of human voice, are classed as broadcast or public-address microphones (cf. Fig. 3-2).

Microphones of relatively small dimensions which exhibit uniform sensitivity with respect to frequency and direction of sound arrival, and which are designed to remain stable with time and temperature, often used for acoustical measurements, are named by the particular intended applications as standard microphones, sound-pressure-measuring microphones, sound level meter microphones, etc. (e.g., Fig. 3-3).

Very small microphones—the size of an aspirin tablet or even smaller—limited generally to the transduction of the relatively narrow frequency band important for speech intelligibility are used in hearing aids and so are called hearing-aid microphones (cf. Fig. 3-4).

EARPHONES

Transducers especially intended for converting electric into acoustic signals and conveying them directly to the listener's ears are called

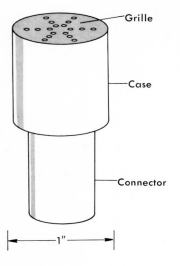

Figure 3-3 Sound level meter microphone.

earphones. Two earphones enclosed in rigid cups provided with ear-cushions to confine the sound from the earphone to the interior volume of the cup and to prevent unwanted external sounds from reaching the ear are called headphones or are referred to as a headset. If each earphone of a headset has an independent connection to each of two signal sources, so that different sounds may be conveyed to each ear, the pair forms a binaural (often, in the vernacular, "stereophonic") headset (cf. Fig. 3-5).

A very stable earphone capable of uniformly reproducing all the important frequencies of speech and music, and especially adapted for the measurement of the characteristics of human hearing, is called an audiometric earphone. An earphone included in a telephone handset for efficiently transmitting the frequency range used in telephone communication is called a telephone receiver. A very small earphone capable of fitting in the ear canal, or adapted to convey sound to the eardrum by a small plastic tube terminated in an ear-canal coupler, is called a hearing-aid receiver (cf. Chapter 4). Finally, a small transducer for converting

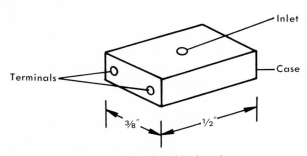

Figure 3-4 Hearing aid microphone.

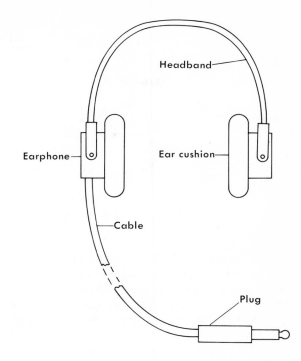

Figure 3-5 Headphone.

electric signals into mechanical vibration intended for attachment in contact with the head, usually over the mastoid bone, and whose vibrations are transmitted to the inner ear via the bony portions of the head, is called a bone-conduction receiver.

LOUDSPEAKERS

A relatively large transducer especially adapted to generate acoustical power in amounts sufficient to fill a room, or to be heard at a distance, is called a loudspeaker or simply a speaker. A loudspeaker generally employs one or more transducers of various sizes—also called loudspeaker motors or drivers (cf. Fig. 3-6)—adapted to efficiently transduce the sound of various parts of the audible spectrum. Each loudspeaker driver is a moving-coil electromechanical transducer attached to a formed diaphragm, usually made of paper or plastic, which has the shape of a cone or spheroidal piston. These various transducers are interconnected by means of electrical dividing networks which allow portions of the total electric signal to reach the particular transducer for which they are especially intended. The largest driver in a loudspeaker, called a woofer, is adapted to transduce signals covering the range from 20 to about 500 Hz. The driver next in size, sometimes called a squawker, reproduces sounds from 500 to 5000 Hz. The sounds above 5000 Hz are reproduced

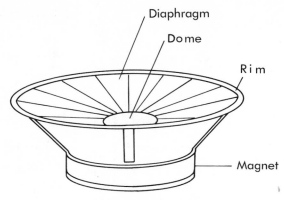

Figure 3–6   Loudspeaker driver.

by the smallest transducer, called a tweeter. Of course, these ranges vary considerably among loudspeakers of different sizes and makes. While the more expensive loudspeakers usually divide the frequency range among three or more transducers, the less expensive ones may employ only one or two transducers which are then required to carry the full range of sounds.

Loudspeaker drivers are housed in an enclosure often called a baffle because it "baffles" or confines the sounds from the back of the loudspeaker cone within the box to prevent them from canceling sounds radiated from the front surface of the transducer cone. Baffles are covered with an acoustically transparent ornamental fabric or "grille." Acoustical engineers have devised many different types of loudspeaker enclosures to satisfy various technical requirements encountered in loudspeaker design.

SPEAKER-MICROPHONES

In many instances a transducer takes on the dual role of microphone and loudspeaker. Examples of this type of application are the transducer used in a dictation machine, a hand-held "walkie-talkie" or "transceiver" radio, a two-way "intercom," and similar devices which allow the user to talk or listen employing the same transducer. Speaker-microphone transducers are usually of a compromise design in order to perform the dual function in reasonably good manner. Obviously, they must use reversible transducers.

TYPES OF TRANSDUCERS

A large variety of electromechanical transducers has been developed over the past hundred years, but only seven types are pre-eminent:

1. carbon-granules transducers

2. magnetic transducers
3. electrostatic (capacitor) transducers
4. electrostatic (electret) transducers
5. piezoelectric transducers
6. moving-coil transducers
7. moving-conductor (ribbon) transducers

With the exception of the carbon-granules transducers, all of these are reversible; they can be used in microphones to convert acoustic into electric signals or in earphones or loudspeakers to convert electric into acoustic signals.

CARBON-GRANULES TRANSDUCERS

Carbon-granules transducers convert vibratory mechanical energy into electrical energy by variation of electrical resistance between specially processed carbon granules contained between two metallic (usually gold-plated) electrodes which are caused to vibrate with respect to each other in response to sound. The varying resistance, in turn, modulates a current which flows through the granules supplied by a local source. Carbon-granules transducers are used almost exclusively in microphones inside telephone handsets.

MAGNETIC TRANSDUCERS

These are based upon the principle that a changing magnetic flux through a coil of wire induces a voltage across the coil terminals. The coil surrounds a magnetic armature, vibrated by a diaphragm in response to sounds, which conducts the flux from a permanent magnet. The armature motions cause a change in flux through the coil. Conversely, applying a current to the coil produces a magnetic flux change which affects the force of attraction between the armature and the magnet, causing the diaphragm to move, thus producing sound.

ELECTROSTATIC (CAPACITOR) TRANSDUCERS

These transducers, also called condenser transducers, consist of two adjacent parallel conductive surfaces, one of which is a thin metallic or metalized plastic foil, which form the electrodes of a capacitor. The application of rather high "polarizing" and signal voltages between these two surfaces results in a motion of foil electrodes generating sound. Conversely, motions of the foil with respect to the other electrode result in a change of capacitance which generates a variable electric signal. Because of its simplicity, an electrostatic transducer is one of the most stable and faithful in quality among those in use today. Therefore, it is frequently found in microphones used for acoustical measurements or for high-fidelity recording.

ELECTROSTATIC (ELECTRET) TRANSDUCERS

A close derivative of the capacitor transducer is one which uses a permanently polarized element called an electret. An electret transducer does not require an external polarizing voltage. In its modern form, an electret is a thin (0.001 inch) mylar or other plastic film upon one side of which a conductive film (usually gold) is evaporated to form an electrode. The plastic film is heated to several hundred degrees Fahrenheit and allowed to cool to room temperature while under the influence of a strong electrostatic field. This process results in a permanent polarization potential equivalent to 100 volts or more.

PIEZOELECTRIC TRANSDUCERS

An important class of transducers is based on the property of certain crystalline substances to generate an electric potential when mechanically stressed. This property is called piezoelectricity, from the Greek *piezoein,* meaning to squeeze. The development of the Rochelle Salt piezoelectric transducer in the 1930's began a quarter-century of dominance for these in low-cost microphones, earphones, and phonograph pickups. Recent researches have led to more advanced piezoelectric transducers using various ceramic materials. These transducers have the shape of a sandwich-like rod consisting of two slabs of piezoelectric material joined into an integral unit with appropriately attached electrodes. The longitudinal stress in the slabs produced by bending the rod results in a differential potential across the electrodes. Conversely, the application of a potential across the electrodes causes a stress to develop in the piezoelectric body which may be used to activate a diaphragm for sound reproduction.

MOVING-COIL TRANSDUCERS

This transducer, which consists of a coil of wire immersed in a magnetic field, was discussed in connection with descriptions of microphones and loudspeakers. The moving-coil transducer is the electroacoustic "workhorse," perhaps used more widely than any other in the popular microphones, earphones, and loudspeakers.

RIBBON TRANSDUCERS

An extremely thin (0.0001 inch) corrugated aluminum ribbon approximately one-eighth-inch wide by two inches long, suspended in a strong magnetic field between two poles, forms an excellent transducer which at one time was widely used, especially in microphones. Ribbon transducers have largely given way to the more rugged moving-coil transducers, as ribbons are easily damaged and are sensitive to air currents.

PERFORMANCE CHARACTERISTICS

One must examine a number of characteristics of a transducer to assess its suitability for a particular application. Most important among them are the electrical impedance, sensitivity or output level, frequency response, and directional response. Additionally, distortion and power-handling capacity also need to be considered, especially in the case of earphones and loudspeakers.

IMPEDANCE

Electrical impedance of a transducer is defined as the voltage needed to cause a unit current to flow through the transducer. The significance of impedance may be viewed as follows: In a microphone, for example, the generated electrical signals must travel through the transducer impedance and the impedance of cable connecting the microphone to the amplifier before amplification can take place. This results in a loss of signal which is a function of transducer impedance. Thus, the impedance of a microphone will determine the length of cable which can be used between it and the amplifier. On the other hand, the amplifier may have been designed for use with microphones of a particular impedance. In the case of a loudspeaker or earphone, the electrical energy from the amplifier, again, must travel through the cable and transducer impedance before being allowed to actuate the transduction mechanism to convert electrical into acoustical energy. Thus, the impedance of a loudspeaker or earphone determines the characteristics of the amplifier or other source of power needed for its efficient operation. Transducer impedance may be measured by the kind of arrangement or apparatus shown in Figure 3–7. While this method is not the most precise, it is simple and may be carried out with ordinary laboratory instruments.

SENSITIVITY LEVEL

Sensitivity is a term which describes the effectiveness of a transducer in transferring one type of energy into another. Microphone sensitivity

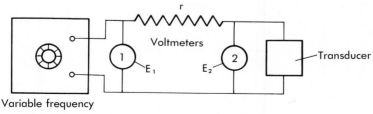

Figure 3–7 The measurement of transducer impedance. (r is chosen so that the voltage at 1 is at least 10 times that at 2. Transducer impedance, $Z = [(E_2/E_1)r]$.

usually is stated in terms of the amplitude of the electric signal resulting from the application of a known acoustical signal. Earphone sensitivity is measured in terms of the amplitude of sound pressure it develops in a cavity of prescribed shape and size (which is intended to simulate a human ear) with the application of a specified electric signal voltage to the earphone terminals. Loudspeaker sensitivity is rated in terms of the sound pressure at a point in space at a specified distance resulting from the application of a given electric signal to the loudspeaker's terminals.

Sensitivity level, or response level, of a transducer in decibels is usually taken to be 20 times the logarithm to the base 10 of the ratio of amplitude sensitivity to a reference sensitivity. For microphones, the reference sensitivity is usually one volt per microbar; whereas for earphones and loudspeakers, it is one microbar per volt.

FREQUENCY RESPONSE

This characteristic describes the sensitivity level of a transducer in dB relative to reference sensitivity as a function of frequency, and is one of the most important descriptors of a transducer from the point of view of fidelity of performance. The frequency response curve of a typical moving-coil dynamic microphone used for public address is illustrated in Figure 3–8. When 0 dB reference is arbitrarily assigned to a particular frequency, say 1000 Hz, this characteristic is called relative frequency response.

Human hearing is capable of sensing sounds in the approximate frequency range of 20 Hz to 20,000 Hz, and this is taken as constituting the range defining "high-fidelity" performance. Microphones intended for making records, and phonograph pickups and loudspeakers in higher

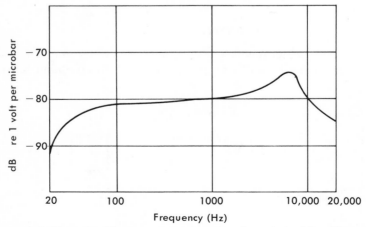

Figure 3–8 Example of frequency response curve of a typical public-address moving-coil dynamic microphone.

price categories, usually cover this range of frequency. Microphones and loudspeakers intended for public-address application cover a narrower range — generally 50 Hz to 12,000 Hz — and often have a frequency response which emphasizes the high frequencies to improve speech intelligibility. An ordinary American telephone covers the range from 200 Hz to about 3200 Hz which is adequate for carrying conversation. Most hearing aids, in which performance usually is subordinated to size, cover a frequency range from about 500 Hz to about 4000 Hz (cf. Chapter 4). An important task for the acoustical engineer today is to improve and expand the performance capabilities of transducers without sacrifice of size, cost, sensitivity, and other performance parameters important to the user.

DIRECTIONAL RESPONSE

Some transducers are designed to perform equally well from all directions, while others are intended to perform preferentially in specific directions. This characterization has given rise to a classification of transducers by directional characteristics.

A directional response pattern (also called a directivity or polar pattern) of a transducer used for sound emission or reception is a description (usually graphic) of the response of the transducer as a function of the direction of the transmitted or incident sound waves in a specified plane and at a specified frequency. A microphone for measuring sound pressure

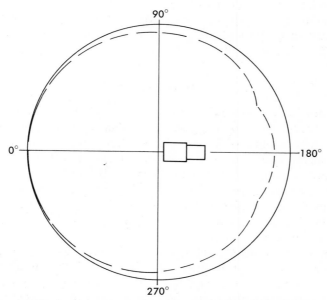

Figure 3–9   Omnidirectional pattern of a sound level meter microphone from 20–5000 Hz; this microphone, however, becomes "semi-directional" at a higher frequency, e.g., 10,000 Hz, as shown by the dashed line.

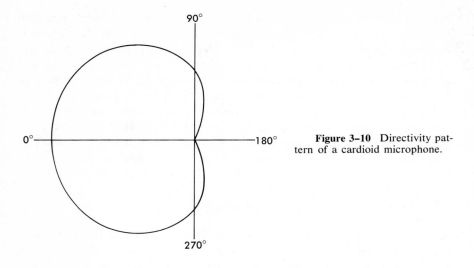

Figure 3-10 Directivity pattern of a cardioid microphone.

levels or for performing other types of acoustical measurements usually is designed to receive sound equally from all directions, in other words, to be omnidirectional; such a pattern is shown in Figure 3–9.

Usually, a microphone for use in public-address applications preferentially receives sounds arriving from the front for efficient transmission of speech and singing. An important class of microphones used in public address, as well as in recording and broadcast applications, is provided with special acoustical networks which allow it to receive sound from the front and to reject it when it arrives from the rear. Such a directivity pattern is called a cardioid (since it resembles the shape of a heart), as depicted in Figure 3–10.

DISTORTION

Distortion in transducers arises from the fact that some of the elements of design may be non-linear, resulting in an output which is not linearly proportional to the input. Distortion may become a problem in loudspeakers where large motions of the voice coil may cause it to traverse non-uniform portions of the magnetic field, or where the loudspeaker cone may develop slightly non-linear mechanical characteristics. Distortion is detected by applying a sine wave input to a loudspeaker and measuring the output with a standard microphone. Distortion may be seen as the presence of harmonic components in the microphone output in addition to the fundamental frequency of the input wave. It can be measured by means of an instrument called a distortion analyzer. Also earphones, especially those using magnetic transducers, may have a tendency to distort which is particularly undesirable in audiometric measurements in that the ear tends to be more sensitive to the higher-frequency harmonic components than to the low-frequency fundamental tones.

TRANSDUCER STRUCTURES

While this chapter is not intended to be a treatise on transducer design, it is clear that every serious user of transducers should have an elementary understanding of how they are constructed so as to utilize them with care and appreciation of their capabilities and limitations. Literally hundreds of different microphones, earphones, and loudspeakers have been produced by various transducer manufacturers. In the following section, a few of the more commonly encountered transducers are discussed.

MICROPHONES

A microphone contains a transducer proper, or cartridge, housed in a suitable enclosure or case for ease of handling, protection, and for convenient incorporation of accessories such as transformers, on-off switches, connectors, etc.

A carbon microphone cartridge, as used in the ordinary telephone mouthpiece, is shown in cross-section in Figure 3–11. It contains a

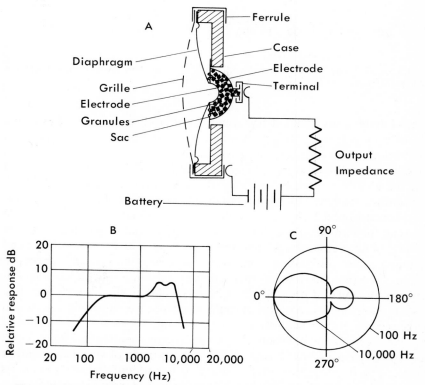

Figure 3–11   A, Illustrative cross-section of a carbon microphone transducer. B, Typical frequency response curve. C, Polar patterns.

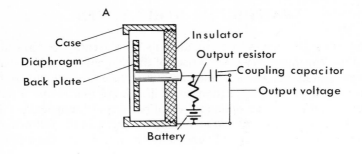

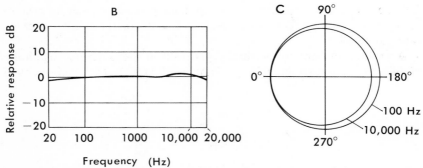

Figure 3–12   A, Illustrative cross-section of an electrostatic (condenser) microphone. B, Typical frequency response curve. C, Polar patterns.

conical diaphragm clamped between a circular case and a grille and held together by a ferrule. The transducer itself comprises a hemispherical electrode, called a button, attached to the diaphragm, concentric with another larger hemispherical electrode attached to the case, between which the carbon granules are located. The carbon granules are made of hard anthracite coal which has been crushed and heated in a hydrogen atmosphere to reduce impurities. They are poured into the cavity formed between the two electrodes and a cloth sac, and sealed with a sealing terminal. Sound pressure acts upon the diaphragm, causing it to vibrate and resulting in an alternating compacting and loosening of the granules, which correspondingly varies their contact resistance and causes a modulation of the current provided by a battery. This results in an alternating voltage developed across an output impedance representing the sound waves which is then transmitted to a receiver.

An electrostatic microphone, shown in cross-section in Figure 3–12, consists of a case which contains a diaphragm made of very thin metal or plastic. The diaphragm is stretched until it is perfectly flat and exhibits a resonance at several thousand Hz. This forms one electrode while a perforated back-plate brought very near the diaphragm forms the other electrode which is connected to an insulated central terminal. A capacitance formed between these two electrodes is charged by an external source (such as a battery). Sound pressure at the front of the diaphragm causes it to move to-and-fro, thereby varying the capacitance between the electrodes, resulting in the generation of an alternating voltage across an output resistance. The alternating motions of the diaphragm cause the film of air between it and the back-plate to be squeezed in and out, resulting in a damping of the diaphragm resonance. Therefore, the frequency response usually is flat and the directivity pattern omnidirectional over most of the frequency range.

An electret microphone is very similar to an electrostatic microphone except that the charge is formed permanently in a dielectric sheet, thus eliminating the need for a battery or other external source of polarizing voltage. With advances in electret technology, current development work is proceeding on microphones based on the electret principle combined with a built-in transistor amplifier for hearing-aid use. These microphones provide a dramatic improvement in hearing-aid quality (this is discussed at greater length in the next chapter).

A piezoelectric transducer, depicted in Figure 3–13, is composed of

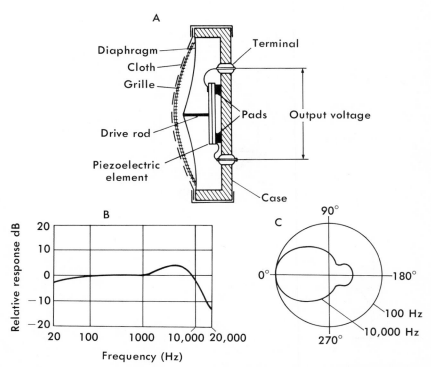

Figure 3–13 A, Illustrative cross-section of a piezoelectric microphone element. B, Typical frequency response curve. C, Polar pattern.

a case and a curvilinear conical diaphragm which is connected to a piezoelectric element by means of a "drive-rod." The element is mounted on insulating pads by a suitable cement, and its electrodes are brought out by means of terminals for connection to an external circuit. The diaphragm is protected by means of a grille to which cloth is typically affixed. The air motion due to a sound wave has to pass through the grille and cloth fabric before striking the diaphragm, and this tends to damp the mechanical resonances. The diaphragm and the element are designed to resonate at around 3 to 4 kHz, which is the point in the frequency range where the ear is most sensitive. The response of a piezoelectric microphone typically rises at resonance, resulting in clear speech transmission. Thus, piezoelectric microphones are satisfactory for home recording, low-cost public-address systems, and amateur broadcast applications.

A moving-coil transducer, shown in Figure 3–14, contains a porous acoustical resistance screen made of fabric or metal cloth which damps and controls the motions of the diaphragm over a frequency range of about 200 Hz to 8000 Hz. By adding a tube which connects the interior of the microphone cartridge with the external atmosphere and produces a low-frequency resonance, and by adding a perforated front grille which encloses a volume of air forming an acoustical resonator in front of the di-

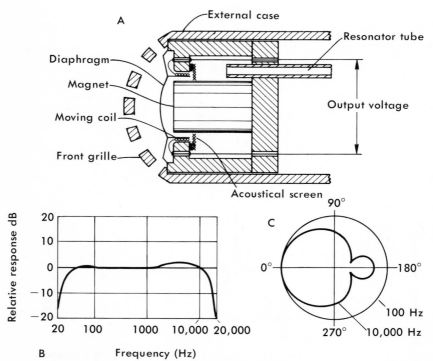

Figure 3–14 A, Illustrative cross-section of a moving coil (dynamic) microphone transducer. B, Typical frequency response curve. C, Polar pattern.

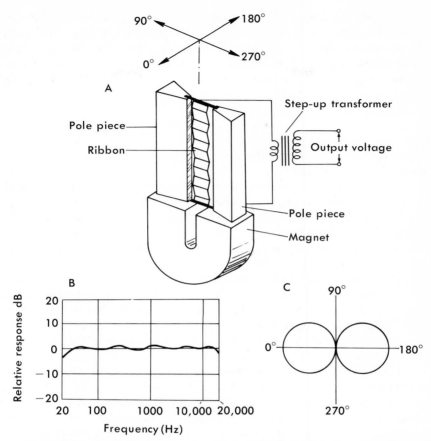

Figure 3–15 A, Stylized view of a ribbon "velocity" microphone transducer. B, Typical frequency response. C, Polar pattern.

aphragm, it is possible to lift the low and high frequency response of the microphone, resulting in wide-band sound transduction. The directivity pattern is omnidirectional over most of the frequency range, becoming semi-directional at high frequencies.

By providing a moving-coil diaphragm with specially designed acoustical networks, it is possible to obtain a cardioid directivity pattern over practically the entire frequency range of the microphone. Because of their excellent ability to reject unwanted sounds, cardioid microphones are used very widely in public-address and broadcast applications.

A ribbon velocity transducer, shown in Figure 3–15, consists of two pole pieces polarized by a strong magnet, so as to form an intense magnetic field between them, and a thin metallic ribbon suspended in the field and free to move as a result of difference of pressure at its two sides. When a sound wave strikes the ribbon from front or rear, it results in a net differential pressure between front and back which produces an electrical output signal; if it arrives from the side, the pressures on the two sides of the ribbon are equal and opposite, resulting in zero output. The directivity pattern has the shape of a "figure-8." A ribbon microphone is a simple device which has excellent frequency response and a uniform pattern at all frequencies, but it is infrequently used because of the fragility of the ribbon.

EARPHONES

Transducers used in earphones differ from those used in microphones in two important respects:

1. The earphone response, with its diaphragm generating a sound pressure in an ear canal, depends upon different acoustical factors than the response of the same transducer receiving sound pressure in open atmosphere. This means that the design criteria are different for microphones and earphones, even if the transducers are reversible.

2. The earphone handles considerably greater amounts of electrical power and develops considerably greater mechanical stresses between the diaphragm and its connection to the electromechanical transducer proper; therefore, in general terms, an earphone must be considerably more robust than the equivalent microphone transducer.

In all other respects, the operating principles of the two types of transducers are the same. Electrostatic, piezoelectric crystal or moving-coil earphone transducers, for example, may be constructed in a manner similar to the corresponding microphone transducers and, therefore, are not discussed further here. Instead, we consider an important class of transducers commonly used in earphones but less frequently used in microphones—the magnetic transducer.

The frequency response of earphones is usually given in terms of sound-pressure-level variations in a 6cc cavity (or a 2cc cavity for hearing-aid earphones) with a constant voltage applied to the terminals of the earphone, adjusted to produce an input of one milliwatt at 1000 Hz. However, the coupler response is not directly related to the sensation of hearing, which must be obtained by a loudness balance (cf. Chapter 7). The coupler is merely a mechanical device for studying earphone behavior and for controlling production quality.

Practically all earphones found in telephone handsets use an "unbalanced" magnetic transducer as shown in Figure 3–16. The unbalance takes the form of a steady attraction between the diaphragm and the magnetic pole-piece polarized by a permanent magnet. Superimposed upon the steady unbalanced force is an alternating magnetic force produced by the signal current passing through coil windings, which causes the to-and-fro force motion of the diaphragm, giving rise to the alternating sound pressure.

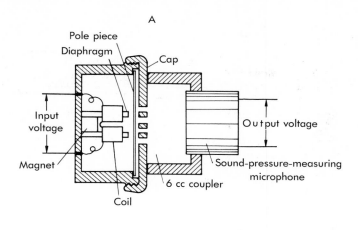

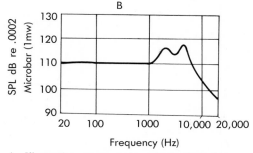

Figure 3–16 A, Illustrative cross-section of simple unbalanced magnetic receiver bearing against a 6 cc coupler with sound-pressure-measuring microphone. B, Typical frequency response.

The unbalanced magnetic receiver has the virtue of great simplicity; however, its diaphragm is rather thick and heavy in order to be able to withstand the steady-state magnetic force. This excess mass results in inefficient operation. In a balanced magnetic transducer, the steady magnetic flow remains within the magnetic structure itself. A balanced magnetic transducer is shown in Figure 3–17, which depicts a hearing-aid receiver in cross-section. The unbalanced flow produced by the electric signal is carried by a thin magnetic reed, called an armature, around which the coil is wound. The reed drives a very light diaphragm. Because the excess mass is eliminated, there is a significant improvement of efficiency which makes the balanced armature transducer suitable for use in hearing aids and other devices where the available power is minimal. In receivers for this latter application, the air displaced by motion of the diaphragm is conducted through a small plastic tube to an ear coupler which is inserted in the ear canal of the user.

LOUDSPEAKERS

A loudspeaker consists of one or more moving-coil drivers of the type described earlier in this chapter installed in a box or baffle which

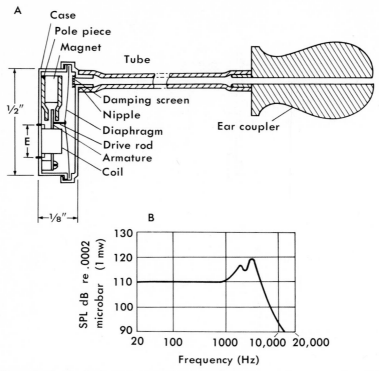

Figure 3–17 A, Stylized cross-section of hearing-aid receiver transducer, balanced magnetic type. B, Response characteristic measured with 1 mw power input at 1000 Hz, into a 2 cc coupler.

prevents the sound radiated from the back surface of the diaphragm from canceling the sound radiated by the front surface. Shown in Figure 3–18, the cross-section is a loudspeaker with three drivers, the woofer, the squawker and the tweeter, attached to corresponding apertures in the front baffle-board mounted in the loudspeaker cabinet. Within the cabinet there is an electrical dividing network which carries to each driver that portion of the signal which the particular unit is designed to handle. In the so-called "acoustical-suspension" type of loudspeaker, the woofer resonance is controlled largely by the cushion of air within the cabinet. Since distortion often is generated by non-linear diaphragm-rim compliance, control by the air cushion results in a significant improvement in loudspeaker performance and freedom from distortion. On the other hand, sometimes a resonator aperture or pipe (shown in Figure 3–18) is added to improve the response of the loudspeaker to very low frequencies. When such a base-boosting device is used, the loudspeaker is called a reflex unit.

A loudspeaker of the type described above is omnidirectional at low

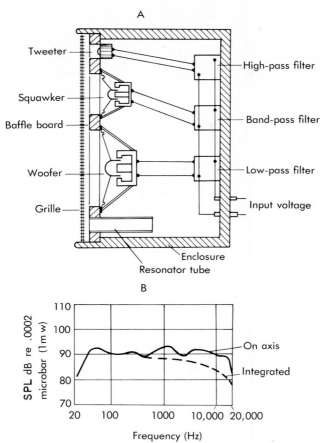

Figure 3–18 A, Cross-sectional view of a high-fidelity loudspeaker. B, Typical frequency response characteristics.

frequencies (up to about 500 Hz), becoming progressively more directional at higher frequencies. In a well-designed loudspeaker, however, the high-frequency polar pattern remains relatively uniform over an included angle of about 90 degrees toward the front. Sometimes loudspeakers for specific applications are designed to embody special directional attributes.

The frequency response of a loudspeaker often is measured at one meter in front of the center of the baffle board. Frequency Response Characteristic, based on integrated performance over an imaginary front hemisphere or sphere surrounding the loudspeaker, often provides a more meaningful criterion of a loudspeaker performance than the head-on response alone.

REFERENCES

Beranek, Leo J. (1954): *Acoustics*. New York, McGraw-Hill Book Co.
Gayford, M. L. (1971): *Electroacoustics*. New York, American Elsevier Publishing Co.
Olson, Harry F. (1957): *Acoustical Engineering*. Princeton, N.J., D. Van Nostrand Co.
The following standards published by the American National Standards Institute (430 Broadway, New York, N.Y. 10018) are useful references:

S 1.1	1960	Acoustical Terminology.
S 1.4	1970	Sound Level Meters.
S 1.5	1963	Practices for Loudspeaker Measurements.
S 1.6	1967	Preferred Frequencies and Band Numbers for Acoustical Measurements.
S 1.8	1969	Preferred Reference Quantities for Acoustical Levels.
S 1.10	1966	Method for the Calibration of Microphones.
S 1.12	1967	Specifications for Laboratory Standard Microphones.
S 3.3	1960	Methods for the Measurements of the Electroacoustic Characteristics of Hearing Aids.
S 3.6	1969	Specifications for Audiometers.
S 3.7	1973	Methods for the Coupler Calibration of Earphones.
S 3.13	1972	Artificial Head-Bone for the Calibration of Audiometer Bone Vibrators.

Chapter Four

AUDIOMETERS AND HEARING AIDS

ROBERT E. SANDLIN AND DONALD F. KREBS

Electroacoustic transducers are employed in two principal ways for clinical purposes: in audiometers and in hearing aids. An audiometer is a device for the measurement of auditory sensitivity, while a hearing aid is a device for the enhancement of auditory sensitivity in those who lost it. There are several good textbooks on audiometry (e.g., Katz, 1972; Newby, 1972) where detailed descriptions of audiometers may be found; hence, the discussion to follow is relatively cursory. The same cannot be said for hearing aids; therefore, the bulk of this chapter is devoted to that topic.

73

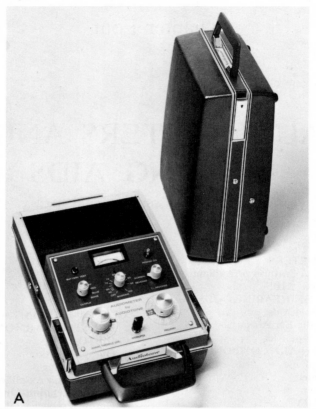

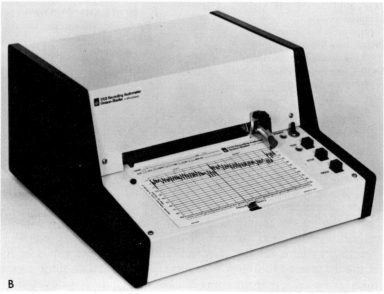

Figure 4–1   Audiometers vary dramatically in size and complexity.

(*Illustration continued on opposite page.*)

AUDIOMETERS

ESSENTIAL FEATURES OF AUDIOMETERS

The single most frequently used clinical tool employed by an audiologist to assess human ear function is the audiometer. Audiometers come in various sizes and configurations with different degrees of complexity (Fig. 4–1). If one were to define the essential features of an audiometer, however, the following must be included:

Frequency Selector. It is the function of the frequency selector to do

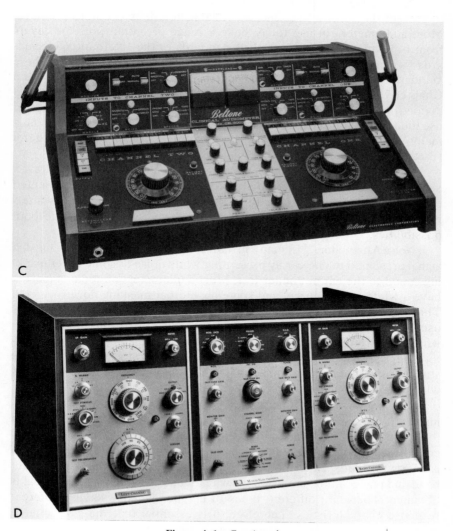

Figure 4–1 *Continued.*

just that, to select the frequency to be delivered to the ear under test. Most audiometers are capable of generating frequencies of 125, 250, 500, 1000, 2000, 4000, and 8000 Hz. You will note that the frequency range is given in steps of one octave; that is, an octave increase for 125 Hz renders 250 Hz, for 250 Hz renders 500 Hz, for 500 Hz renders 1000 Hz, etc. In more sophisticated audiometers (the so-called "clinical" audiometers), half-octave values in the discrete frequencies of 750, 1500, 3000, and 6000 Hz, in addition to those mentioned above may be available. Obviously, the range of frequencies available does not cover the entire range of human hearing, but rather covers the range which is felt to be critical for understanding speech and for social functioning.

Hearing Level Selector. It is the purpose of the hearing level selector to present the several frequencies available at a defined output pressure. Most audiometers in use today have a range of output pressure levels from 0 dB to 110 dB calibrated to standards of the International Standards Organization or the American National Standards Institute. These standards set 0 dB hearing level to the minimum audible pressure (cf. Chapter 7) for healthy young ears. Usually, the hearing level selector is divided into five-decibel steps, although there are some audiometers in use today which provide one-decibel increments. This is finer than is normally needed to adequately assess hearing, but can be justified for research purposes.

Interrupter Switch. This switch is used to present or to withdraw a signal at the ear. The switch may be so positioned that a tone is presented only when it is depressed, or the tone may be continuous and is interrupted when the switch is depressed. Many audiometers provide both possibilities.

Noise Attenuator. In many instances, it may be necessary to mask a signal presented to one ear by presenting white noise or some other masking sound to the ear not under test. Most audiometers on today's market have a white noise source, and some have other masking noises as well. The dial is marked in decibels and, like the hearing level selector, is usually calibrated in five-decibel steps. One must be careful to observe to what standard the noise generator is calibrated as the hearing level selector and the noise control dial are usually calibrated differently. The student must familiarize himself with the different calibration standards which may exist together in the same audiometer.

Earphones. While the foregoing are essential features of audiometers, it is apparent that there must be a way of presenting these signals to the ear; that is, there must be an electroacoustic transducer. This is accomplished by earphones, although clinical audiometers typically have a capacity for loudspeaker output. The earphones are mounted on a headband and placed at the ear in such a way that a reasonably effective seal is obtained. There are different types of earphones, each having different response characteristics. Therefore, it is essential that the earphone be calibrated to the audiometer with which it is being used.

Power. It is obvious that there must be a means to energize or provide power to the audiometer. This is done by a simple switch, but there are two kinds of power sources which may be used. The most commonly employed power supply is alternating current (AC); that is, the kind of electrical power provided by a wall receptacle found in the home, school, or office, generated by the local power company and supplied to the community. The other kind of power supply is direct current (DC) supplied by a battery. The advantages of a DC-powered audiometer are that it is highly portable and does not depend upon the availability of AC power for operation. Very few audiometers offer the user the choice of AC or DC; the power source is in the design.

Speech Circuit. Some audiometers will have a speech circuit which enables the audiologist to assess the patient's ability to understand speech stimuli. Like all of the other signal inputs to the earphones, speech stimuli must also be calibrated to some standard. The student would be wise to know the calibrated level of speech input.

Bone Conduction Circuit. Most audiometers with which the student will become familiar will have a bone conduction circuit which permits the testing of hearing by stimulation to the skull. That is, the pure-tone energy is transmitted to the cochlear structures by means of bone conduction rather than by air conduction as is the case when earphones are used as the energy source.

Certainly, this very basic description of an audiometer is only to familiarize the student with that which he will observe when he uses an audiometer for the first time. Obviously, there are audiometers which are indeed basic and will only supply a generated, controlled pure tone at a calibrated level at the earphone. This rather simple audiometer can be contrasted to the so-called "clinical audiometer" which can do a number of functions in determining the status of the human ear. The advanced audiometer is a significant diagnostic tool in the hands of a competent audiologist.

HEARING AIDS

'Twas brillig, and the slithy toves
Did gyre and gimble in the wabe;
All mimsy were the borogoves,
And the mome raths outgrabe.
Lewis Carroll

Certainly, Carroll's phonologically valid, but meaningless, verse is not unlike the confusion experienced by some hearing-impaired individuals straining to understand the intended message of the speaker. It wasn't until rather recent times that man had usable and efficient electroacoustic systems in the form of wearable hearing aids to bring the intended messages of speakers into sharper focus. Histories of the development of electroacoustic devices worn by the hearing-impaired have been

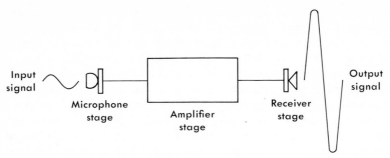

Figure 4–2 The basic schema of the three significant stages of a hearing aid.

reported by Davis and Silverman (1970), Katz (1972), and Newby (1972). A chapter dealing with advances in design and utilization of electroacoustic devices is of specific and general interest to those concerned with the problems of impaired hearing. While one is in sympathy with the myriad of problems associated with hearing loss and the evaluation of hearing aid amplification, such is not the purpose of this chapter; we described briefly our biases relative to hearing aid evaluation and the successful fitting of electroacoustic devices.

The reader will discern the absence of controversial issues dealing with the non-technical, but equally important, issues of successful hearing-aid utilization. Included are the technical parameters of electroacoustic amplifying systems which merit consideration: essential components, response characteristics, limitation of responses, methods of limiting response, distortion, slope amplification, and application of electroacoustic devices to types of hearing impairment.

Basically, in any amplifying device, the primary purpose is to take a generated signal, pass it through an amplifying system, and make it louder. Figure 4–2 simply suggests that the input signal is "picked up" by the microphone, put through the amplifier, and sent to the receiver where the output signal is of greater intensity than the input signal. The sophistication of hearing aid circuitry has undergone significant technological advance during the past few decades. From the very basic carbon type amplifier to the transistor operated instrument, a rather sustained and useful advance has been forthcoming from the hearing aid industry. The resultant miniaturization of component parts has contributed significantly to design advance.

TYPES OF HEARING AIDS

A primary diagnostic decision which an audiologist must make is whether a patient is a candidate for monaural or binaural hearing aid amplification. It is safe to assume that in the presence of a bilateral hearing loss, maximum compensation can most often be obtained by binaural fitting. Although there is controversy as to whether or not binaural amplification is superior to monaural, clinical experience suggests that binaural fitting is, indeed, superior in appreciably ameliorating such problems as loss of discrimination in the presence of noise, sound localization, and the subjective feeling of circumferential hearing. The decision to fit monaurally or binaurally is ultimately based on the acceptance of the patient and his ability to purchase the recommended instrument. However, assuming that these are not of major concern, binaural fitting should always be considered when the audiometric configuration is such as to suggest hearing aid amplification at all. Whether monaural or binaural, the hearing aid is available in four types: conventional (or body-worn), eyeglass, in-the-ear, or behind-the-ear.

EAR-LEVEL AIDS

When considering ear-level amplification, there are three types of hearing aid design which may resolve the patient's problem, the first of which is the post-auricular (behind-the-ear) aid. The post-auricular hearing aid fits behind the external ear and a small plastic tube coming from the nubbin of the receiver to the earmold is inserted into the external ear canal. In some instances the microphone is forward-facing, in others it is rear-facing or rear-mounted. The forward-facing microphone is superior in most listening situations. Figure 4–3 shows a schematic diagram of a post-auricular hearing aid. You will note that contained within the rather basic circuit are the three essential components which comprise any hearing aid and which were shown in Figure 4–2. All of the electronic components and subsequent circuitry are contained within a common plastic housing, the hearing aid case. Within the last decade, the post-auricular

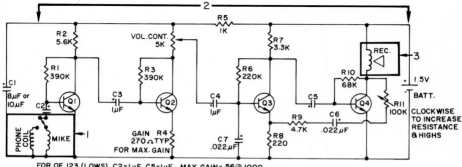

FOR OE 123 (LOWS) C2=1µF, C5=1µF, MAX. GAIN=56@ 1000
FOR OE 124 (NO LOWS) C2=.1µF, C5=.022µF, MAX.GAIN=53@ 1000

Figure 4–3   Circuit diagram of a four-transistor post-auricular hearing aid. (Courtesy of Vicon Instrument Co.)

hearing aid has become the instrument of choice for the vast majority of hearing aid users.

There are other considerations which should be taken into account when conducting a comprehensive hearing aid evaluation. Chief among these is the age of the patient. Special care must be given to the very young child to make certain that the hearing aid is not only the appropriate one, but is one which can be worn with a minimal amount of difficulty. It has been our experience, for the very young child on whom we have placed post-auricular devices, that we must have some means of securing the instrument to the head, perhaps by a band across the head or some other method. If such security is not provided, the hearing aid can be dislodged and fall from the ear. However, this is not an insurmountable problem and can be resolved with a reasonable amount of creativity and observation. The task is somewhat easier for the adult patient, although one encounters cosmetic considerations more often than in the younger patient. For the most part, the vast majority of hearing loss types among the adult population can be successfully fitted with post-auricular instruments; however, there are several possibilities which one may consider.

There are those patients who would prefer that ear-level hearing be achieved by the eyeglass hearing aid. In the eyeglass instrument the microphone, amplifier, and receiver are mounted in the temple of the eyeglass, again with a polyethylene tube going from the receiver nubbin to the earmold inserted into the external canal. Although one can find very little acoustic advantage between the postauricular hearing aid and the eyeglass instrument, experience has shown that, from a cosmetic point of view, many patients will prefer the eyeglass instrument. This preference is true whether the instrument is binaurally or monaurally fitted. Although, acoustically, we have no real preference for one or the other, from a utilitarian standpoint the post-auricular aid seems to be most beneficial. The obvious reason for this preference is that the patient can remove the hearing aid without having to remove his glasses. For those patients preferring only part-time use of amplification, it would seem somewhat unwise to recommend hearing aid amplification applied through the eyeglass-type instrument. However, the converse may very well be true for those patients who desire full-time amplified experience and who also wear glasses during their waking hours. It should be made reasonably clear that the decision again is the patient's because one does not have to compromise the acoustic response of the instrument.

ALL-IN-THE-EAR AIDS

The only advantage of this variety of hearing aid is that it is, indeed, contained within the earmold which is inserted into the ear. If one is considering this type of hearing aid, he must be willing to accept the compromises which are imposed. These include a smaller microphone, a smaller receiver, and an amplifier which has limited gain and output response. Gain, maximum power output, and frequency response are limited when compared with those that can be achieved in the post-auricular, eyeglass, or body-worn hearing instruments. From a clinical point of view, little support is found for recommendation of the all-in-the-ear hearing aid in that it is most difficult to modify once the unit is made to conform to the peculiarities of the external canal of the patient. It is less difficult in ear-level aids to modify response characteristics in that they lend themselves to easy manipulation by hearing aid engineers at the factory.

BODY-TYPE AIDS

The body-type, or body-worn, instrument has several distinct advantages which are denied to ear-level instruments. In general, greater acoustic gain and maximum output values can be generated in a body-worn aid simply because it is larger. Because the physical space in which hearing aid components can be placed is appreciably greater than that of ear-worn instruments, much more sophisticated circuitry can be utilized to modify the shape of the output envelope. In general, however, the current use of body-worn instruments is limited to those who have severe to profound hearing losses and who require greater maximum power output and acoustic gain than can be achieved in an ear-worn device. Also there are those who routinely select the body-type instrument for the very young child in that they feel it is less subject to damage or failure than ear-level devices. There is no reasonable argument against this practice other than to suggest that the reliability, durability, and stability of ear-worn devices are greater than they were a few years ago. Therefore, one may con-

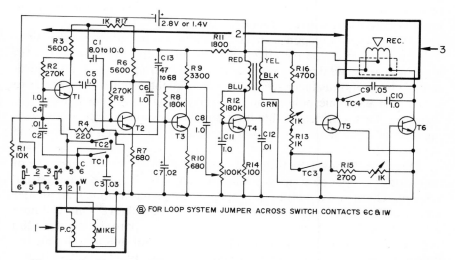

Figure 4-4 Circuit diagram of a six-transistor body-type hearing aid. (Courtesy of Vicon Instrument Co.)

sider the ear-level hearing aid the instrument of choice if appropriate acoustic properties can be achieved.

Figure 4–4 shows a somewhat more complicated hearing aid schematic diagram representative of the body-type hearing instrument. With the exception of the receiver, all components and associated circuitry are contained within a common space. Since the body-type aid can accommodate more component parts, more sophistication of output signal control can be exercised as that control relates to frequency bandwidth, maximum power output, method of output limiting, and the slope of amplification. Body-type hearing aids are still frequently employed for those individuals having amplification demands which cannot be met by post-auricular instruments. Many congenitally deaf children are candidates for the body-type hearing aid.

HEARING AID COMPONENTS

Let us take a brief look at each of the major parts of a hearing aid — microphone, amplifier, and receiver — and see what each contributes to the total operation of the instrument.

MICROPHONE

The primary purpose of the hearing aid microphone, regardless of type and construction, is to respond to changes of sound pressure. As a result of this response to pressure change, a rather weak but sufficient current is generated at the microphone level and input to the amplifier where its current (measured in milliamperes) is greatly magnified. Either crystal or magnetic microphones may be used in hearing aids, but the magnetic type is preferred and used in modern aids.

The frequency response curve of hearing aid transducers determines in large measure the output envelope (what the output signal looks like) of a given hearing aid device. Manufacturers of hearing aids will often institute methods of transducer selection in their quality-control procedures to insure that each microphone or receiver will have a defined frequency response. This is critical in that the frequency response of the transducer must be of a pre-determined value to achieve the desired output of the hearing aid.

Figure 4–5 shows the frequency response curve of a common type of magnetic microphone used in post-auricular aids. It is obvious that the response characteristic of the microphone shown has a somewhat greater emphasis for the frequency region located above 500 Hz. One will note also that the range of frequency response extends approximately to 3200 Hz. Although there are hearing aid microphones of different design and construction which yield greater frequency range, Figure 4–5 is illustra-

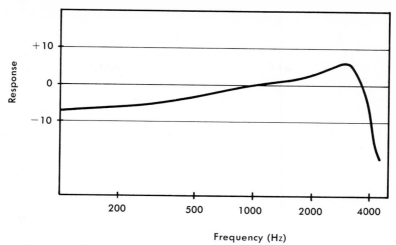

Figure 4-5 The frequency response of the hearing aid microphone. Note the slight emphasis of the frequency range above 1000 Hz.

tive of typical microphone response. The electret microphone has been introduced recently into hearing aids and has largely eliminated the effects of clothing noise and modified the range of frequency response. The smoothness of the frequency response has been signficiantly improved with the introduction of the microphone's modification.

AMPLIFIER

The hearing aid amplifier takes a rather weak electrical signal, generated by the microphone, and amplifies it most significantly. The degree to which the signal is amplified is a function of design. Amplifiers can be designed to yield only minimal amplification of the input signal to very great changes of amplification of the input signal. The amplifier is where significant changes can be brought about in controlling and shaping the input signal to the desired output signal.

Figure 4-6 shows the frequency response of a hearing aid amplifier. It is immediately apparent that the amplifier has a flat response throughout its spectrum; that is, the amplifier is linear with respect to frequency response. There is no apparent emphasis of high- or low-frequency ranges as is found in microphones and receivers. In the electronics of the hearing aid amplifier, many dramatic changes have come about which were not imagined a decade ago. The miniaturization of components, the introduction of highly stable transistors, the utilization of various crystals in developing integrated circuitry, and a host of other innovations serve to make today's commercial hearing aid a highly versatile and useful amplifying device.

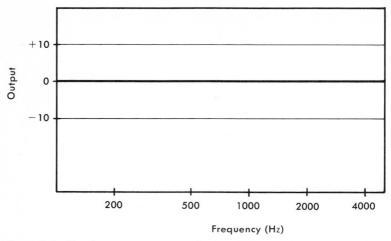

Figure 4–6 The frequency response of a hearing aid amplifier. Note the absolute linearity of the response.

RECEIVER

The purpose of the hearing aid receiver, regardless of type and construction, is to respond to changes of voltage generated by the hearing aid amplifier. When the changes occur, the diaphragm of the receiver moves and in so doing converts electrical energy into acoustic energy. Hearing aid receivers, like hearing aid microphones, are usually of the magnetic type.

Figure 4–7 displays the frequency response of a hearing output

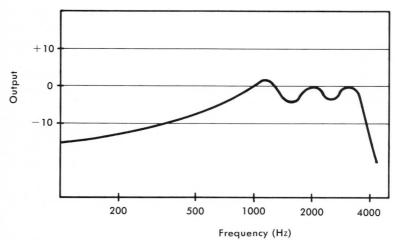

Figure 4–7 The frequency response of a hearing aid receiver.

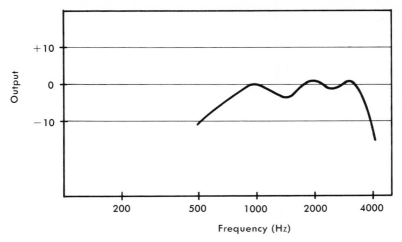

Figure 4–8 The combined effect of the hearing aid microphone, receiver, and amplifier.

transducer, i.e., a receiver. Again, it is apparent that the frequency range above 1000 Hz is slightly more amplified than the range below 1000 Hz. Note also that the response of the receiver, as was also apparent for the microphone, falls off rather sharply above 3200 Hz. Certainly, the reader is aware that there are receivers having frequency response extending beyond 3200 Hz. Here, again, the response characteristic of the receiver is a function of design. The smaller the actual size of the receiver, the greater is the limitation of the response. Hence, the receiver used in ear-level instruments does not have the same performance characteristic as the receiver used in a body-type instrument.

Figure 4–8 shows the resultant output of the hearing aid when all its parts are functioning as an amplifying unit. Note that the output envelope clearly shows the influence of the microphone and the receiver response characteristics. The shaping of the output envelope of a hearing aid can frequently be obtained by careful selection of microphone and receiver; however, when greater emphasis of high or low tonal regions is desired, it can be effectively achieved by appropriate electronic changes within the amplifier.

SUMMARY

Technological advances in hearing aid design have been realized mainly through significant breakthroughs in component design and the introduction of new materials in their manufacture. Although the complexity of design and production is more demanding, the advantages accruing to the hearing aid user have been substantial. There have been significant advances in hearing aid size, design, components, and associated circuitry. In the transducer field alone, tremendous advances have added substantially to patient utilization and acceptance of amplification.

The reader is reminded that useful information about the current status of hearing aid development can be obtained from many of the leading hearing aid manufacturers. As a matter of fact, many hearing aid companies employ audiologists who, in part, are responsible for the dissemination of information about the current state of the art as well as contributing their skill and knowledge to the development of superior products. Additionally, the student may wish to contact local hearing aid dispensers who, in large measure, are responsible for demonstrating to the hearing-impaired person the advantages provided by technological development.

The basic functions of a conventional hearing aid are summarized as follows: The hearing aid microphone (input transducer) responds to sound pressure changes. These pressure changes create movement of the microphone diaphragm which is directly proportional to the pressure changes. As a result of this diaphragmatic movement, a weak electric current is generated which is greatly increased by the hearing aid amplifier which also exercises control over the magnitude of amplification as well as the shape of the output signal. The signal, thus electrically amplified, is then fed to the hearing aid receiver (output transducer). This causes its diaphragm to move and thereby converts the electric signal back into acoustic energy at an intensity significantly greater than that which impinged upon the diaphragm of the microphone. The efficiency and fidelity with which this is accomplished determine the quality of the instrument and the success of its utilization.

PROPERTIES OF HEARING AIDS

It is useful to define some of the commonly used terms referring to parameters of hearing aid response. Additionally, it is interesting to look somewhat more closely at the several output configurations of hearing aids. There are several performance parameters which are accessible to instrumental measurement. From these several measurements we can gain a great deal of information about the efficiency of the hearing aid in responding to pressure changes as well as an excellent idea of whether or not the hearing aid is the one most appropriate for a given loss of hearing. Obviously, all hearing losses are not identical in their severity or type. It would seem just as obvious, therefore, that hearing aid amplification which best resolves the deficit created by hearing loss cannot be expressed by one instrument having a fixed response. That is, different losses require different hearing aid amplified responses.

ACOUSTIC GAIN

Acoustic gain is best defined as the output of the hearing aid minus the input. Let us assume that at 1000 Hz the output of the hearing aid is 100 dB and the input to its microphone is 60 dB sound pressure level. Following the basic formula, we subtract the input (60 dB) from the output (100 dB) and state that the gain of the instrument at 1000 Hz is 40 dB. The Hearing Aid Industry Conference (HAIC) has agreed to a standard input of 60 dB SPL for obtaining basic frequency response information. HAIC has also agreed upon a method of arriving at an expression of acoustic gain. This is accomplished by averaging the actual acoustic gain at 500, 1000, and 2000 Hz. The resulting single gain figure then expresses the HAIC gain. For example, consider the following:

Frequency	Acoustic Gain
500 Hz	35 dB
1000 Hz	50 dB
2000 Hz	65 dB
	150 dB ÷ 3 = 50 dB

Therefore, the HAIC gain would be 50 dB.

FREQUENCY RESPONSE RANGE

The frequency response range of a hearing aid is the one to which it is sensitive and over which it will provide some degree of amplification. Although several attempts have been made to meaningfully display

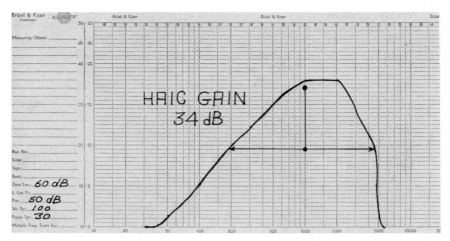

Figure 4–9 A demonstration of the method by which the HAIC frequency response range is determined. The HAIC gain (34 dB) is plotted at 1000 Hz; 15 dB down a horizontal line is drawn until intersecting the response curve. The frequency range is determined by the points of intersection.

frequency response range, the only generally accepted method is that adopted by HAIC. The HAIC method is illustrated in Figure 4–9 wherein one plots the average acoustic gain (computed by the HAIC method) on the vertical axis at 1000 Hz. A horizontal line is drawn 15 dB below that point extending until it intersects the two extremes of the frequency response curve. In Figure 4–9, then, the acoustic gain at 500 Hz is 30 dB, 36 dB at 1000 Hz, and 36 dB at 2000 Hz. The average of these three—and, therefore, the HAIC gain—is 34 dB; this is plotted at 1000 Hz. A line is drawn 15 dB below this point and continued to the intersection of the frequency response curve at each end. Thus, the frequency response of the hearing aid shown in Figure 4–9 has a range from approximately 180 Hz to about 4200 Hz.

MAXIMUM POWER OUTPUT

This measurement is defined as the maximum acoustic output that the hearing aid is capable of producing, regardless of how intense the input signal may be. Let us assume that we have a hearing aid with a maximum power output of 130 dB and an acoustic gain of 40 dB. Remembering that the level of the input signal is generally accepted as 60 dB, we would get the following result:

Input Level	Output Level
60 dB	100 dB
70 dB	110 dB
80 dB	120 dB
90 dB	130 dB
100 dB	130 dB

It now becomes reasonably clear that when a 90 dB input signal impinges upon the face of the microphone, the maximum power output of the hearing aid has been accomplished. Input signals greater than 90 dB would not result in greater power output. It is at this point that the instrument is said to be "in saturation." That is, it can no longer amplify inputs greater than 90 dB. It is our contention that control of the maximum power output is critical. A defense of this contention is found later in this chapter when we review methods of output limiting.

CONVENTIONAL LINEAR AMPLIFIER

Amplifiers of this type were among the earliest to be developed in the hearing aid industry. A "conventional" amplifier implies simply that there is a one-to-one relationship between the input signal and the result output level. Therefore, if we were to increase the level of the input signal by 10 dB there would be a like increase in the output signal.

That is, if we went from a 60 dB input signal to a 70 dB input signal, we would go from an output of 100 dB to 110 dB, assuming an acoustic gain of 40 dB.

NON-LINEAR AMPLIFIER

Amplifiers of this type perform in such a manner that there is not a linear relationship between the input signal and the output. That is, for an increase of 10 dB in the input signal, there may be something less than a 10 dB increase of output. For example, let us assume an output pressure of 100 dB; suddenly there is an increase of 10 dB in the input signal at the microphone. In a conventional linear amplifier the output would increase to 110 dB; but in a non-linear amplifier the output would be something less than 110 dB but still more than 100 dB. The degree of non-linearity between the input signal and the output is a function of engineering design. A general term applied to this type of non-linearity is *compression amplification*.

Figure 4–10 shows a basic response curve of a hearing aid rather like that of many post-auricular instruments. Recalling that the zero level is 60 dB, and knowing that the standard input level is 60 dB, we can quite easily compute acoustic gain per frequency. Keeping in mind that acoustic gain is defined as output minus input, we arrive at the following acoustic gain values:

Frequency	Acoustic Gain
500 Hz	30 dB
1000 Hz	40 dB
2000 Hz	40 dB
3000 Hz	43 dB

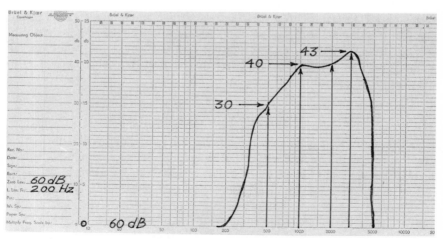

Figure 4–10 The acoustic gain of a typical post-auricular hearing aid.

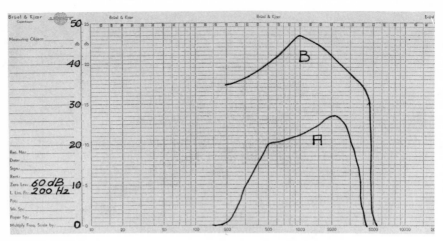

Figure 4–11   A basic response curve (A) and a maximum power output curve (B).

Our current view is that control of acoustic gain is essential if we are to optimally fit the hearing-impaired individual. Technological advances in hearing aid engineering and production capabilities now make it a relatively routine procedure to achieve specified response characteristics as they relate to acoustic gain per frequency. At the moment, it is most difficult to realize acoustic gain values per octave greater than 18 to 20 dB. That is, we may have a gain of 20 dB at 500 Hz and would be unable to reach an acoustic gain greater than 38 to 40 dB at 1000 Hz, thus giving an 18 to 20 dB rise for the octave lying between 500 and 1000 Hz.

Figure 4–11 shows a basic gain curve (A) and the maximum power output curve (B) of a post-auricular hearing aid. You will note that the zero level (baseline) is 60 dB. These response curves are reasonably representative of present-day instruments which have power limiting at approximately 110 dB. This kind of information is most important for those who are making decisions about the most appropriate hearing instrument. Unless the maximum power output is specified at some point on the graph, or by an actual maximum power output curve, there is no way to compute it by measuring the basic response curve.

FREQUENCY-SHAPING

One cannot stress too strongly the need for definitive information about the specific hearing aid being considered for a given person. Intelligent attention to the objective information given by the response curve and other hearing aid performance data can greatly reduce needless error and unreasoned guesswork. Attention to the reported acoustic data is certainly not all that is needed to successfully fit a hearing aid, but just as certainly these data are most important and helpful in arriving at decisions.

Figure 4–12 portrays the effects of frequency-shaping upon the out-

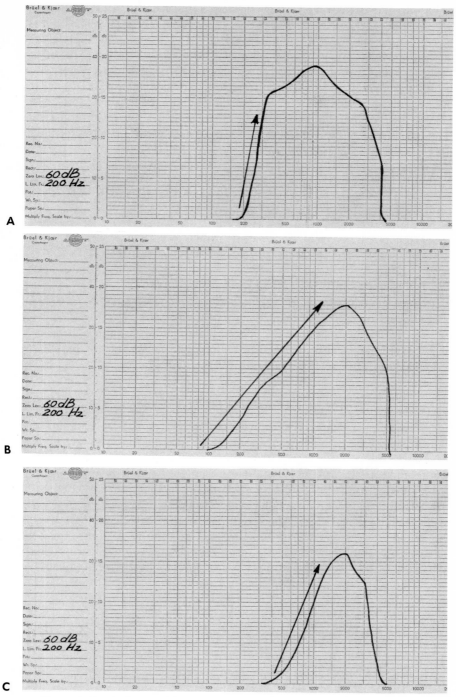

A

B

C

Figure 4–12 A shows minimal frequency shaping as suggested by the angle of the arrow. B shows the effects of frequency shaping (slope amplification) suggested by the angle of the arrow. Note the appreciable suppression of the lower frequencies when compared with A. C also demonstrates the effects of frequency shaping. Note that there is little or no gain at 500 Hz but appreciable gain at 1000 Hz and above with the maximum at 2000 Hz.

put envelope. You will immediately note that low-frequency suppression is pronounced as you go from Figure 4–12A to 4–12C. Sandlin (1969) has suggested that appropriate frequency-shaping (or slope amplification) is of significant benefit in dealing with certain kinds of hearing losses. Frequency-shaping would appear to be indicated when, for example, the hearing-impaired individual has better hearing for the low frequencies than for the highs. The rationale is rather simple and implies that for those tonal regions where minimal gain is needed, the hearing aid output response should be controlled by appropriate shaping of the response. Reddell (1966) has also found slope amplification to be of benefit to the majority of those having hearing loss configurations which indicate the need for controlled response of the hearing aid.

EXTRA-CIRCUITRY MODIFICATIONS

While the output envelope of the hearing aid is determined primarily by the interdependent function of the microphone, amplifier, and receiver, it can be appreciably modified by other means. In some instances, the extra-circuitry modifications are intentionally accomplished; in others, it may be a rather arbitrary process without full awareness of the effects upon the output envelope as a result of the modification.

EARMOLD-VENTING

Figure 4–13 displays a conventional earmold used for coupling the hearing aid to the ear. The fact is that the earmold, too, introduces acoustic modifications to the signal which can be altered by "venting" or making holes in the mold. Figure 4–14 shows the effects of earmold-venting upon an output envelope. Response curve A in that figure indicates the shape of the frequency response curve when a .016-inch diameter bore is drilled in the earmold canal, thus creating a vent from the earmold canal to the outside air. Note that the acoustic gain at 1000 Hz is approximately 34 dB. For comparison, observe curve B when the vent size is increased to a diameter of .083 inch and there is an appreciable change of the acous-

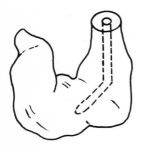

Figure 4–13 An earmold is the plastic piece which couples the hearing aid to the ear.

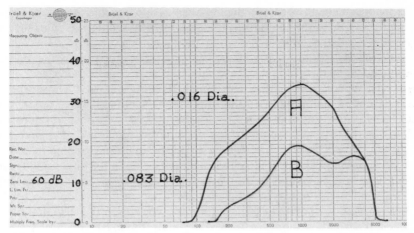

Figure 4–14 The effects of earmold venting upon the output envelope of a hearing aid.

tic gain at 1000 Hz. The magnitude of the difference is about 19 dB. In effect, the increased vent size will cost about 15 dB acoustic gain at 1000 Hz. Vent sizes larger or smaller than these would alter the output envelope correspondingly. One would seriously question the practice of arbitrarily venting an earmold to relieve client discomfort without being fully aware of the effects which such venting may have upon the output characteristics of the instrument.

INSERT FILTERS

Filters inserted into the tube leading to the earmold are another method of achieving modified acoustic response. Normally, these insert filters can be grouped into three commonly used types:

1. Mechanical Filters. Generally, these are small, metallic cylinders having rather small internal diameters. The size of the diameter will determine the effect which the filter will have on the output of the hearing aid.

2. Sintered Filters. These filters have been fairly recently introduced to the hearing aid industry. The sintered filter consists of small, metallic balls sintered together. The number and size of the balls determines the effect upon the output response of the instrument.

3. Lamb's Wool Filters. These filters are simply what the name implies. Effective filtering is achieved by "packing" lamb's wool into the polyethylene tubing of the post-auricular aid. The density with which the tubing is packed will determine the degree of filtering which takes place. Lamb's wool is used as the packing substance because it resists moisture retention more effectively than other substances. However, lamb's wool is probably the least desirable means of selective filtering in that it is very difficult to control the amount of the density with which it is packed into the polyethylene tubing.

Figure 4–15 shows the effects of sintered filters upon the output response of the hearing aid. Response curve A shows the basic, unfiltered, function of the hearing instrument. Response curve B shows the effects of a no. 4 sintered filter upon the output envelope. One of the advantages which the sintered filter provides is that of the consistency of the effect. In that no. 4 implies a type of sintered filter having a specified number of small metallic balls, one can predict with reasonable accuracy that all such no. 4 sintered filters would have essentially the same filtering effect. The use is increasing in the industry and does lend an additional dimension to the control of the hearing aid output.

Figure 4–16 shows the effect of lamb's wool upon the response characteristics of a hearing aid. Curve A shows the basic response curve before the introduction of the lamb's wool filter. Response curve B shows the drastic effect of lamb's wool filtering upon the output envelope. It is immediately apparent that the effect of the lamb's wool filter is most dramatic. Since such significant changes can occur which may adversely affect the performance of the hearing aid and render it of questionable benefit to the user, great care should be exercised. Unless one can measure the filtering effect of the substance employed to externally modify the hearing aid, one must proceed with prudence and caution.

While one may not be opposed to the use of filters to externally modify the response of a hearing aid, their use demands some general knowledge of the predictable effects. The need for any external modification can be appreciably reduced by careful attention to parameters of investigation

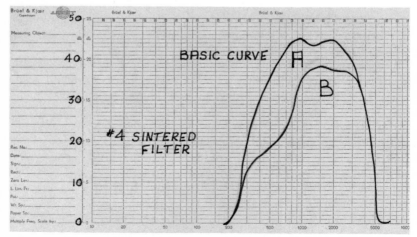

Figure 4–15   The effects of sintered filters upon the output envelope of a hearing aid. Curve A shows the basic, unfiltered response, while curve B shows the effects of the sintering.

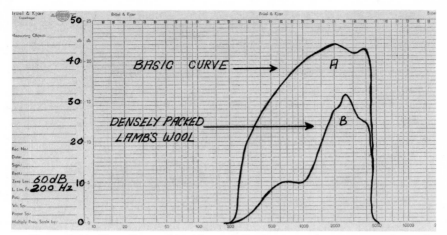

Figure 4–16 The effects of lamb's wool filtering upon the output envelope of a hearing aid. Response curve A shows the basic, unfiltered response, while curve B shows the effects of the filtering.

during the hearing aid evaluation process. One must be certain that user acceptance does not come at the expense of hearing aid efficiency, if such efficiency could have been accomplished by hearing aid design following appropriate hearing aid evaluation procedures.

OUTPUT-LIMITING AND RELATED HARMONIC DISTORTION

One of the important aspects of electroacoustic analysis has to do with the description and measurement of the various methods of output-limiting. One must be aware that any attempt to control the output of a hearing aid introduces a number of problems. Some of these attendant problems may be amplitude or harmonic distortion, attack, recovery and release times, and others affecting output response characteristics.

OUTPUT-LIMITING

Hearing aid dispensers, audiologists, and hearing aid manufacturers have realized for some time that control of maximum power output (MPO) in meeting the individual's needs is an important function in getting the hearing-impaired to accept amplification. Observations of hearing aid users confirm that the individual who makes maximal use of his hearing aid and does not place it in the dresser drawer is the one who has been correctly fitted with respect to MPO. There are, of course, other factors influencing user acceptance, such as (1) uniformity of frequency response, (2) frequency correction, (3) distortion, (4) gain, and (5) the physical appearance of the aid. However, these factors do not play nearly as great a role in user acceptance as does that of appropriate MPO.

The next question of the inquiring student is: How does one most closely approximate the person's required MPO? This is where a gray area exists. MPO, it is felt, should be directly related to the person's tolerance to loud sounds. But what physiological sensation, if any, can be used as a reliable means of assessing tolerance? Does one employ a sensation level for tickle, pain, or dizziness? Obviously, the prospective hearing aid user is not going to be comfortable with sound pressures causing dizziness, tickle, or pain. Therefore, a need exists to establish a level which the user accepts as loud and would deny further increase of loudness. That level of maximum loudness which the individual is willing to accept can be referred to as the functional tolerance level or level of discomfort (cf. Chapter 7).

Although investigation must continue for the best stimulus by which one can establish a functional tolerance level, narrow bands of white noise seem to best serve this need. One must keep in mind that measurement of a functional tolerance level cannot be considered absolute, in that the individual's evaluation of acceptable levels may change over time. Experience leads one to believe that these changes are minimal. Ideally, however, the hearing aid should have the capability of being adjusted to the changing amplification needs of the client as they are manifest. Relatively few hearing aids, however, are internally adjustable to any large degree with respect to maximum power output (MPO). All instruments can be adjusted externally, but this also affects gain and frequency response. In general, there are two methods by which MPO can be controlled. One is by means of "peak clipping" and the other is through the use of "peak limiting" or, as it is more commonly referred to, compression amplification.

PEAK CLIPPING

A hearing aid amplifier is designed to saturate at some pre-determined level. When an amplifier saturates, a resultant peak clipping of the output signal occurs and harmonics are added to the signal which were not present initially, whether it be odd or even harmonic distortion, the result is nearly the same, that is, unwanted and unneeded signal distortion. In an effort to prevent peak clipping at low input levels, hearing aids are designed to produce an MPO which is at least 65 dB, and preferably 70 dB, above the maximum acoustic gain of the instrument. By this method, normal conversational sound pressures will generally not cause the system to saturate if the hearing aid is set at full gain. In Figure 4–17 stylized drawings suggest the appearance of a pure tone sine wave showing the effects of various methods of output-limiting.

Illustration A of Figure 4–17 shows a sine wave of an audio frequency. It is symmetrical in every respect and has the expected ap-

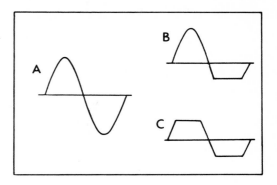

Figure 4–17 Two methods of peak clipping as a means of output limiting. A shows a normal, unaltered sine wave. B shows the effects of unsymmetrical peak clipping upon the sine wave. C shows the sine wave appearance when symmetrical peak clipping is present.

pearance of a pure tone; that is to say, it is undistorted. Illustration B shows an asymmetrically limited sine wave. This configuration indicates that both odd and even harmonic distortion are present, with the second harmonic dominating. Although the tone may sound similar to the wave of illustration A with respect to frequency, its harmonic structure differs appreciably; it is rather like the phenomenon experienced when we listen to tones of the same fundamental frequency on two different musical instruments. Observation of B will clearly show that the upper half of the wave is undisturbed, while the lower half shows the effect of asymmetrical peak clipping.

A symmetrically clipped sine wave is shown in illustration C of Figure 4–17. In addition to the fundamental frequency, all of the odd harmonics are also included. There are no even harmonics present in an absolutely square wave. Note that each half of the wave clearly shows the effects of symmetrical peak clipping.

Figure 4–18 presents a series of response curves for a hearing aid which limits the output by means of peak clipping. For this series of curves, the hearing aid was set to maximum output; the zero level (base line) is 80 dB SPL, and the input signal levels are 50, 60, 70, 80, and 90 dB SPL. Frequency response is from 100 Hz to approximately 5000 Hz. One will note that above 70 dB the output curves flatten and tend to converge. In a peak clipping hearing aid, the point at which the curves evidently begin to flatten and converge is the point at which harmonic distortion is introduced as an output product. All conventional linear amplifiers use peak clipping as a method of MPO control.

A further illustration of this effect is shown in Figure 4–19 with plots of the resultant output when an input signal of 70 dB SPL is applied. Utilizing a spectrum analyzer and related measuring equipment, one can measure the second and third harmonic contained within the output envelope. Notice in Figure 4–19 that the second harmonic predominates, but that the third harmonic is nearly as great for certain frequencies. The regions of high second harmonic distortion are centered at 1000 Hz and 1700 Hz where the second harmonic distortion is about 15 dB below the

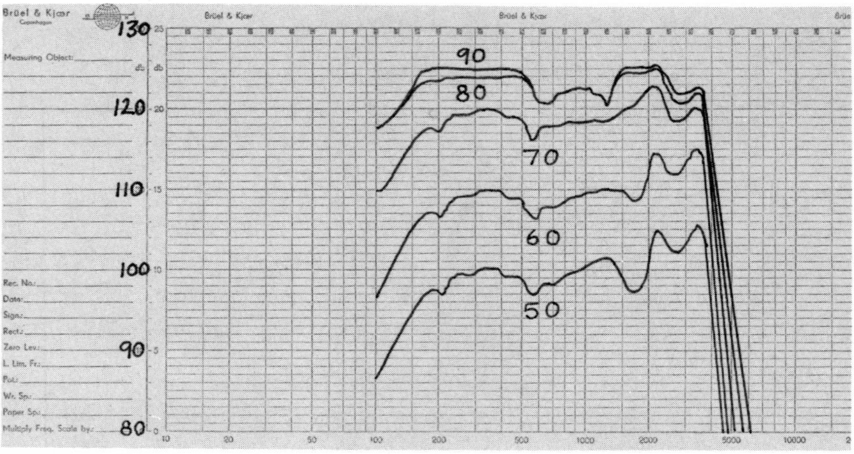

Figure 4–18 A series of output curves for a conventional linear amplifier which achieves output limiting by means of peak clipping.

basic response curve. Using Table 4–1, we can compute the percentage of second harmonic distortion for those particular frequencies; it is approximately 18 per cent. The greatest third harmonic distortion occurs at 650 Hz and is 23 dB below the basic curve. Again, using Table 4–1 as a guide, the computed third harmonic distortion value for 650 Hz is 7 per cent.

Figure 4–20 shows a 1000 Hz tone via the same hearing aid at input levels of 60, 70, 80, and 90 dB SPL. Note how the sine wave increasingly distorts as the input signal level increases; for purposes of illustration, the

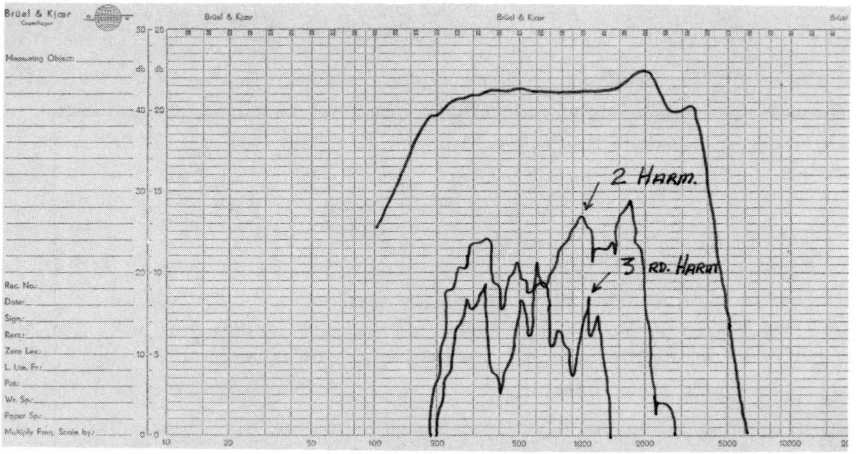

Figure 4–19 The basic response curve of a hearing aid. Second and third harmonic distortion curves are also shown.

TABLE 4–1 *Harmonic Distortion*

Difference (in dB) Between Basic Response and Harmonic Display Curve	Per Cent Harmonic Distortion
0 dB	100
1	90
2	80
3	71
4	63
5	56
6	50
7	45
8	40
9	36
10	32
11	28
12	25
13	22.4
14	20
15	18
16	16
17	14
18	12.5
19	11
20	10
21	9
22	8
23	7
24	6.3
25	5.6
26	5
27	4.5
28	4
29	3.6
30	3.2
31	2.8
32	2.5
33	2.2
34	2
35	1.8
36	1.6
37	1.4
38	1.3
39	1.1
40	1

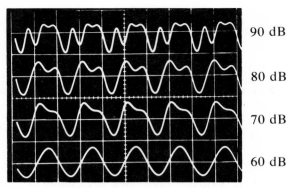

90 dB

80 dB

70 dB

60 dB

Figure 4–20 Oscilloscope tracings showing the effects of an asymmetrically peak clipping hearing aid. The bottom sine wave shows no effect of peak clipping. As the level of the signal increases from 60 dB to 90 dB, the effects of the asymmetrical clipping become evident.

vertical size of the sine waves was maintained by adjusting the oscilloscope controls. Note also that the upper half of the sine wave is significantly distorted, while the lower half is relatively free of distortion, thereby indicating asymmetrical peak clipping.

On the other hand, Figure 4–21 represents hearing aid output-limiting by means of symmetrical peak clipping. The third harmonic is predominant and falls 11 dB below the basic response curve at 430 Hz and 14 dB at 1000 Hz. Again referring to Table 4–1, 11 dB down represents 28 per cent harmonic distortion at 430 Hz, and 14 dB below the basic curve represents 20 per cent harmonic distortion at 1000 Hz. The second harmonic is 34 dB down from the basic response curve at 1500 Hz; a dif-

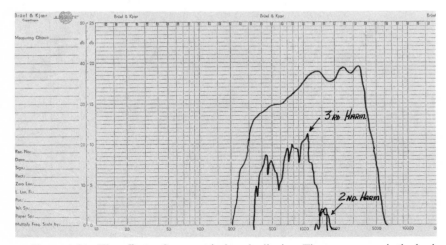

Figure 4–21 The effects of symmetrical peak clipping. The upper curve is the basic curve; the lower curves show second and third harmonics. Note the relative dominance of the third harmonic.

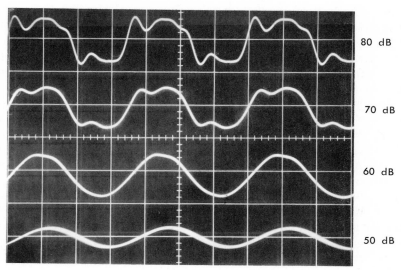

Figure 4–22 Oscilloscope tracings showing the effects of symmetrical peak clipping when a 1000 Hz tone is presented at 50, 60, 70, and 80 dB SPL inputs. Note that vertical size has been instrumentally controlled to keep the wave excursions within the grid lines.

ference of this magnitude represents two per cent harmonic distortion. Although in severe symmetrical peak clipping the resulting sine wave would have assumed the shape of a square wave, the response shown is something less than that. Figure 4–22 shows the effects of symmetrical peak clipping upon the sine wave. Notice how each half of the cycle is distorted when symmetrical peak clipping is the method of choice for output-limiting. For signal input levels at 50 and 60 dB, there is little or no symmetrical distortion. However, for inputs of 70 and 80 dB, the effects of symmetrical peak clipping are evident.

COMPRESSION AMPLIFICATION

Another frequently used form of output-limiting is referred to as *compression amplification.* In this type of controlled output amplification, the hearing aid is freed of certain distortion problems in that output-limiting is achieved through the use of an automatic volume control (AVC). With AVC, a sensing circuit within the hearing aid amplifier system reacts to sound pressures which exceed some pre-determined level. When these sound pressure levels are exceeded, the circuit quickly responds to the increase and automatically limits the intensity of the output signal at a level consistent with the design capabilities of the amplifier. This unique circuit function takes place without producing significant harmonic distortion at the output stage.

An everyday illustration of automatic volume control is suggested when one listens to a sports event broadcast. When the sports commentator is speaking, the general overall noise level of the crowd is suppressed. This obvious reduction of the crowd noise occurs as a result of the more intense signal (the commentator's voice) activating the AVC circuit which attenuates the output, thus lowering the level of all sound passing through the amplifier and thereby making the commentator's voice relatively louder. One of the unfortunate limitations of compression amplification is that more intense sounds cause weaker sounds to be made still weaker by the same amount that the louder sound is reduced by the AVC action. The function may become debilitating when one considers the size of the amplitude envelope for a given speech sound.

An AVC circuit which functions to control sudden and unwanted changes of the intensity of the input signal must deal with real-time functions. A limitation of compression amplification is found in the attack, recovery, and release times which, if not properly designed and controlled, could interfere with speech discrimination. If the system reacts too slowly to sudden increases of signal level, much of the loud sound will get to the ear before the AVC starts to operate. On the other hand, if the AVC reacts quickly, but over-reacts in amount of signal control, the output level may be so attenuated that the person cannot hear it sufficiently well to identify it. Additionally, after the intensity of the signal is controlled by the AVC circuit to the desired level, the input signal may suddenly decrease. When this occurs, the AVC must release the signal which was previously being controlled.

Figure 4–23 shows the essential features of AVC reacting to a sudden change of input signal level assuming, in the example displayed, that the input signal level goes abruptly from 60 dB to 80 dB SPL. The output signal (left side of photograph) suddenly increases in level, thereby activating the AVC circuit to bring the output to the desired level. The time (in milliseconds) required for the AVC to sense the change of input level and react to it is called the *attack* time (upper part of photograph). Sometimes, however, the AVC may "over-control" the input signal and drive the output down to a level below that which is desirable for the listener.

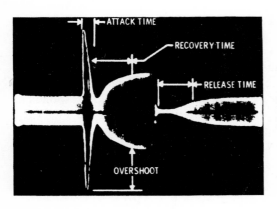

Figure 4–23 The attack, recovery, and release times of a hearing aid with compression amplification.

When that occurs, the signal begins to approach the desired output level; the time required to get from maximum attack to the desired output signal level is called the *recovery* time. If the input signal level were suddenly reduced, it would again take time for the AVC to sense the change and react to it; this is referred to as *release* time. The error ("undershoot") on release is somewhat like the undershoot on the attack sequence, and can result in so-called "blackout" of the sound.*

In modern hearing aids, these time constants (attack, recovery, and release) vary from instantaneous (no delay) to time delays as long as 150 msec. Extremely short time constants may result in harmonic distortion which, of course, reduces the benefits of compression amplification. On the other hand, extremely long time constants may result in discomfort and/or loss of information. Optimally related attack, recovery, and release times have yet to be adequately established. Most undesirable time-related phenomena can be avoided if the compression circuit operates fast enough; however, if it functions too fast, harmonic distortion appears. In general, an attack-recovery time of five to 10 msec and a release time of 20 to 60 msec would not create significant distortion and are sufficiently fast to offer minimal interference with speech stimuli.

EFFECTS OF OUTPUT-LIMITING

At this point in our analysis, we examine the input and output curve relationships to better understand what happens as a function of various kinds of output-limiting. Figure 4–24 displays what happens to input/output relationships in conventional linear, non-linear, and linear compression hearing aids. The majority of instruments on today's market limit MPO by symmetrical or asymmetrical peak clipping and have input/output gain ratios of 1:1. This means that, for every 10 dB increase of level at the input stage, there is a corresponding 10 dB increase at the output stage. This increase continues to the point of saturation, as suggested by the uppermost curve in Figure 4–24.

Hearing aids in which the output is limited by non-linear compression present a broad array of input/output curve relationships ranging from a very sharp knee (bend), where compression is first apparent, to a very broad knee. For a normal range of inputs (up to 100 dB SPL), saturation output is never completely accomplished. Linear compression may have input/output ratios at pre-determined constants less than the 1:1 as in conventional amplifiers. In a linear compression hearing aid the output

---

*To date, standards have not been set regarding the reporting of acoustic phenomena associated with compression amplification. The time-related sequence described here as attack, recovery and release may be referred to by others as attack and recovery or attack and release. That is, what has been described in Figure 4–23 as release may be defined by some as recovery. That which is described as attack and recovery has been referred to as attack time. Although general consensus has not been reached, it is probable that standard terminology will be forthcoming to describe these acoustic phenomena.

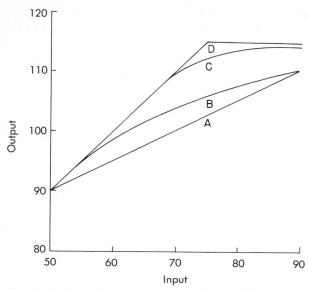

Figure 4–24 The input/output response of different amplifiers. Curve A is a linear compressor. Curve B is a non-linear compressor with a broad knee (bend). Curve C is a non-linear compressor with a sharp knee. Curve D is a conventional linear amplifier.

may, for example, increase 10 dB for every increase of 20 dB at the input stage, and this compression ratio of 2:1 may be maintained throughout the normal range of inputs. A curvilinear amplifier input/output characteristic falls somewhere between the peak-limiter amplifier curve and the linear compressor curve.

There are those who support the thesis that harmonic distortion introduces minimal interference with the discrimination of speech signals, but most will agree that it is an undesirable product in the output signal of a hearing instrument. A recent study by Hartman (1971) showed that 30 per cent harmonic distortion significantly reduced sentence intelligibility as compared to a condition free of all harmonic distortion. He reported further that sentence intelligibility scores were higher under conditions of second-harmonic distortion than under third-harmonic distortion, but not significantly so. His test population consisted of 30 subjects with cochlear hearing impairments.

Davis et al. (1947) found that both normal and hearing-impaired listeners performed better on speech discrimination tests under conditions of compression amplification than under conditions of peak clipping. Hudgins et al. (1948) similarly concluded that limiting hearing aid output by compression amplification "reduced distortion to a minimum, thus maintaining, in most cases, the maximum level of performance over a wide range of speech-input levels." In spite of these findings, during the early 1950's wearable hearing aids incorporating compression amplification were marketed by only a few manufacturers. They were generally unsuccessful as some manufacturers were apparently not fully cognizant of all the acoustic variations inherent in compression amplification. This led to an evaluation by Krebs (1961) who found that the manufacturers had overlooked overshoot and undershoot problems of the attack-recovery-release sequence. Subsequently, Krebs (1964) reported that listener fatigue was created by attack times of 20 msec or longer and that release times in excess of 100 msec were noticeable and distracting.

Several studies in the 1960's demonstrated the superiority of amplitude compression with respect to methods which produce harmonic distortion. These include the work of Krestinger and Young (1960), Harris et al. (1961), and Jerger, Speaks, and Malmquist (1966). The effects of various time constants were investigated by Lynn and Carhart (1963), while linear compression was studied by Caraway and Carhart (1967). Much more recently, Rintlemann (1972) showed the improvement of discrimination accomplished by a compression ratio of 2:1, as compared to 1:1 and an even further (but very small) improvement at 3:1.

There are other output signal distortions which could contribute to speech interference. Among them is amplitude distortion: any time there is AVC, amplitude distortion is present in the output waveform. One may also find frequency distortion in any hearing aid where the slope of amplification has been altered by design. Finally, intermodulation distortion may be reflected in the output of a hearing aid (Olsen and Wilber, 1967). Output distortion, whatever the type, must be offset by the advantages of the circuit design. If overall performance and patient utilization of the instrument are augmented, then they may well outweigh the deleterious effects of distortion.

OUTPUT PRESSURES

In the final analysis, hearing aids are designed to deal with sound pressures. The efficiency with which this is accomplished is a matter of design engineering, production, and costs. Compromises made any place along the line must have some trade-off in the finished product. All of the design features which have been discussed in this chapter were engineering attempts to amplify, modify, or alter those sound pressures which impinge upon the face of the hearing aid microphone. Whether controlling maximum power output by symmetrical or asymmetrical peak clipping, by automatic volume control through linear or non-linear compression amplification, the purpose is to deal effectively with sound pressures. Whether one extends the frequency response range of a hearing aid or restricts it, whether the aid has sloped amplification or flat amplification, the concern is still with output pressures.

The human ear deals with the same sound pressures as does the hearing aid. However, when the human ear becomes impaired, it fails to deal efficiently with sound pressures. The extent to which it does handle them efficiently depends upon the nature and degree of impairment.

The most efficient hearing aid that one can design for any impaired ear is the one which best approximates the user's need for controlled pressures at the drum membrane. All persons with impaired hearing do not have the same amplification needs; sound pressures at the output of the aid must be controlled differentially, depending upon the loss. Victoreen (1960) suggested that the one basic fact which must be paramount in intelligent utilization of hearing aids is attention to the objective measurement of sound pressure to provide appropriate hearing enhancement. While hearing aid size, configuration, and cost may be factors to consider, the essential obligation in decision-making must ultimately be related to control of sound pressures. It is the appearance of the output envelope which is of greatest importance.

HEARING AID EVALUATION

The most effective hearing aid is that which permits a person with a hearing loss to use amplification as efficiently as his impairment will permit. No chapter concerned with the electroacoustical analysis of hearing aids can be complete, then, without a description of the parameters of investigation for assessing a given patient's need for amplification. Certainly, the literature suggests an abundance of information relative to the opinion of those having developed hearing aid evaluation procedures. While this chapter is not intended to definitively analyze those current procedures, we do profess to offer some reasonable information relating to that which should be important to any hearing aid evaluation procedure.

While everyone likes to consider himself an expert in the professional discipline which he represents, it is highly unlikely that real objectivity is to be achieved in hearing aid evaluation. The patient's subjective reaction to amplification is often the final determinant as to whether or not the hearing aid is used. These subjective reactions can range from color and type of hearing aid to the place where it is worn. It is singularly amazing, in spite of the obvious superiority of certain electroacoustic devices for particular hearing loss types, that patients will reject them for purely cosmetic or other subjective reasons. However, assuming that this is something over which one exercises little control, what are some of the objective considerations which must be taken in account when undertaking a hearing aid evaluation?

FREQUENCY RESPONSE

Hearing aids have limited frequency range when compared with the average response of the human ear. Response is limited not only by the amplifier, but also by the construction of the transducers employed. The maximum response which can be achieved in today's commercially available hearing aids probably extends from 100 Hz to 5000 Hz. This is adequate for most hearing-impaired individuals who require amplification.

Another important aspect of appropriate hearing aid evaluation is to determine the slope of amplification needed by the patient. By "slope of amplification" is meant the acoustic gain per frequency within the frequency response range of the hearing aid. In many instances, the audiometric configuration of a given hearing loss would indicate adequate hearing for the lower frequencies with an appreciable loss for the higher. Obviously, the amount of acoustic gain needed for the lower frequencies, where better hearing is found, would be significantly less than the acoustic gain needed for the higher frequencies. In such a case, the hearing aid should have a slope of amplification whereby these different acoustic gain requirements are met. One cannot over-emphasize the need for intelligent consideration to be given to the gain per frequency, as it often means the difference between patient utilization or rejection of the hearing aid. Available evidence suggests that hearing enhancement is in large part determined by the slope of the output envelope.

GAIN REQUIREMENTS

Although related to the concept of slope amplification, the overall gain requirements of the hearing aid should be strongly considered in assessing hearing aid needs. It is possible to provide a great deal of acoustic gain or minimal gain depending upon the design requirements. Careful investigation of the gain-handling capacities of a hearing aid is required to determine if it is appropriate for the type of loss demonstrated by the patient.

We are convinced that one of the errors which has been perpetuated in hearing aid selection is that of too much maximum power output. Other investigators seem to agree. McCandless (1972), for example, has shown that there is a positive correlation between the patient's subjective evaluation of tolerance and the maximum power output required of the hearing aid, and he has demonstrated the physiological correlates of the patient's subjective tolerance to sound. Sandlin (1969) has suggested that, regardless of the auditory pathology demonstrated, the average maximum output required by the vast majority of hearing aid users approximates 112 dB SPL. These data are somewhat greater than those suggested by McCandless (107 dB), but are in close enough agreement to support the notion of the importance of ascertaining maximum power output requirements. Certainly, if one were to review the literature published by the hearing aid manufacturers, as well as some of the current practices by hearing aid dispensers and audiologists, one would find that in many instances the maximum power output requirement specified may exceed 130 dB. While there is no argument that hearing aids can now be designed to yield maximum power outputs exceeding 130 dB SPL, it is doubtful that this kind of power is indicated for the vast majority of hearing aid users.

ASSESSMENT

The body-worn hearing aid is an essential instrument for many persons, and in no way do we intend to deny its importance. However, it is apparent that the trend in hearing aid selection and fitting, through hearing aid evaluation processes, is truly to ear-level instruments having specific response characteristics meeting the individual need. Table 4–2 shows hearing aid sales by type in one year. More than half of the aids sold were the post-auricular type, and another quarter was in eyeglasses. With the small proportion of all-in-the-ear models, the ear-level aids constitute nearly 90 per cent of all aids sold in the United States.

The measurement of a patient's tolerance to sound stimuli as a means for specifying maximum power output of the hearing aid is of critical importance. We submit, however, that the patient's response is a function of the instructions given to him (cf. the Introduction of this text). An appropriate instruction is to have the patient say when the intensity of the signal approaches the point where he would not want to listen even for short periods of time were it made louder. By this method, one would (rather subjectively) assess the point at which the maximum power output should be set for the recommended instrumentation.

Similarly, if one were to measure a patient's assessment of a most comfortable listening level (MCL) as a critical parameter for hearing aid evaluation, one would give instructions which would assist in arriving at an answer approximating the use-gain requirement of the aid. It would seem, therefore, that something approximating the following instruction would be appropriate. The patient is to let you know when the sound stimulus to which he is listening reaches that intensity level most comfortable for him. That is, if the signal were made louder it would be beyond that most comfortable level and, if made softer, would be below that most comfortable level. By assessing the MCL requirements in this manner and converting these data into appropriate use-gain specification, instrument choice is made easier. In determining acoustic gain per frequency, it

TABLE 4–2 *Hearing Aid Sales by Type for the Year Ending June 30, 1973**

Model	Per Cent
Post-auricular	64.8
Eyeglass	23.8
Body-worn	9.2
All-in-the-ear	2.3

*During this period, a total of 616,310 hearing aids were produced in, or imported to, the United States (see *National Hearing Aid Journal,* November, 1973).

would seem rather straightforward to first select those frequency points to be measured. Normally, octave or half-octave points are selected within the frequency response of the instrument. By establishing MCL values for those frequency points selected, one can achieve the desired slope amplification for the hearing aid.

This discussion of the hearing aid evaluation process is not exhaustive, but rather points out the need for intelligent consideration of the patient's response to several stimuli. From the patient's response, the most appropriate hearing aid amplification may be selected. There is no question that, within the past decade, hearing aid technology has advanced greatly and has lessened the need for clinical guesswork. With the introduction of ceramic and electret microphones, as well as the stabilized performance of transistors, and the obvious space-saving provided by semi-conductor substances, much control can now be exercised over the performance characteristics of a given hearing aid. With reasonable attention to the parameters of hearing aid acoustics essential to the hearing-impaired, specified performance can now be achieved.

In final analysis, the efficiency with which one uses amplification and the acceptance of the electroacoustic device will determine the efficacy of any given hearing aid evaluation procedure. As one examines existing "rules of thumb" and discards them in favor of better measures and specific evaluation processes, the needs of the acoustically deficient individual will be more effectively met. The psychology of the hearing-impaired person is as complex as it is for any handicapped individual. To ignore the psychological needs of the person or to treat them lightly in any final hearing aid evaluation process would be less than intelligent. The student must become familiar with the psychological aspects of hearing impairment; in so doing he will enhance his ability to provide effective treatment.

SUMMARY

One must marvel at the contribution which technological development has brought to the hearing aid industry. The last decade encompassed significant advances in transducer and amplifier design. The miniaturization of components without unreasonable sacrifice of quality has greatly added to public acceptance. The transistor has given the hearing aid engineer a latitude which he had never enjoyed before its introduction. With the transistor came the post-auricular hearing aid and the all-in-the-ear instrument. Their acoustic characteristics, though somewhat reduced in gain and power output, were successfully utilized by a number of hearing-impaired persons. Continued experimentation with various means of output-limiting and frequency-shaping (slope amplification) led to new and useful techniques in the art of hearing aid fitting. With advanced circuit designs came additional problems of performance control. For example, compression amplification yielded attendant problems of adequately controlling attack and recovery times to the point where speech intelligibility was not adversely affected. The introduction of the ceramic microphone responsible for extending the lower frequency range of post-auricular aids also gave rise to seismic effects introduced into the output of the instrument. Continued experimentation eliminated the adverse effects and gave rise to general acceptance and use of the ceramic microphone.

The wearable hearing aid has become an accepted device in today's culture. Nevertheless, there may be more than 600,000 persons in the United States today without aids who might benefit from them. Clearly, more experimentation, more advance, and more acceptance are required.

REFERENCES

Caraway, B. J., and Carhart, R. (1967): Influence of compressor action on speech intelligibility. *Journal of the Acoustical Society of America, 41*:1424–1433.

Davis, H., and Silverman, S. R. (1970): *Hearing and Deafness* (3rd Ed.). New York, Holt, Rinehart, & Winston.

Davis, H., Stevens, S. S., Nichols, R. H., Jr., Hudgins, C. V., Marquis, R. J., Peterson, G. E., and Ross, D. A. (1947): *Hearing Aids, An Experimental Study of Design Objectives.* Cambridge, Mass., Harvard University Press.

Harris, J. D., Haines, H. L., Kelsey, P. A., and Clack, T. D. (1961): Relation between speech intelligibility and the electroacoustic characteristics of low fidelity circuitry. *Journal of Auditory Research, 1*:357–381.

Hartman, P. W. (1971): *The Effects of Harmonic Distortion on Sentence Intelligibility of Hypoacousic Adults.* Unpublished doctoral dissertation, University of Southern California.

Hudgins, C. V., Marquis, R. J., Nichols, R. H., Jr., Peterson, G. E., and Ross, D. A. (1948): The comparative performance of an experimental hearing aid and two commercial instruments. *Journal of the Acoustical Society of America, 20*:241–258.

Jerger, J. F., Speaks, C., and Malmquist, C. (1966): Hearing aid performance and hearing aid selection. *Journal of Speech and Hearing Research, 9*:136–149.

Katz, J. (1972): *Handbook of Clinical Audiology.* Baltimore, Williams & Wilkins Co.

Krebs, D. F. (1961): Compression amplification and its use by the hard of hearing. Unpublished report, Research Division, Zenith Radio Corporation.

Krebs, D. F. (1964): Considerations in the design and use of hearing aids. *Audecibel, 13*:90–95, 114.

Krestinger, E. A., and Young, N. B. (1960): The use of fast limiting to improve the intelligibility of speech in noise. *Speech Monographs, 27*:63–69.

Lynn, G., and Carhart, R. (1963): Influence of attack and release in compression amplification on understanding of speech by hypoacousics. *Journal of Speech and Hearing Disorders, 28*:124–140.

McCandless, G. (1972): Unpublished paper given to the meeting of the International Hearing Aid Seminar.

Newby, H. A. (1972): *Audiology* (3rd Ed.). New York, Appleton-Century-Crofts.

Olsen, W., and Wilber, S. (1967): Physical performance characteristics of different hearing aids and speech discrimination scores achieved with them by hearing impaired persons. Paper given to the meeting of the American Speech and Hearing Association, Chicago.

Reddell, R. C. (1966): Selecting hearing aids by interpreting audiologic data. *Journal of Auditory Research, 8*:445–452.

Rintlemann, W. F. (1972): Effects of amplitude compression upon speech perception—a review of research. *Oticongress 2*, Copenhagen.

Sandlin, R. E. (1969): The Physician and Sensori-Neural Hearing Loss, Sense of Sound Series. Phoenix, Audiotone, Inc.

Victoreen, J. A. (1960): *Hearing Enhancement.* Springfield, Ill., Charles C Thomas, Publisher.

Victoreen, J. A. (1972): *Prosthetic Hearing Evaluation.* Unpublished manuscript.

Part Three

PSYCHOACOUSTICS

In the third part of this text, we are able to see how all the preceding chapters apply. In Part One, we learned a little about the receiver, and in Part Two, we learned about the transmitter. Now, we are ready to discuss what is received during the hearing process. In Chapter 5, we will study the human response to acoustic events. The succeeding chapters of this part deal with those responses to stimuli which give rise to sensations of pitch, sensations of loudness, sensations of events distributed in time, and sensations which arise simultaneously or differentially in both ears. This part deals first (Chapter 6) with those acoustic phenomena which allow us to order them by a system extending from high to low. The next chapter (Chapter 7) treats the system which extends from loud to soft, and Chapter 8 considers the system ranging from slow to fast. Chapter 9, finally, deals with the fact that we have two ears; a very interesting fact, indeed, as two ears are only sometimes better than one.

Our approach is at once historical and experimental. We have considered the questions which one might ask about our perception of acoustic events, the questions which have been asked, the answers which we have, and those which we don't have. Thus, in Part Three, we face the matter of how we function in the audible world.

Chapter Five

ABSOLUTE AND RELATIVE THRESHOLDS

SANFORD E. GERBER

INTRODUCTION

At the beginning of the book we reminded ourselves that most of us have some concept of a sensory threshold. We noted that we regard some lights as not bright enough to be seen, while others are; some sounds are not loud enough to be heard, while others are; some physical events, therefore, are below the sensory threshold and some are above. Our contemporary idea of the sensory threshold is essentially one articulated by Gustav Theodor Fechner (1801–1887). The idea did not originate with Fechner; it had appeared in early Greek philosophy and in the works of such distinguished theorists as Leibnitz. In fact, some 75 years before Fechner, the notion had been discussed by Johann Friedrich Herbart (1776–1841). Nevertheless, it is essentially to Fechner that we owe most of our modern concepts of a sensory threshold, however correct or incorrect they may be. Fechner's historical position is discussed in the next section.

113

In the succeeding chapters, various thresholds are discussed. Implicit in all discussions of threshold is the concept that sensation can be measured, and this concept essentially originated with Fechner. Furthermore, it has been agreed that such measurement is possible; by "measurement" we mean "assign numbers to, according to certain rules" (Hirsh, 1952). However, it is not the numbers which concern us, but rather the insight which the search for sensory thresholds might give us into human behavior and action. A threshold is a quantity, that is, an amount or a number of something which leads to some kind of action. Research for thresholds is of fundamental importance in every field. Physiologists, for example, seek that stimulus which would just cause a nerve to fire or a muscle to contract. Pharmacologists titrate certain drugs by finding the effective dose at which some specified proportion of experimental animals shows the symptoms chosen as signs of the effect. Designers of educational tests assess the difficulty of a question by specifying the proportion of responders who pass it. It should be obvious that human beings do behave as threshold detectors of a kind.

Research for a sensory threshold in a given observer implies some very peculiar things. It implies that somehow we can "get into the head" of that observer. Even Fechner worried about this kind of problem, i.e., how to determine what is going on inside someone else's head. Ruesch (1956) summarized that "we are not interested in the way nature is constructed but in how the observer perceives it, and his method of perceiving." In other words we are interested in what the observer tells us about the stimuli. Fechner thought that he could write an equation that would relate stimuli to the reports of stimuli.

When we speak of a sensory threshold, we use the term "threshold" in its literal sense, that of a barrier. For some kinds of barriers we continue to prefer the Latin equivalent of threshold, *limen*. Often, when we want to speak of the absolute threshold, we use the term threshold; but, more often, when we wish to speak of a relative threshold, we use the term difference limen. If we don't know what goes on in the observer's head, and if we have to rely on his verbal report of a stimulus, and if we want to assign numbers to these properties with respect to the verbal reports, it follows that we have to acquire some numbers. The threshold has been traditionally viewed as varying randomly in time about some average value. Therefore, it has had to be defined statistically as that signal value reported by the subjects on half of the occasions on which it was presented. That is to say that the threshold is reported in terms of the properties of the stimulus, rather than the properties of the observer. Specifically, it refers to that stimulus value that an observer claims to detect only half of the time. Of course, one doesn't know how this occurs and so one must be "willing to leave unanswered all questions as to the process mediating between the stimulus and its central effect or conscious accompaniment," but "one can still attempt to correlate the physical stimulus energies and receptor process, on the one hand, with the experience as reported by the subject on the other" (Allport, 1955). Even then we will have succeeded only in reporting the past (Macksoud, 1973).

In spite of these kinds of abstract difficulties, it does remain possible to measure reports of thresholds. In fact, we are aware of two kinds of reports: additive and substitutive. Some thresholds we report in an additive manner; that is, we report that we now have more of something than we had before by using such terms as brighter or louder or warmer. On the other hand, some thresholds we report as being substitutive; that is, we report that a certain sensation has replaced another, as, for example, when we say one tone is higher than another, it is not that we hear more of it but that we hear the higher one instead of the lower one. With these kinds of reports we can make an amazingly accurate picture of one's sensory world.

HISTORICAL DEVELOPMENT

The history of threshold research can be divided into three parts. Simply stated they are before, during, and since Fechner. We have touched upon what led to Fechner's monumental contribution, and so the first part of this section reviews that briefly. The second part of the section discusses in some detail Fechner's psychophysical methods. The third part foreshadows, to a certain extent, what is to come later.

BEFORE FECHNER

As early as Aristotle, and probably before, the notion had been expressed that one comes to know the world through his senses. Of course, this is a truism, but not a total truism. Nevertheless, this view of the source of human knowledge dominated philosophy through the nineteenth century. In that era it was learned that different nerves served motor functions than served sensory functions. As a result of this discovery, the physiologists of the time turned their attention to the physiology of sensation. Most notable among them was Johannes Müller, and it was he who originated the doctrine of *specific nerve energies*. This doctrine we know to be true, in a general way, to the extent that a given sensation is determined by which nerve fibers are stimulated. A familiar illustration of this fact occurs when we rub our eyes. This apparently tactile stimulus gives rise to a visual response; usually a transitory flash of red spots. But no red-spot stimulus is present. One of Müller's disciples was H. L. F. von Helmholtz, one of the most important figures in the history of auditory science. Helmholtz extended Müller's doctrine of specific nerve energies to apply to each separate auditory fiber. "He held not only that auditory nerve fibers were responsible for auditory experience, but also that the quality of a given auditory sensation depended on which of the auditory fibers were stimulated" (Hirsh, 1952). Helmholtz was wrong in particular but not in general. Another of Helmholtz's observations, this time fully correct, was that some time intervenes between the occurrence of a stimulus and its corresponding sensation. It was Helmholtz who, in 1850, measured the velocity of the nervous impulse.

The dominant philosophy of the nineteenth century, and indeed for a couple of preceding centuries, had been the dualism of Descartes. It was Descartes who first stated the so-called "mind-body problem," a doctrine that the mind and body are parallel, and that a parallel exists between the physical world and bodily processes. This dominant dualistic philosophy led G. T. Fechner to seek an equation, a mathematical relationship, between the world of physics and the world of psychology.

Fechner, of course, was not the first. While Fechner's monumental work was published in 1860, he was familiar with the work published in German in 1848, and previously published in Latin in 1834 by E. H. Weber (1795–1878). Weber observed that for an increment in a stimulus to cause it to be just noticeably different from the one preceding it, it would have always to be a constant fraction of the original. It is to Weber that we owe the notion of the *just-noticeable difference* or the *jnd*. For a century or more, the jnd was the unit of measurement employed in psychophysics. Weber considered it to be a difference noticed 50 per cent of the time. That is consistent with our definition of threshold. Weber's law said that the amount of increase divided by the value to be increased should yield a constant ratio. He thought, therefore, that a just-noticeable difference of any stimulus could be obtained from constant increments of the stimulus, provided they were expressed as ratios between the size of the change and the magnitude from which the change was made:

$$\frac{\Delta I}{I} = K$$

This equation has come to us as Weber's law, and it implies that the magnitude of a sensation could be measured by counting a number of $\Delta I/I$'s. The fact of the matter is that Weber's law is not generally true, but is true for only certain parts of the sensible spectrum. Fechner's great contribution initially was to observe the universality of Weber's law. In fact it was Fechner who first called it a law. We know today that Weber's law applies for a considerable part of the range of intensive stimuli in hearing. There is something wrong with this formulation, and it was Fechner who corrected it. Also, as we pointed out above, it was Fechner who first gave to Weber's formulation the status of a law. Weber had not suggested that his conceptualization was in any way necessarily a psychophysical universal. His own observations, although supplemented in 1848, were limited to the sense of touch. Weber's great contribution, one unaltered by time, was the introduction of the just-noticeable difference as a unit of measurement. However, it was Fechner who first employed it in that way.

G. T. FECHNER

Gustav Theodor Fechner was one of those persons who is characteristic of the "great-man" approach to history. He was at once physicist and philosopher, while also being somewhat of a mystic. Perhaps it was his mysticism which led him to retire largely from the world of academe and to devote his efforts to quantizing the relationship between the world of physical events and the world of psychological perception. In a very real way, Fechner was the father of psychophysics. Ever since the time of Fechner, the term *psychophysics* has been used "to describe the relationship between sensation and stimulation" (Engen, 1971). Engen pointed out further that "the problem of classical psychophysics . . . was the relation between stimulus and response, but the stimulus variable received most of the emphasis. The basic purpose of the classical method was to determine a threshold, measured as a transition point on the physical dimension." Fechner was the first to develop some methods to ascertain threshold which are now called the classical psychophysical methods. Fechner's notion of threshold is pervasive to this day: that it is a barrier which must be crossed in terms of the physical properties of the stimulus. On one side of that barrier human observers fail to respond, and on the other they do respond. In point of fact, Fechner's initial purpose was to develop methods for measuring not the absolute but the relative threshold, which is historically sensible. Fechner's logic was that one could count just-noticeable differences and in that way would be summing equal sensory units. Fechner's version of Weber's law was that the just-noticeable difference is a logarithmic one rather than one of constant percentage. Thus, where Weber's law states that

$$\frac{\Delta I}{I} = K,$$

Fechner's version says that

$$S = K \log I$$

where S is sensation. Moreover, we know that Weber's law is sometimes true, but even then only approximately true. There are problems, however, with Fechner's law as well. We will return to these after we describe Fechner's methods.

Earlier we displayed a table showing seven psychophysical methods as described by Stevens (1951). Essentially, all of these had been described by Fechner. He proposed three methods: the method of adjustment (or of average error, or of reproduction); the method of serial exploration (or of limits, or of minimal changes); and the method of constant stimuli (or of right and wrong cases). Again, since no idea is original, these too did not originate with Fechner. In fact, Green and Swets (1966) suggested that the methods "had been introduced for various purposes from five to 150 years before Fechner began his work." Whether or not they originated with Fechner is of little importance; it was he who first saw them as expressly psychophysical methods.

The method of adjustment is one in which the observer has control over the stimulus. He is instructed to adjust stimulus magnitude in order to satisfy some criterial instructions he had received. The essential nature of this method is that it is the observer, and not the experimenter, who controls the stimulus value. In a method of adjustment, for example, a listener may be instructed to adjust one tone to be equal in loudness to another.

Fechner's method of serial exploration comes to us most frequently as the method of limits. It differs in only one major way from the method of adjustment and that is that the experimenter controls the value of the stimulus. In this method, the experimenter repeatedly varies some property of the stimulus in a given direction, and solicits a report from the observer. This procedure may be repeated several times and several reports received until some average report is determined. The method of limits is the one most characteristically employed for clinical audiometry.

What Fechner called the method of right and wrong cases is today more often called the method of constant stimuli. In this method, stimulus differences are presented constantly in time, and the subject is instructed to report such things as "right or wrong" or "more or less" in similar events. What the experimenter does, then, is to get the percentage of correct judgments.

There were and are some problems with Fechner's conceptualizations. One of his problems was his central concept, the idea that there is a sensory threshold. Fechner's own experiments showed that the sensory threshold was unstable, "that it varied randomly over time" (Green and Swets, 1966). A particularly wise observation was made in 1950 by Lawson and Uhlenbeck: ". . . it is important to emphasize that one can speak of a *minimum* detectable signal only (1) when the number of observations is limited or (2) when the time of observation is limited." Within these limitations, it is apparent that a so-called threshold must be alterable by variations of either the stimulus or the responder. Licklider (1960) reminded us that "human beings change their modes of reaction as they pass from one situation to another. Even within a homogeneous situation, their characteristics 'drift.'" Anyway, the so-called threshold varies, depending upon whether we approach it from above or below. We get different thresholds as a function of whether we ascend or descend to it (Mueller, 1965; Gerber, 1967). And, even if we keep the stimuli constant, we can cause an observer to change his behavior by changing our instructions to him, or for that matter, "by varying the relative values and costs" of his responses (Pollack, 1961). So that, finally, we must agree with Ruesch (1956) that "observer-bound properties . . . influence our picture of nature."

Fechner was in trouble from the start. This "cut" which divides stimuli between those to which a subject does or does not respond, or those to which a subject responds differentially, seems to move about in time. As a result, the so-called threshold is only a measure of dispersion of response. Engen (1971) reminded us that a subject's sensitivity, motivation, and attention can and do vary from moment to moment. Moreover, Licklider (1951) raised the issue of "trying to distinguish between normal variations in the absolute threshold and partial deafness," for example.

AFTER FECHNER

If we now jump ahead about 75 years, we come to the time of S. S. Stevens, who undoubtedly was the outstanding figure of twentieth-century psychophysics. It is to Stevens that we are indebted for yet another version of the Weber-Fechner law: the power law. Stevens' variation of the fundamental psychophysical law was that sensation varies as some measurable exponent of the stimulus. It was he who first strenuously underlined the significance of statistical evaluation of sensory and perceptual reporting. He said (1951), "we trap the threshold value of a stimulus by means of statistical devices for interpolating in the gap between stimuli that are definitely below threshold and stimuli that are definitely above threshold." He also said (1961) that "the jnd is a statistical concept, a measure of the dispersion or variability of a discriminatory response, in short, a measure of error." But he believed that the traditional psychophysical methods were such statistical procedures and that they could be employed appropriately for the kinds of sampling and interpolating that he had in mind. In a way, Stevens was to Fechner as Fechner was to Weber. He saw both the truth and the error of Fechner's law; unfortunately, he never really saw the error of his own law. In a symposium to which Stevens himself contributed, Pollack (1961) claimed that ". . . a sensory threshold detector is not tenable. The experimental evidence indicates strongly that the sensory information about the environment is preserved in a form such that a continuous range of information is available for subsequent decision making." This is in contrast to Stevens' (1951) claim that "the threshold is a value that divides the continuum of stimuli into two classes: those to which the organism reacts and those to which it does not." Stevens, like Fechner, defined the threshold statistically as that value of the stimulus reported by the subject on half of the occasions on which it was presented. Alternative interpretations of a subject's performance have been proposed, all of which view the subject as using more than the immediate sensory information to determine his response on each trial.

If we define the sensory threshold in terms of the properties of the stimulus leading to a response half of the time, what will we call those stimuli to which an observer responds less than half of the time? Fechner himself had considered the possibility of what he called "negative sensations," but he felt that such signals had no effect on an organism. However, we must consider with Licklider (1960) that human beings "do not give identical responses to identical stimuli." The notion that the threshold is related in some definable way — whether a percentage à la Weber, a logarithm à la Fechner, or an exponent à la Stevens — neglects the peculiarities of human observers. Macksoud (1973) reminded us that "not even the best magician can produce a rabbit out of the hat unless there is already a rabbit in the hat." Therefore, he pointed out, "to draw a stimulus-response pattern is to say *more* than that a certain sort of behavior is highly correlated with another occurrence." After discussing, in the next two sections, some traditional ideas about the sensory threshold, we introduce quite a different one.

THE ABSOLUTE THRESHOLD

When we approach the matter of the absolute threshold, we must ask first if there is one. All the preceding may suggest that there is not, but let us, for the purposes of this section, assume that there is. What then is meant by an *absolute* threshold? Stevens (1951) claimed that "for each animal reaction there is a finite value of the stimulus below which nothing happens." This conceptualization is quite in line with the one stated at the beginning of this chapter as well as the one in the introduction to the book. It appeals again to those literal definitions of a threshold as a barrier that must be crossed. The barrier below which nothing happens is the absolute threshold.

Bartley (1951) offered the notion that adding or subtracting some "neural effect" to an amount which already exists leads to crossing the threshold in either direction. This is a very important concept, especially in clinical audiometry. How do we decide that a person's hearing is impaired? By "impaired" hearing, we mean that the absolute threshold of hearing for a given person is (in some physical sense) poorer than that for a large number of similar people. The threshold of hearing, in a clinical sense, implies that the barrier not only exists but is movable as a function of disease or injury or age. The fact is that we could not deal clinically with auditory events were it not for some notion of absolute threshold. So, when we are speaking of audition, the absolute threshold may also be called the "threshold of hearing" or the "threshold of audibility." We may employ the threshold of audibility as a measure of the sensitivity of the auditory system. A hearing loss implies a diminution of sensitivity. In other words, if a person is insensitive to a particular acoustic stimulus, we say that his threshold is high; whereas, if he is especially sensitive to that stimulus, we say that his threshold is low.

METHODS FOR MEASURING

In hearing, the absolute threshold which is of usual concern is the threshold of audibility. This threshold, like most other traditional psychophysical thresholds, is determined by the physics of the stimulus. Specifically, it is the minimum sound pressure of a signal which evokes a response some number of times, usually 50 per cent. Typically, we measure a threshold of audibility with a method of limits. Data derived from such procedures are reported in Chapter 7 under the general heading of loudness. It is our purpose in this brief section to see how we proceed to make such a measure. Meaningful measurement cannot be made with a presentation of only a single stimulus. Instead, many presentations need to be made over a period of time. For purposes of audiometry, we typically instruct our listener to raise his hand or push a button whenever he hears a tone and to lower his hand when he cannot hear the tone. Furthermore, we typically begin with a tone which we expect to be well above his threshold and then reduce it until he lowers his arm. We might continue reducing the tone to be sure that we really are below threshold and then increase the signal level until our listener raises his hand again. This process, repeated several times, is the one traditionally used for clinical audiometry, although it is indeed suspect. Remember that earlier we pointed out that the threshold differs as a function of the direction from which it is approached. One might even say that there are two different methods of limits, ascending and descending.

One might also measure an absolute threshold by a method of adjustment. In fact, a method of adjustment is employed in automatic audiometry. In this procedure the listener is given a push-button which operates an attenuator. He is told to hold the button for as long as he can hear the tone and to let go of it when he no longer hears the tone. When the tone reappears, he is to push the button again. In this way he is provided with control over the signal level. Threshold determined in this way varies somewhat with the rate of change of signal level, but not a great deal. The method of constant stimuli, another of Fechner's classical methods, may also be employed for the measurement of the absolute threshold, including the threshold of audibility. With such a method, we may present to an observer a group of tones at random intensities and ask him to report how many there were in the group. Or we might ask for a yes-or-no response following each stimulus presentation. The yes-no technique is discussed later in the section on signal detection.

The absolute threshold may be influenced by a number of stimulus variables, not to mention the observer variables which we discussed earlier. One of the principal stimulus variables is the matter of ascending vs. descending procedures. This has been shown to make a considerable difference, not only in the threshold of audibility but also in other psychoacoustic thresholds as well (cf. Chapter 8). It has been shown that the direction of approach renders considerably different thresholds. Another influence is whether or not the stimuli are continuous or interrupted: the threshold of audibility will vary as a function of stimulus duration when employing interrupted tones. Furthermore, the rate at which interrupted stimuli are presented also affects the threshold of audibility. And finally the nature of the instructions given to the listener will affect what *appears* to be the absolute threshold. If we define the desired stimulus for him as a clear and obvious tone, we get a higher threshold than if we ask him only to distinguish if something occurred.

And sometimes we see "off" responses: the listener realizes that the stimulus occurred only when it stops occurring. It is not unusual to present a tone to an observer and have him not raise his hand until the presentation is withdrawn. This is an "off" response. So, while the classical psychophysical methods apply to the measurement of absolute threshold, and indeed have been applied for over 100 years, they are subject to the variability of the physics as well as the psychology of the situation.

THE RELATIVE THRESHOLD

In many ways the relative threshold is more interesting and important than the absolute threshold. We communicate by making discriminations not between something and nothing, but between something and something else. There are two kinds of thresholds, substitutive and additive; this means that we hear something other than what we heard before, or we hear something more than we heard before. In the next chapter, which deals with pitch, we discuss substitutive differential or relative thresholds with emphasis on the problem of pitch discrimination. The following chapter is concerned with loudness phenomena which are additive differential thresholds, namely, what causes us to say that one signal is louder than another.

WHY THE DIFFERENTIAL THRESHOLD?

The importance of measuring differential thresholds, especially in hearing, was exemplified by Hirsh (1952), who stressed the importance of detecting "a difference in telling apart the voices of friends, telling a car horn from a train whistle, telling one word from another, telling a child's laugh from his cry. . . ." Our ability to communicate, our ability to survive in the acoustic world, depends upon our ability to make differential judgments.

When measuring the absolute threshold, we are concerned with the smallest physical value discriminable from silence. Similarly, in the measurement of the differential threshold for hearing, we are concerned with the smallest physical value of a stimulus whereby we may discriminate it from another stimulus. How small a difference can exist between two signals such that we can tell them apart? This is essentially the question that Fechner himself had raised. The data on auditory differential or relative thresholds are found in the next several chapters; we have data on pitch discrimination, loudness discrimination, temporal discrimination, and binaural discrimination.

METHODS FOR MEASURING

If one assumes a classical point of view, then the differential threshold is viewed in a manner essentially identical to the view of the absolute threshold. Hence, for example, Stevens (1951) could say, "here the problem is to locate on the continuum of *stimulus increments* the point that divides the increments into two classes: those to which the organism reacts and those to which it does not. Thus the differential threshold, like the absolute threshold, is a cut that divides a physical continuum." This means, then, that the classical methods are applicable here too. And, furthermore, the same methods employed for the measurement of the absolute threshold are employable for differential or relative thresholds. In obtaining a relative threshold, each stimulus may be presented along with some standard, either simultaneously or sequentially. The subject's task is to judge whether one is greater or louder or higher or in some other way different from the other. And, again, we will express that difference which leads the subject to make this judgment half of the time. For measurement of relative thresholds, we might employ a somewhat different paradigm or psychophysical method. This would be the method of comparison, or the "same-different" paradigm. The same-different paradigm is to differential measurement as the yes-no paradigm is to absolute measurement. In the yes-no case, we want to know only if our observer observed something. In the same-different case, we know he observed something — we want to know if he observed more than one something. A method of comparison is a psychophysical procedure derived from classical methods which permits this to be done. In a method of comparison, the listener is asked to compare some test stimulus with some different stimulus and to report his judgments. We might go a step beyond same-different and ask for more or less, or even further, more or less or equal. Again, these are derived from the classical method of constant stimuli.

While other methods lead to the traditional jnd, the just-noticeable difference, modern psychophysics has introduced some other methods, for example, the ratio methods. In a ratio method, the subject would be asked not only to report which of two stimuli was larger but how the two stimuli were related, that is, how much larger. Other modern methods would include magnitude estimation and magnitude production, which may be based on the method of single stimuli. In this case, for example, we might present a tone of some sound pressure level to a listener and ask him to assign a number to it, giving him some "anchors" such as telling him that a magnitude of 10 is painfully loud, and a magnitude of 0 is inaudible. Given these anchors, he is expected to make an estimate of the magnitude of the loudness of this particular stimulus on a scale from 0 to 10. We might ask him instead to sing a tone having a magnitude of, say, 7 on the scale; this is a method of magnitude production. These methods, of course, are not limited to psychoacoustics. Magnitude production, for example, has been found to be useful in studies of muscle control or tension.

Carterette (1973) has suggested that reaction time itself may be a psychophysical method useful for the measurement of relative thresholds. He has observed that "the stimulus range over which reaction times vary may be twice as large as the range of probability of direct response, and about the same as the range of confidence judgments." For example, an intensity difference between two stimuli may be sufficiently great so that an observer could always tell which was the louder. But reaction time would continue to decrease as the intensity differences increased. In such a case, the study of reaction time itself becomes a psychophysical method.

SIGNAL DETECTION

The notion of signal detection and the theory on the subject did not originate in psychophysics. The psychophysical theory of signal detection (sometimes called detectability) dates from the late 1950's. It arose from work in engineering which had gone on for 20 or 25 years. That work, in turn, arose partly from statistics, probability theory, and decision theory, going back still further. The essential problem is if a signal and a noise occur simultaneously, how can we detect the signal in the noise background?

HISTORY

Probably, the publication which most clearly marks the birth of the psychophysical theory of signal detection was Tanner's 1956 paper, "Theory of Recognition." In that paper, and in other papers written about that time, Tanner and his associates developed the following syllogism: all communication systems are noisy; the human nervous system is a communication system; therefore, some noise is always present in the nervous system. Adopting this point of view obviated the need for the classical concept of the absolute threshold. It is not necessary in this sense to ask questions having to do with whether or not signals can be heard; instead, one asks questions having to do with whether or not signals can be discriminated from noise. In this sense, then, all psychophysical questions become questions of relative threshold. But there is a more important philosophical notion which derives from the study of signal detection. Classical psychophysics depends upon a "stimulus bias." By that is meant that all thresholds and all psychophysical behavior are described in terms of the stimuli which give rise to the behavior, rather than in terms of the organism which exhibits the behavior. These classical ideas can be examined in signal-detection terms; thus, Green and Swets (1966) were able to describe the traditional notion of an absolute threshold as follows: "Either the stimulus produces a sensory event of sufficient magnitude for the observer to think a stimulus was there (a detect state), or the sensory

event is so weak as to produce the opposite state (a non-detect state)."
Signal-detection theory is not concerned with non-detect states but rather
with responses of observers, and only then with the stimuli that lead to the
responses. The theory of signal detection seeks to determine what causes
an observer to respond as though he detected a signal, whether or not a
signal was actually present.

COSTS AND VALUES

One of the most important contributions of the psychophysical
theory of signal detection to our understanding of psychophysics in general has been the introduction of the notion of costs and values. If we assume, and we should, that an observer's response is determined by some
things in addition to the properties of the stimulus, then we must raise
questions of the costs and values of the response to the observer. What
we are saying here, in essence, is that a human observer is a probability
machine. This is easily demonstrated in our everyday activities. For example, when we want to cross a busy street, we look to see what are the
odds of getting run over by a truck. If we determine that the probability of
being hit by a truck is very small, then we proceed to cross the street; if,
on the other hand, we determine that there is a high probability that we
will be struck, we wait on the curb. Not only have we determined the
probabilities, we have determined them based on the value of getting
across the street with respect to the costs of getting hit by a truck. The
value of getting across the street remains the same, but the cost of getting
hit by a truck is considerably more than the cost of being struck by a
tricycle. And so our determination of the probability can be influenced by
the relative costs and values of the situation. These notions of probability,
cost, and value apply in the psychophysical case.

Imagine the following very simple experiment. We say to a listener
that he is going to hear 100 bursts of noise, 50 of which contain a
sinusoidal stimulus. We can do this experiment using a yes-no paradigm;
that is, after each noise burst, we can have the observer respond, "yes,
there was a tone in that noise" or "no, there was no tone in that noise
burst." Prior to the introduction of the first noise burst, the probability of
the tone occurring therein is, of course, .5; that is, the odds that there will
be a tone are equal to the odds that there will not. Let us suppose, then,
that after the first noise burst, the subject responds, "yes." Now, what are
the odds that a tone will occur in the second noise burst, and how does he
decide? His decision is based on two kinds of things: on what he decided
the first time (which varies as a function of whether or not he was told
about the correctness of his response), and on the relative costs of making
an error to the values of making the correct response. We can adjust the
costs and values. Let us suppose, for example, that we provided our observer with 100 pennies. We then told him that for each correct response
we would give him an additional penny, while for each incorrect response

we would take a penny from him. We have now placed monetary costs and values on his responses, and they are equal. We could make them unequal as in the example of the truck and tricycle. We could say that he gets one penny for each correct response and loses five pennies for each incorrect response. We will find in this case that his performance will change. If his performance changes by a forced change of his response criterion due to alterations of costs and values, what has become of the sensory threshold? Green and Swets (1966) claim that "there is little evidence to support the old, classical theory of the threshold . . ." Things in addition to the stimuli influence a subject's response. Therefore, ". . . a principal advantage of modern detection theory is that is shows how to compress a host of factors which affect the observer's attitude into a single variable, called the decision or response *criterion*. . . ."

RESPONSE BIAS

We must assume a bias in favor of a response rather than a bias in favor of a stimulus. Green and Swets (1966) have assumed that "sensory events caused by noise can exactly duplicate any sensory event caused by the signal and that the observer, therefore, is constitutionally incapable of determining whether any given sensory event was caused by noise or by the signal." The point is that there are certain things which cause subjects to respond. When the subject does not respond, we are not interested in what else may have occurred. In other words, assuming again the yes-no paradigm, we are interested only in those conditions which lead to a yes response. There are two such conditions, called "hit" and "false alarm." A hit occurs when the observer says "yes, there was a signal in that noise package" when, in fact, that was the case. A false alarm, on the other hand, occurs when the observer says, "yes, there was a signal in that noise package" when, in fact, the stimulus consisted of noise alone. Another way of putting this is in the words of Engen (1971), who said that detection theory "puts the emphasis on judgmental rather than sensory aspects of the psychophysical experiment."

CONCLUSION

And now we have come back to the beginning. Earlier we argued that there may be room for considering the properties of the responder separately from the properties of the stimulus. The classical traditional assumption of a stimulus bias has led us to report human behavior in terms of the stimuli which lead to the behavior. Signal detection theory permits us to report response behavior, and, after all, responses are what psychophysics is about. Responses to acoustic stimuli are what psychoacoustics is about. In the succeeding chapters, the point of view of signal detection is not usually explicit. Nevertheless, the reader must always be aware that the response-bias interpretation is always possible and is usually preferable.

REFERENCES

Allport, F. H. (1955): *Theories of Perception and the Concept of Structure.* New York, John Wiley & Sons.

Bartley, S. H. (1951): The psychophysiology of vision. *In* S. S. Stevens (ed.): *Handbook of Experimental Psychology.* New York, John Wiley & Sons.

Boring, E. G. (1950): *A History of Experimental Psychology* (2nd Ed.). New York, Appleton-Century-Crofts.

Carterette, E. C. (1973): Personal communication.

Engen, T. (1971): Psychophysics I. Discrimination and detection. *In* J. W. Kling and L. A. Riggs (eds.): *Woodworth and Schlosberg's Experimental Psychology* (3rd Ed.). New York, Holt, Rinehart & Winston.

Gerber, S. E. (1967): Flutter perception in normal listeners. *Journal of Speech and Hearing Research, 10:*319–322.

Green, D. M., and Swets, J. A. (1966): *Signal Detection Theory and Psychophysics.* New York, John Wiley & Sons.

Hirsh, I. J. (1952): *The Measurement of Hearing.* New York, McGraw-Hill Book Co.

Lawson, J. L., and Uhlenbeck, G. E. (1950): *Threshold Signals.* New York, McGraw-Hill Book Co.

Licklider, J. C. R. (1951): Basic correlates of the auditory stimulus. *In* S. S. Stevens (ed.): *Handbook of Experimental Psychology.* New York, John Wiley & Sons, Inc.

Licklider, J. C. R. (1960): Quasi-linear operator models in the study of manual tracking. *In* R. D. Luce (ed.): *Developments in Mathematical Psychology.* Glencoe, Ill., The Free Press.

Macksoud, S. J. (1973): *Other Illusions.* Binghamton, N. Y., privately published.

Mueller, C. G. (1965): *Sensory Psychology.* Englewood Cliffs, N. J., Prentice-Hall.

Pollack, I. (1961): Selected developments in psychophysics, with implications for sensory organization. *In* W. A. Rosenblith (ed.): *Sensory Communication.* Cambridge, Mass., The M.I.T. Press.

Ruesch, J. (1956): The observer and the observed: Human communication theory. *In* R. R. Grinker (ed): *Toward a Unified Theory of Human Behavior.* New York, Basic Books.

Stevens, S. S. (1951): Mathematics, measurement, and psychophysics. *In* S. S. Stevens (ed.): *Handbook of Experimental Psychology.* New York, John Wiley & Sons.

Stevens, S. S. (1961): The psychophysics of sensory function. *In* W. A. Rosenblith (ed.): *Sensory Communication.* Cambridge, Mass., The M.I.T. Press.

Stevens, S. S., and Davis, H. (1938): *Hearing, Its Psychology and Physiology.* New York, John Wiley & Sons.

Tanner, W. P., Jr. (1956): Theory of recognition. *Journal of the Acoustical Society of America, 28:*882–888.

Chapter Six

PITCH*

DONALD G. DOEHRING

The term *pitch* has been customarily defined as one of the psychological attributes of tones, a quality or dimension of tonal perception that corresponds most closely to the physical dimension of frequency within the range 20 to 20,000 Hz. Pitch perception has been studied with reference to pure tones, complex tones, speech, and music. For many years the psychology of hearing was mostly concerned with pitch perception, an interest engendered by the work of von Helmholtz (1863). A great deal of attention, beginning well before the time of von Helmholtz and extending into the present century, has been devoted to explaining how complex

---

*This chapter was prepared while the writer was on leave at the University of Cambridge as a Visiting Scientist of the Medical Research Council of Canada. The assistance of Jean Doehring and the comments of G. B. Henning are gratefully acknowledged.

tones are perceived; furthermore, within the past two decades there has been renewed interest in studying complex tone perception by modern methods of psychology, physiology, and electronics. This work, which was stimulated by the research of Schouten (1940) and von Békésy (1960), was largely aimed at determining the relative contributions of two psychological mechanisms — frequency analysis and periodicity detection — and two corresponding physiological mechanisms — the place and volley principles — to the perception of complex tones. Recent findings have been reviewed in books edited by Tobias (1970) and Plomp and Smoorenberg (1970). This type of research continues to be a major focus of interest in the study of pitch perception.

During the present century there has also been a well-integrated series of psychophysical investigations of how pitch as a dimension or attribute of pure tones is related to other dimensions such as loudness and duration, how the pitch dimension can be quantified by psychophysical scaling procedures, and with what degree of precision pitch changes can be discriminated. At present there is much less emphasis on the study of pitch as a single psychophysical dimension of pure-tone perception, probably because of increased interest in studying the types of complex sounds and sound patterns which carry more important adaptive information.

Knowledge regarding the psychophysics of pure-tone perception, however, has contributed to the study of speech perception, and there has recently been a great deal of work concerned with the frequency characteristics of speech signals. This research, which has also been influenced by linguistic theories of distinctive feature analysis, provides the very important suggestion that speech perception involves a limited sampling of selected features rather than an exhaustive analysis of the entire acoustical speech signal.

The role of pitch in musical perception and performance has always interested psychologists and musicians, but there has been relatively little systematic research on this aspect of pitch perception. Elaborate theories of musical perception have developed independently of psychological research, perhaps because music seems to serve an esthetic rather than an adaptive function. However, the recent interest in complex pitch perception and speech perception referred to above suggests that the study of pitch in relation to music perception could help to determine whether there are separate mechanisms involved in the perception of complex speech and nonspeech sounds.

Research on pitch perception in the last quarter of the twentieth century must take cognizance of major reorientations in perceptual theory during the first three quarters of the century. Traditional psychophysical approaches have tended to describe pitch perception in terms of the frequency or periodicity analyzing power of the "ear" of a passive, specially trained laboratory observer who listens to isolated, artificially produced sounds. More recent theories of perception postulate an active, decision-emitting listener who busily constructs a perceptual model of his world by selectively abstracting information regarding the invariance or regularity of the acoustical signal in the context of his previous adaptive experience. It is important that these two approaches be reconciled, the first of which lends itself more easily to systematic experimentation and the second of which bears more obvious relevance to the human perceiver in the real world.

In the present chapter we attempt a necessarily selective review of traditional and contemporary concepts of pitch perception, indicate where the reader may go for more detailed information, and try to provide a general framework by means of which the rigorous (but narrow and static) approach of the psychophysicist can be equated with the more dynamic and global (but intuitive) approach of the perceptual theorist. Some major findings of "traditional psychophysics" with respect to pure and complex tones are reviewed first, with a sometimes artificial distinction between what are considered "traditional" findings and what are later discussed under "current" concepts. Pitch perception in music is then discussed, followed by a brief mention of the relation between pitch perception and speech perception. Then current concepts are considered, with some final speculations regarding the possible directions of further research on pitch perception.

PSYCHOPHYSICAL CONCEPTS

THE PITCH OF PURE TONES

The psychophysics of pitch perception for pure tones can be described in a fairly straightforward manner. The perceived pitch of pure tones varies largely as a function of tonal frequency, but may also be affected to some extent by the duration and intensity of tones. The amount of frequency change necessary for detection of a pitch change varies systematically as a function of duration, intensity, frequency, and acoustic background.

Duration. All audible pure tones of sufficient duration are perceived as having pitch (cf. Chapter 8). Very short tones are heard as clicks, longer tones as a click with some tonal quality, and still longer tones as having definite pitch preceded and followed by clicks (Licklider, 1951). The clicks result from the necessarily rapid turning on and off of the tone, which introduces additional frequencies that are generally referred to as "transients." The pitch of short tones can be assessed by having the listener adjust a relatively long comparison tone until its pitch matches that of the short tone. The shortest duration that a pure tone of moderate intensity can be perceived as having pitch varies as a function of frequency below 1000 Hz. Longer durations are required as frequency decreases to a duration of about 25 msec at 125 Hz. Above 1000 Hz

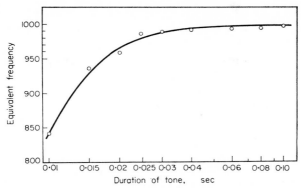

Figure 6-1 The variation of the pitch of a tone as a function of its duration. (From Littler, T. S.: The Physics of the Ear. Elmsford, N. Y., Pergamon, 1965.)

tones of about 10 msec are heard as having pitch. It can be generalized that below 1000 Hz two or three cycles of a sinusoidal signal are required for pitch perception, thus involving an increase of minimum duration with decreasing frequency; whereas, above 1000 Hz only a fixed minimum duration is required for the observer to report a distinct pitch. As the duration of tones approaches the minimum for pitch perception, there is also a systematic change of the apparent pitch as indicated in Figure 6-1. The apparent pitch of low-frequency tones becomes higher and that of high-frequency tones becomes lower.

Intensity. Changes of the intensity of pure tones have also been said to result in systematic changes of pitch (Fig. 6-2), with the largest changes occurring for high and low frequencies and relatively small changes in the region 1000 to 3000 Hz. However, recent research (Cohen, 1961) has demonstrated much smaller changes (two per cent or less) for high frequencies and no consistent change at all for low-frequency pure tones. Furthermore, the pitch of complex tones such as those produced by most musical instruments is even less affected by changes of intensity. Thus, changes of pitch as a function of intensity are not very important in most practical situations.

Frequency. The pitch of pure tones does not vary linearly as a function of frequency; that is, a given amount of frequency change in two different parts of the frequency range does not necessarily involve an equal amount of change of apparent pitch. The relationship of pitch to frequency has traditionally been investigated by psychophysical scaling procedures rather than by the matching procedures used to investigate the effects of duration and intensity. Pitch scales have been constructed by asking the subject to adjust a variable tone until its pitch appears to be half that of a fixed tone (fractionation) or to adjust a variable tone to a pitch halfway between those of two fixed tones (bisection). The resulting scale

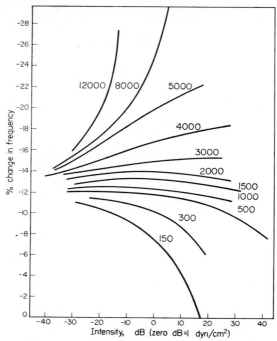

Figure 6–2 Contours showing how pitch changes with intensity. (From Littler, T. S.: The Physics of the Ear. Elmsford, N.Y., Pergamon, 1965.)

is expressed in units called *mels,* with a given difference in any part of the mel scale representing an equal change of apparent pitch (Stevens and Davis, 1938). The extent to which the mel scales deviate from the frequency scale can be seen in Figure 6–3. With linear frequency, an equal distance along the horizontal axis of the graph represents an equal frequency change. As pitch increases, a given amount of pitch change is associated with larger and larger increases of frequency; thus, apparent subjective pitch increases more and more slowly with increases of linear frequency. On a logarithmic frequency scale, a doubling of frequency represents an equal interval; e.g., the distance from 10 to 100 Hz equals that from 100 to 1000 Hz, or from 1000 to 10,000 Hz. As pitch increases along the logarithmic frequency scale, a given amount of pitch change is associated with larger and larger increases of frequency; thus, apparent subjective pitch increases more and more rapidly with increases of logarithmic frequency. The relation of pitch to logarithmic frequency is particularly important for music, since musical scales are based on logarithmic frequency scales. An increase of an octave involves a doubling of frequency. For example, middle C is 262 Hz, high C is 524 Hz, and C above high C is 1048 Hz. The relationship between pitch and

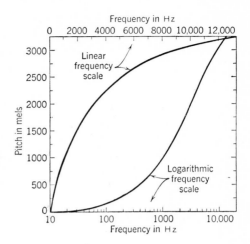

Figure 6-3 Pitch as a function of frequency. The upper curve shows that subjective pitch (in mels) increases less and less rapidly as the stimulus frequency is increased linearly. The lower curve shows that subjective pitch increases more and more rapidly as stimulus frequency is increased logarithmically. (The musical scale is a logarithmic scale.) The pitch of a 1000 Hz tone, 40 db above threshold, is defined as 1000 mels. (From Stevens, S. S. (ed.): Handbook of Experimental Psychology. New York, John Wiley and Sons, Inc., 1951, p. 1003.)

logarithmic frequency, then, seems to provide an important paradox regarding pitch perception: musical intervals that are responded to by performers and listeners as equal do not necessarily involve equal changes of pitch as defined by the mel scale, since intervals in the lower part of the frequency range involve much smaller changes of pitch than those in the higher part of the frequency range. This is discussed further in the section on music.

Discrimination. As described in the previous chapter, a differential threshold (or difference limen) is obtained by changing the stimulus along a given dimension by an amount just sufficient for the subject to reliably detect the change. The differential threshold for frequency can be expressed in terms of the absolute change of frequency (ΔF) or the amount of change relative to the initial frequency ($\Delta F/F$). The difference limen (DL) for frequency varies as a function of both frequency and intensity (Licklider, 1951), as well as duration and background noise (Henning, 1967; 1970). Frequency discrimination tends to be quite poor (large DL) for very soft tones, but to approach a stable minimum for sufficiently loud tones at any given frequency. Earlier studies indicated that the relative DL ($\Delta F/F$) remained constant above 1000 Hz and became larger as frequency decreased below 1000 Hz. However, in certain frequency ranges the discriminations could have been based on changes in both pitch and loudness.

When random-amplitude tones are used to prevent discrimination on the basis of loudness change, it is found that the relative DL remains fairly constant below 4000 Hz and increases rapidly above 6000 Hz. It is possible to construct another form of pitch scale by determining the number of DLs that fall between each series of discrete frequencies within the frequency range. Although early studies indicated a very good agreement between this type of scale and the mel scale (Stevens and

Davis, 1938), there is no close correspondence between the two types of scale when random-amplitude tones are used to determine the DL (Henning, 1966).

THE PITCH OF COMPLEX TONES

Sounds that are composed of more than one sinusoid are justifiably called complex tones, because the perceived pitch quite often seems to involve something other than the component frequencies. One of the earliest laws dealing with hearing, Ohm's acoustic law, stated that the "ear" can separate a complex tone into its sinusoidal components, enabling the listener to perceive the individual pure tones that go to make up the complex tone. Or, expressed in a somewhat different way, any pitch perceived by the ear must correspond to a sinusoidal component of the physical stimulus. Ohm's law has generated over a century of research, largely aimed at demonstrating its limitations (see Plomp, 1966; Tobias, 1970; Plomp and Smoorenberg, 1970). Not only is the listener unable to hear all the components of many complex tones, he may report hearing tones that are not even present.

Nonlinear Distortion. Not long after Ohm formulated his law, von Helmholtz proposed that frequency analysis was limited by a less-than-perfect sensory transduction of the air-conducted sound. When a sinusoidal tone is distorted by nonlinear transmission, the resulting tone contains additional frequency components of relatively low intensity called aural harmonics. For a pure tone of sufficient intensity, then, nonlinear distortion may add detectable high-pitched components. Thus, the listener cannot function as an ideal analyzer even when listening to a single tone.

Two-Tone Combinations. When tones of relatively low intensity which differ considerably in frequency are presented together, they are perceived as two distinct tones, in accordance with Ohm's law. However, some very interesting additional sounds are heard when the two tones are louder or more similar in frequency. When the tones are only a few Hertz apart, they are perceived as a single tone that waxes and wanes in loudness at a rate equal to the difference between their frequencies; e.g., combined tones of 1000 Hz and 1003 Hz will result in a tone that is perceived as "beating" three times per second. When two fairly loud tones that are more widely spaced are presented together, a number of *combination* tones of much lower intensity may be heard in addition to the two original components. If loud tones of 700 Hz and 1000 Hz are presented, the listener may hear a *difference* tone of 300 Hz and a much weaker *summation* tone of 1700 Hz. Because of the nonlinear distortion involved in the transduction of the original component tones, he may also hear their second harmonics (1400 and 2000 Hz, respectively) and even their third harmonics (2100 and 3000 Hz). These harmonics may in turn become involved in the production of difference and summation tones; e.g., the second harmonic of the 700 Hz tone may combine with the fundamental of the 1000 Hz tone to produce a difference tone of 300 Hz; and, to complete the auditory confusion, some of the plethora of tones thus produced might be close enough in frequency to result in perceptible beats. For certain two-tone combinations, then, pitch perception may involve much more than the elegant two-tone frequency analysis postulated by Ohm's acoustic law (Ward, 1970).

Combinations of More Than Two Tones. Pitch perception of multicomponent tones can be considered from several different aspects with reference to Ohm's law. When the listener is asked to identify the components of complex tones, he very seldom performs perfectly. His frequency analysis may be impeded by combination tones; and in the case of many components, perfect analysis could be beyond his limited span of perception. But an even more curious exception to Ohm's law occurs when the listener perceives a complex tone as having a fundamental that does not correspond to any of its components. If a complex tone consisting only of higher harmonics of a 100 Hz tone (e.g., 700, 800, 900, and 1000 Hz) is presented, many listeners may hear the complex tone as having a pitch of 100 Hz. This is seemingly beyond Ohm's law. Although the perceived pitch in the above example could be interpreted as a difference tone, a pitch of 100 Hz is also heard when only the odd higher harmonics of 100 Hz (300, 500, 700, 900 Hz) are presented. In this case, a pitch corresponding to 200 Hz would be reported if a difference tone were responsible for the perceived pitch. Furthermore, a pitch corresponding to the "missing fundamental" is reported for complex tones whose intensity is sufficiently low to rule out the possibility of audible difference tones.

Discovery of the missing fundamental—or rather its rediscovery, since the concept originated from the work of Seebeck in 1841—has led to the formulation of a somewhat different explanation of pitch perception. Pitch is not perceived by a spectral analysis of component frequencies in a simple or complex sound wave, but rather by an analysis of the *periodicity* of the sound wave; that is, the most prominent period of waveform alternation. This period corresponds to the fundamental frequency in complex tones which contain a fundamental frequency (Plomp, 1966).

For complex tones which contain only the higher harmonics of a fundamental, the most prominent periodic component of the complex wave form still corresponds to the fundamental. A great deal of research in recent years (cf. Small, 1970; Plomp and Smoorenberg, 1970) has been devoted to periodicity pitch. The work of Schouten (1940) is usually credited with leading to this renewal of interest. In general, it has been found that, within certain limits, any sound that varies in intensity at a regular rate can give rise to a pitch corresponding to the rate of alternation, regardless of the spectral composition of the fluctuating sound. Thus, periodicity or time analysis has been postulated as an alternative to the explanation of pitch perception in terms of frequency or spectral analysis. It should be noted that periodicity analysis would predict the same pitch as frequency analysis for a simple tone since the period of a pure tone is the reciprocal of its frequency. The difference between the two explanations of pitch perception relates to complex tones where period- icity analysis would predict perception of a single pitch corresponding to the fundamental, and frequency analysis would predict perception of the pitch of all spectral components of sufficient intensity. Neither type of analysis can by itself explain the variety of phenomena occurring in the perception of complex tones. Frequency analysis and periodicity pitch are discussed at greater length in the section on current concepts.

MUSIC

The term pitch is encountered in matters dealing with music. Al- though music is more than a sequence of pure tones of different frequency, we can gain insight into the factors that affect pitch perception if we consider this rather skeletal aspect of music. It is enlightening to consider the special abilities of musicians to perceive and produce very precise gradations of pitch. Listening to music provides an impressive demonstration of the ability to perceive the components of complex sounds. Discussions of music in relation to pitch perception can be found in Seashore (1938), Winckel (1967), and Ward (1970).

MUSICAL PITCH SCALES

Virtually all music involves notes with easily perceived fundamental frequencies, and most orchestral and choral music seems to require the perception of more than one note played or sung at the same time. Figure 6–4 shows the octaves covered by the piano along with the average ranges of singing voices and musical instruments. It can be seen that the piano and several other instruments approach the lower limits of the human frequency range, but the highest notes, even those of the piccolo, do not extend much beyond 4000 Hz. However, these represent only the fundamental frequencies. The harmonics or overtones of many instru- ments, which help to give the instruments their characteristic quality, ex- tend considerably higher, presumably justifying the expense of high- fidelity amplification systems with a frequency response extending to 20,000 Hz or more.

MELODIC STRUCTURE

Tonal sequences in a musical composition usually take the form of easily identifiable melodies. The melodic structure is partly defined by the duration of notes, intervals between notes, and accents produced by in- tensity variation, but the pitch of the notes is probably the most crucial feature of melodic definition. Any given melody does not depend upon a

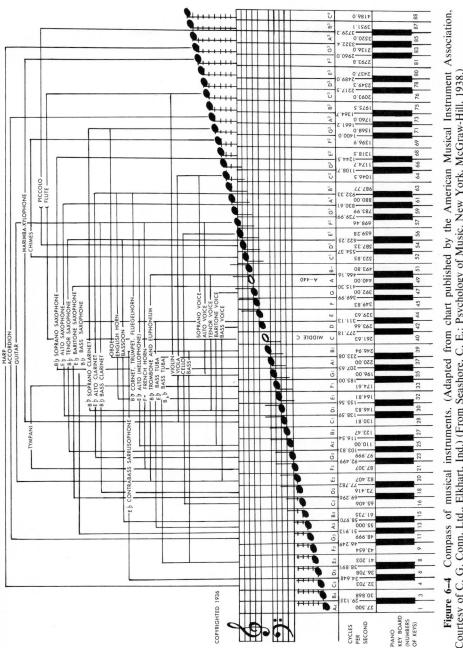

Figure 6-4 Compass of musical instruments. (Adapted from chart published by the American Musical Instrument Association, Courtesy of C. G. Conn, Ltd., Elkhart, Ind.) (From Seashore, C. E.: Psychology of Music. New York, McGraw-Hill, 1938.)

specific set of pitches, but only upon the relationships among pitches. As long as the logarithmic frequency differences within a melody are preserved, it does not matter in what part of the frequency range the melody is played. The most common example is musical transposition where changing a composition from one key to another does not change the melody. The frequencies of the notes in a transposed melody do not even have to correspond to those of the musical scale. Thus, one can alter the speed of a phonograph or tape recorder by a sufficient amount to produce notes that lie somewhat between those shown in Figure 6–4, and the melody will still sound like the same melody. The recognition of melody involves perception of relationships among a temporal sequence of sounds whose fundamental frequencies differ in semitone steps. This process cannot be explained in terms of psychophysical investigations of single sounds.

COMPLEXITIES OF MUSICAL PITCH

It is also instructive to consider the phenomena which occur when musical notes are played together. In conventional Western music there is a fixed number of common three- and four-note combinations designated as chords. Each chord has not only a basic set of notes or "root" positions, but two or three "inversions" in which one or more of the component notes is transposed to a different octave. The pianist must learn to perceive and play many combinations of three or four notes in a large number of pitch ranges which are designated as Keys or Scales (see Karolyi, 1965, for an introduction to the "grammar" of music).

The root positions of chords are identified in terms of musical intervals which, in turn, are defined by the number of notes in the scale from the lowest note in the chord, with the third being two notes above and the fifth four notes above the lowest note. This is not quite as simple as it sounds, because the chromatic scale of eight notes (do, re, mi, fa, sol, la, ti, do) does not consist of equal distances in terms of logarithmic frequency. Six of the intervals are separated by two semitones, and the remaining two are separated by only one semitone. These discrepancies, interestingly enough, may not be apparent to the casual listener to whom the eight notes may appear to involve equidistant intervals of pitch.

The musician thus makes use of a set of complicated scales of relative pitch when he plays and listens to chords and tonal sequences. The various scales begin at different frequencies and have unequal frequency differences in various parts of the scale. Moreover, most compositions involve several changes of scale during a composition. To the musician this does not seem a particularly difficult task because he is proceeding according to a definite set of rules. But the listener who relates the perception of meaningful sets of simultaneous and successive pitches to the complex logarithmic frequency relationships involved in scales, intervals, and chords can congratulate himself on performing a rather staggering feat of complex pitch perception. Of course, the recognition of chords can be explained in terms of Ohm's acoustic law, and seems to provide a good example of the operation of frequency analysis. An equally impressive accomplishment is the ability of music lovers, musicians, and particularly symphony conductors to separately perceive instruments played together. Somehow the distortions and complexities involved in harmonics, beats, summation tones, and difference tones do not often coalesce the orchestral sound into either a totally confused tonal mass or a singly perceived waveform. However, the type of ability needed to perceive separate instruments and melodic themes in a musical ensemble probably involves a process that cannot be easily explained in terms of some combination of frequency analysis and periodicity detection. It is tempting to speculate that musical perception involves a rule-governed process of feature extraction analogous to that which is said to occur in speech perception (cf. Chapter 12).

MUSICAL CONSONANCE AND DISSONANCE

Consonance and dissonance are concepts that have excited lively controversy among music theorists for many centuries. Pairs of tones are judged to be consonant or dissonant on the basis of an esthetic judgment as to whether they sound well together (consonant) or not (dissonant). Not surprisingly, there is much less agreement among listeners regarding consonance and dissonance than there is regarding the relative pitch of tones. A number of theorists have postulated that consonance is related to the ratios of the frequencies of the two tones. Simple ratios such as 1:1 (unison), and 1:2 (octave) would be the most consonant, whereas more complex ratios such as 8:9 or 9:10 would tend to sound most dissonant. Some of the explanations for this apparent correspondence between frequency ratios and esthetic experience invoked a sort of internal spiritual harmony for tones with simple frequency relationships. Others have postulated the occurrence of beats and combination tones that prove disturbing to the listener in tonal pairs having complex frequency ratios, thus providing an objective explanation for an esthetic judgment involving pitch perception. However, listeners without musical training do not tend to judge the simpler ratios such as octaves as most consonant, selecting instead more complex ratios such as 5:7 or 5:8.

The criterion for consonance is not as closely related to the frequency scale as is the criterion for pitch, and thus may be more affected by musical training and changing subcultural values with regard to musical form. A given individual's criterion of consonance may also change from time to time. Most musicians and listeners would consider a composition that involved only "consonant" tones throughout as colorless and boring. This is particularly true for most forms of modern music.

ACOUSTIC CHARACTERISTICS OF MUSICAL TONES

It must be emphasized that very few musical notes approach the simplicity of sustained pure tones. Each instrument has a particular pattern of harmonics, and the instrumentalist may further "color" the tone by the use of vibrato or trills, both of which involve relatively rapid oscillations of frequency. In addition, many musical notes are quite brief and consist almost entirely of complex frequency spectra associated with on-off transients. The particular form of the transient serves as another means of distinguishing between musical instruments, and the musician adds another dimension to his performance by his "attack," which effectively varies the transients. Thus, the perception of the pitch of individual musical notes, which most listeners and performers seem to find not at all difficult, takes place in spite of a variety of additional acoustic trappings which probably actually assist in the selective comprehension of musical meaning.

ABSOLUTE PITCH

The ability to name a note played in isolation or to produce a given note by singing, whistling, or blindfolded adjustment of a pure-tone generator is termed "absolute" or "perfect" pitch and is one of the aspects of pitch perception which has excited the most discussion over the years (Ward, 1963). This ability is not surprising if we classify it as analogous to the naming of isolated colors, smells, and tastes. Since relative pitch is much more important than absolute pitch for the performance and identification of melodies, the ability for absolute pitch identification may be trained out of us in early life. In any case, it is a rare accomplishment that is not at all well understood. Seashore (1938) cited an example of a member of a family which included several highly accomplished musicians who disliked music himself because he had such "perfect" pitch that he could not stand hearing any note that deviated in the slightest from the required frequency. Although such anecdotal evidence is difficult to evaluate, absolute pitch is a very interesting concept. Further study of this phenomenon may elucidate some of the processes underlying pitch perception, particularly with regard to similarities and differences between music perception and speech perception.

RELATION BETWEEN PITCH PERCEPTION AND SPEECH PERCEPTION

Speech perception is dealt with at length in Chapter 12. Here we consider only the role of pitch perception in speech recognition and some of the apparent similarities and differences between music perception and speech perception.

SPEECH RECOGNITION AND PITCH PERCEPTION

A major point made by modern investigators (e.g., Liberman et al., 1967) is that speech perception cannot be explained entirely in terms of acoustic analysis. Once again, Ohm's law proves insufficient, and this time for the most important type of auditory perception. Speech perception depends upon the perception of a specific set of phonemic sounds. As was the case for complex nonspeech sounds, the listener perceives both more and less of the frequency components than one might predict from acoustic analysis. Because of "categorical perception" (see Chapter 12), he may not be able to distinguish among a variety of slightly different complex sounds, all of which are responded to as the same consonant, but makes very precise discrimination of the "boundaries" between consonants. As was also the case for complex nonspeech sounds, the listener identifies speech sounds on the basis of changes of temporal patterning that would not be revealed by spectral analysis. Speech perception is characterized by a dynamic "parallel processing" of sets of "features" of phonemic sounds. This involves the perception of rapid frequency changes in relation to sustained frequency bands and noise bursts, and probably is better described in terms of pattern perception than either frequency or periodicity analysis.

Speech perception, like melody recognition, involves the recognition of relationships among simultaneous and successive sounds rather than the perception of a fixed set of pitches. This is exemplified by the fact that we recognize the same sentence spoken by a child and a male adult, and both the words and the melody of a song anywhere within the frequency range of the singing voice. Both speech and music, then, require the listener to perform a complicated series of relational abstractions for accurate recognition of sentences and melodies. Speech perception appears to be the more perceptually demanding of the two processes, even though "good" speech perception seems a much more universal phenomenon than good music perception.

The two types of perception seem to differ in several respects. The perception of rapid frequency transitions is more crucial for speech recognition than for music recognition. Categorical perception is said to be unique to speech perception, but may operate in music to the extent that musicians and listeners do respond to slightly different frequencies as equivalent in pitch. However, it is most interesting that the traditional musical concepts of absolute and relative pitch involve a very precisely tuned perception of specific frequencies and specific frequency differences that seem diametrically opposed to the concept of categorical perception.

SEQUENTIAL CONSTRAINTS IN SPEECH AND MUSIC

Just as important as pattern recognition *per se* in speech perception is the listener's implicit knowledge of the probabilities that a particular phonemic sound is more likely to be followed by some classes of phoneme than others, and that a particular class of words is more likely to be followed by some classes of words than others. Since these probabilistic constraints on sequences of speech sounds can be regarded as a product of perceptual learning, we can make use of Gibson's (1966) description of perception as an active, self-guided search by a listener who is tuned to anticipate invariances in his environment. According to Gibson, the individual does not construct his awareness of the world from bare intensities and frequencies of energy, but detects the world from invariant properties in the flux of energy, a notion that is very much in accordance with the concept of categorical perception. Thus, the listener brings to the listening situation a repertoire of implicit learned expectancies regarding the probabilistic constraints of speech that are just as important as the acoustic input in determining what he perceives.

The characterization of perception as an active process involving previously learned probabilities of stimulus patterning has been described by terms such as "set," "expectancy," "decision strategy," and "response bias." This aspect of perception must be included in any explanation of how pitch is perceived. In music perception the listener's past experience in anticipating what note may follow another is crucial to his esthetic experience. He applies a different set of expectancies to Bach, Mozart, Beethoven, and Stravinsky, because each composer applied a different set of constraints upon chordal structure and tonal sequences. Some compositions, such as those of Stephen Foster, contain highly predictable tonal sequences that would be judged by most music lovers as very uninteresting. At the other extreme, the contemporary composer John Cage advocates compositions involving randomly selected notes, thus depriving the listener of any expectancy whatsoever regarding tonal sequences. In a very general sense, then, the perception of frequency changes in speech and music can be said to involve a common process, but there appear to be important differences as to certain details. The temptation to make a direct analogy between the two processes must also be tempered by their apparent differences in function. Speech perception is part of a communicative process whose primary function is to transmit information, whereas music perception serves an apparent function of esthetic enrichment.

HEMISPHERIC LATERALIZATION

There is no need to further belabor the point that pitch perception in both speech and music involves much more than a passive frequency or periodicity analyzer. The perceiver of pitch is an adaptive organism who uses all available acoustic cues and experiential clues to proceed efficiently toward his goal of optimizing the perception of speech, music, and other auditory events. Does the perception of music and other nonspeech sounds entail a somewhat simpler process of less adaptive value than speech perception, but involving essentially the same mechanism? The research of Milner (1962), Kimura (1967), and others has demonstrated a striking difference between speech and music perception with respect to cerebral functioning. Speech perception is mediated primarily by the left cerebral hemisphere, whereas the perception of both melodies and chords is mediated primarily by the right cerebral hemisphere (cf. Chapter 9). Exactly what this means with regard to the processes involved is not yet clear, but Liberman and his associates (1967) have used this type of evidence as support for a theory that speech perception is a unique form which differs from all others, both auditory and non-auditory. Only the speech system is said to be capable of effectively analyzing the complicated dynamic changes that constitute the acoustic cues of speech perception. Further study of pitch perception for speech and nonspeech sounds in relation to hemispheric asymmetry may reduce some of our uncertainty about how pitch perception takes place in the adapting organism.

CURRENT CONCEPTS

PERCEPTION OF COMPLEX TONES

A considerable amount of research within the past decade has been directed toward the traditional problems of pitch perception for complex tones — the roles of frequency analysis, periodicity analysis, and nonlinear distortion in the perception of pitch, timbre, and combination tones. Although the exact details are still being studied, there is general agreement that the perception of pitch and other phenomena related to the frequency characteristics of acoustic stimuli involves both frequency and periodicity analysis. Detailed discussions have been presented by Licklider (1959), von Békésy (1963), and Plomp (1966), and in books edited by Tobias (1970) and Plomp and Smoorenberg (1970). The conclusions of Plomp are summarized here.

The listener does have a limited ability to "hear out" the components of complex tones, although he does not always use it. Plomp found that his subjects could discriminate the first five to eight harmonics of complex tones. Frequency-resolving power is said to be limited by the *critical bandwidths* of the tonal components. The concept of critical bandwidth, which was formulated by Fletcher (1940), is central to Plomp's theory of complex tone perception: it refers to the frequency range within which white noise can reduce the audibility of a pure tone (Fig. 6–5). Like other variables which affect pitch perception, the width of the critical band on a linear frequency scale varies as a function of frequency, having a fairly constant width of about 90 Hz below 200 Hz, and increasing in width with increasing frequency thereafter. As stated previously, the harmonics of a complex tone are equidistant in frequency, being separated by an

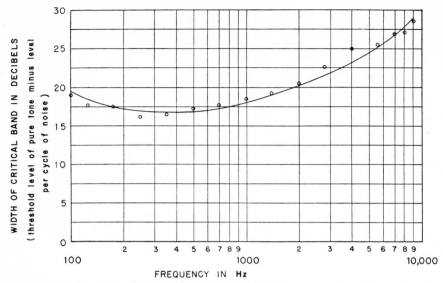

Figure 6–5 Width of a critical band as a function of frequency. The width, in decibels, is equal to $10 \log_{10} W$, where W is the width of the critical band in cycles per second. The smooth curve is from data obtained at the Bell Telephone Laboratories. (From Hirsh, I. J.: The Measurement of Hearing. New York, McGraw-Hill, 1952.)

amount equal to the frequency of the fundamental. Since the critical bandwidths become wider for higher frequency tones, there comes a point in the frequency range where the higher harmonics are separated by less than a critical bandwidth, and the tones cannot be heard separately. The listener can indeed function as a frequency analyzer for lower harmonics but often does not.

If imperfect frequency analysis were the sole mechanism for pitch perception, we should, when listening to a complex tone, hear separately the fundamental and all other components whose frequency separation was greater than a critical bandwidth, along with some residual sound arising from the components that cannot be separately resolved. Instead, complex sounds consisting of harmonic components (such as notes played on musical instruments) are characterized by one definite pitch even when the fundamental is absent, and despite the fact that the separate audibility of lower harmonics can be demonstrated under certain experimental conditions. From Plomp's own research and that of others, he concluded that the pitch of complex tones is dependent upon periodicity analysis rather than frequency analysis. He found that the periodicity pitch of complex tones with fundamental frequencies below about 1400 Hz is dependent upon the higher harmonics rather than the fundamental, and for complex tones with higher fundamental frequencies, the periodicity pitch is largely dependent upon the frequency of the fundamental.

Although an explanation of pitch perception by periodicity analysis is in accord with the findings of experiments by Plomp and others, it does not account for the limited ability to hear out the components of complex tones in a particular experimental situation or the ability to easily discriminate among complex tones of identical fundamental frequency and periodicity produced by the singer, the violinist, and the pianist. Plomp accounted for the discriminability of such differences in complex tones by invoking once more the limited frequency-analyzing mechanism of the ear.

Although the single perceived pitch of a complex tone is always dependent upon its most prominent periodicity, variations of harmonic structure are perceived as differences in *timbre*. Timbre and pitch are said to be two separate dimensions of auditory perception. Complex sounds such as spoken vowels are actually discriminated in terms of timbre variations rather than variations of fundamental frequency.

A final objection to the concept of periodicity pitch is that periodicity cannot be preserved in the auditory nerve for frequencies above 4000 Hz. Plomp pointed out that the highest notes produced by musical instruments and by the human voice do not greatly exceed 4000 Hz. He postulated that simple tones and complex tones whose fundamental exceeds 4000 Hz, although audible, are not perceived as having pitch, but have a noise-like character. Thus, pitch perception occurs only in the frequency range of 20 to 4000 Hz, and the information gained from audible sounds above this limit involves a different form of perception.

Plomp, then, felt that periodicity analysis leads to the perception of a complex tone as a unity having a characteristic pitch that "overshadows" the individual pitches of the first five to eight harmonics, that limited frequency analysis contributes a distinctive quality or timbre to the unitarily perceived pitch, and that differences in timbre help us to recognize speech sounds and to separately perceive certain sets of complex tones, as in an orchestra or a social gathering. He would insist, of course, that the resolution of different complex tones spoken or played simultaneously is still subject to the limitations of the relative strength of spectral components in successive critical bands.

Plomp also used the critical band concept to explain tonal consonance and dissonance. Subjects were asked to judge the degree of consonance or dissonance of pairs of simultaneously presented pure tones, where consonant tones were defined for the subject as beautiful and euphonius. He found that for the frequency range of 125 to 2000 Hz, tones were judged as consonant when their frequency difference exceeded the critical bandwidth at that part of the frequency range, and as most dissonant when they differed by about one quarter of the critical bandwidth. Although this finding fits well with his concept of the critical band, the basis of the consonance-dissonance judgment remains much more subjectively insubstantial than that of pitch, and is more likely to be disputed by musicians and others.

Plomp directly confronted the traditional problems of pitch perception and attempted to fit them within a single explanatory scheme. This largely involved a modification, integration, and reinterpretation of previous theories. Only a bare outline of his work has been given here, and it is impossible to indicate within the scope of this chapter the great proliferation of work by psychologists, physiologists, and physicists on the frequency analysis-periodicity detection problem (cf. Tobias, 1970; Plomp and Smoorenberg, 1970) which will undoubtedly be the subject of many erudite investigations for a number of years to come. The final definition of the term "pitch" must probably await the outcome of such investigations.

OTHER VARIABLES INFLUENCING PITCH PERCEPTION

The pitch of a sound is usually perceived or recalled in relation to the pitch of another sound or sounds. This must involve some processes in addition to those resulting from a single tonal *input*. Wickelgren (1969) has proposed a theory that separates perception, storage (memory), and retrieval (decision strategy). Other investigators have also begun to investigate such factors in relation to pitch perception. Massaro (1970) proposed a storage interference model to explain storage and decay of pitch memory. Elliott (1971) found that memory for one tone and for two successive tones involved at least two factors, frequency analysis and memory. Discrimination of simultaneous tones appears to involve a somewhat different process than the discrimination of successive tones (Doehring and Ling, 1971), and listeners make use of a variety of strategies for discriminating among successive tones, depending upon the exact requirements of the discrimination task (Doehring, 1971). Much more work on memory and decision processes in pitch perception can be anticipated.

Musical perception seems to involve factors other than the perception of exact relationships among a set of pitches. Dowling and Fujitani (1971) report that listeners judge melodies as similar in terms of the direction of change of pitch from one note to another in addition to making similarity judgments based on absolute or relative pitch, and describe this as the recognition of melodic contours. Bregman and Campbell (1971) found that rapid sequences of tones containing alternate notes in a high- and low-frequency range are perceived as two separate streams or tunes, and conclude that the listener habitually segregates co-occurring auditory sequences which are sufficiently different in frequency range. Attneave and Olson (1971) confirmed the importance of relational judgments in musical pitch perception. When both musical and nonmusical listeners were asked to reproduce tonal patterns, they preserved the logarithmic frequency differences between component tones but tended to transpose the patterns to another part of the frequency range. This was interpreted as evidence that, in the normal situation of being stimulated by tonal patterns rather than isolated pitches, the listener responds on the basis of the musical frequency scale rather than the mel scale. Most interestingly, accuracy of transposition deteriorated above 5000 Hz, the upper limits of conventional musical instruments, and the region beyond the extent of periodicity detection.

Not only is the ability to discriminate differences of frequency important, but also the discrimination of differences of the amount and the duration of frequency transitions. Pollack (1968) found that frequency transitions were discriminated by two different processes, one operating for fast changes involving large frequency differences and the other for slow changes involving small differences. He interpreted this finding with respect to frequency and periodicity analysis, as an example of the manner in which the auditory system solves the problem of successfully processing a wide range of transition conditions by employing different modes of operation. The "trade off" between frequency and time analysis in the discrimination of frequency changes occurs in such a way that a sharp frequency analysis is accompanied by a coarse time analysis and a sharp time analysis is associated with a coarse frequency analysis. Nabelek and Hirsh (1969) also investigated the discrimination of frequency transitions and emphasized their importance in speech discrimination. Their ultimate goal was to find out whether phoneme identification depends upon changes of the magnitude, the duration, or the rate of frequency change. They found the same type of dual mechanism reported by Pollack. Optimal discriminability was associated with large frequency changes for relatively short transition durations, leading the writers to conclude that this aspect of the discrimination of frequency change is a general property of hearing and is not unique to speech perception.

Finally, Broadbent (1971) has speculated about a possible biological basis for the dual mechanisms of frequency analysis and periodicity detection proposed by Plomp. He hypothesizes that the relatively low fundamental frequency of voiced sounds is processed by periodicity detection, and the higher-frequency formants and formant transitions are processed by frequency analysis. The consonants and vowels emitted by a given speaker are bundled together into a single, identifiable package by the periodic modulation of his fundamental frequency. The listener is thereby assisted in selectively attending to one particular speaker and "filtering out" other speakers. Broadbent has thus demonstrated that an apparently paradoxical duality of the hearing mechanism can be meaningfully applied to a rigorously formulated explanation of human perception.

SUMMARY

Our present knowledge suggests that pitch perception is not a unitary process. The dual processes of frequency and time analysis are associated with other dualities that have been mentioned. The ability to detect a wide range of audible frequencies might seem to imply that we respond to all frequencies within this range by the same process. However, we have seen that low-frequency information is processed differently from high-frequency information with respect to the minimum tonal duration for perceived pitch, the effects of intensity on pitch, frequency discrimination, critical bandwidth, and perception of the pitch of complex tones. It must be concluded that responses to auditory frequency do not involve a simple unitary process. Perhaps what we normally perceive as pitch consists of periodic modulations from which we obtain information about the identity of speakers and the melodic content of music, and the residual sounds associated with the complex spectra which are modulated provide information about the verbal content of speech and the identity of musical instruments. If so, the two mechanisms would be employed in an opposite manner to extract the message and the source of the message in speech and music perception. This could suggest a basis for the apparent specialization of the left cerebral hemisphere for speech perception and the right hemisphere for music and other nonspeech perception. However, such speculation is probably premature, particularly since the left hemisphere seems to be dominant for both verbal message extraction (Kimura, 1967) and speaker identification (Doehring and Bartholomeus, 1971).

Some precautions must be advanced about the interpretation of past research and the planning of future research on pitch. Lawrence (1968) was concerned about the exact form of the acoustic signal reaching the tympanic membrane in psychoacoustic experimentation. The signal is subject to a number of sources of potential distortion after it leaves the tone generator, is transformed from electrical to acoustical energy, and transmitted to the listener. Precise knowledge of the resulting auditory stimulus is necessary before there is any definite speculation regarding wave patterns of the basilar membrane or coding patterns of nerve fibers. Lawrence also wondered about the meaningfulness of subjective reports concerning the specially constituted auditory input that is presented to the listener in a psychoacoustic experiment. We normally respond or fail to respond to auditory input as part of our overall adaptation, and select those aspects of auditory and other sensory input that are meaningful and rewarding. In the experimental situation, the listener may have to invent a sort of explanation for the artificial listening task that is largely based on his interpretation of the experimenter's expectations. Thurlow and Hartman (1959) found a variety of individual differences in investigating the "missing fundamental." Some listeners reported hearing the missing fundamental, while others heard the higher harmonics but not the fundamental. The writers speculated that perception of the missing fundamental may be the most prominent part of a complex perceptual process that is based on the past experience of listeners in listening to the complex tones produced by singing voices and musical instruments. This could be interpreted as a form of auditory "closure" based on previous auditory learning, in contrast to the assumption of many previous investigators that the "ear" — in splendid peripheral isolation — performs a frequency or periodicity analysis of the acoustic input. The reservations of these writers and others about the generality of experimental findings regarding pitch perception must be taken seriously. Many of the data of psycho-acoustics are based upon the subjective reports of trained listeners, often the experimenters themselves, and we do not know the extent to which their mode of perceiving pitch in the experimental situation is character-istic of populations of trained and untrained listeners making adaptive responses to speech and music outside the laboratory.

The most challenging frontiers of research on pitch perception, in the opinion of the present writer, relate to the broad and poorly defined ques-tions about how the human listener actually uses pitch information as an adaptive cue. The traditional theoretical approach has not been con-cerned with this aspect of pitch perception. Licklider (1959) pointed out that theories of pitch perception are concerned with processes rather than outcomes, whereas theories of speech perception have been concerned with the result or effect of perception rather than how it is brought about. Recent investigators of speech perception have become more concerned with process, and there is now some indication that systematic study of the adaptive outcomes of pitch perception will be undertaken. One major question is whether pitch perception should be studied in isolation or as an integral aspect of dynamic changes of the amplitude, duration, and spectral characteristics of complex acoustic stimuli. Another question relates to the concurrent operation during pitch perception of processes other than those traditionally studied, such as memory, decision strategy, selective attention, expectancy, and distinctive feature extraction. Methods must be devised to permit a more cogent scientific explanation of the richness and complexity of musical experience. Neurophysiological mechanisms of pitch perception are only beginning to be understood. There have been very few investigations related to the development of pitch perception in infants and young children. Theoretical models that will encompass the potential range of relevant variables are essential, but must probably await the accumulation of more empirical knowledge. The pitch perceiver does not seem to be ideal, and whether he is best charac-terized as actively seeking to tune himself to invariance, as performing a hierarchy of feature analyses, as an information processor who uses a pe-ripheral sensory filter and a central comparator to extract relevant fea-tures of the acoustic stimulus, or as some even more esoteric type of analyzer remains to be seen.

REFERENCES

Attneave, F., and Olson, R. K. (1971): Pitch as a medium: A new approach to psychophysi-cal scaling. *American Journal of Psychology 84*:147–166.

Bregman, A. S., and Campbell, J. (1971): Primary auditory stream segregation and percep-tion of order in rapid sequences of tones. *Journal of Experimental Psychology 89*:244–259.

Broadbent, D. E. (1971): *Decision and Stress*. New York, Academic Press.

Cohen, A. (1961): Further investigations of the effects of intensity upon the pitch of pure tones. *Journal of the Acoustical Society of America 33*:1363–1376.

Doehring, D. G. (1971): Serial order effects in auditory discrimination by oddity and matching to sample. *Perception and Psychophysics 10*:137–141.

Doehring, D. G., and Bartholomeus, B. N. (1971): Laterality effects in voice recognition. *Neuropsychologia* 9:425–430.

Doehring, D. G., and Ling, D. (1971): Matching to sample of three-tone simultaneous and successive sounds by musical and non-musical subjects. *Psychonomic Science* 25:103–105.

Dowling, W. J., and Fujitani, D. S. (1971): Contour, pitch, and pitch recognition in memory for melodies. *Journal of the Acoustical Society of America* 49:524–531.

Elliott, L. L. (1971): Auditory memory for one and two tones. *Journal of the Acoustical Society of America* 49:450–456.

Fletcher, H. (1940): Auditory patterns. *Review of Modern Physics* 12:47–65.

Gibson, J. J. (1966): *The Senses Considered as Perceptual Systems*. Boston, Houghton Mifflin Co.

Henning, G. B. (1966): Frequency discrimination of random-amplitude tones. *Journal of the Acoustical Society of America* 39:336–339.

Henning, G. B. (1967): Frequency discrimination in noise. *Journal of the Acoustical Society of America* 41:774–777.

Henning, G. B. (1970): A comparison of the effects of signal duration on frequency and amplitude discrimination. *In* R. Plomp and G. F. Smoorenberg (eds.): *Frequency Analysis and Periodicity Detection in Hearing*. Leiden, A. W. Sijthoff.

Karolyi, O. (1965): *Introducing Music*. Baltimore, Penguin Books.

Kimura, D. (1967): Functional asymmetry of the brain in dichotic listening. *Cortex* 3:163–178.

Lawrence, M. (1968): Audition. *Annual Review of Psychology* 19:1–26.

Liberman, A. M., Cooper, F. S., Shankweiler, D. P., and Studdert-Kennedy, M. (1967): Perception of the speech code. *Psychological Review* 74:431–461.

Licklider, J. C. R. (1951): Basic correlates of the auditory stimulus. *In* S. S. Stevens (ed.): *Handbook of Experimental Psychology*. New York, John Wiley & Sons.

Licklider, J. C. R. (1959): Three auditory theories. *In* S. Koch (ed.): *Psychology, A Study of A Science*. Vol. 1. New York, McGraw-Hill Book Co.

Massaro, D. W. (1970): Consolidation and interference in the perceptual memory system. *Perception and Psychophysics* 7:153–156.

Milner, B. (1962): Laterality effects in audition. *In* V. B. Mountcastle (ed.): *Interhemispheric Relations and Cerebral Dominance*. Baltimore, The Johns Hopkins University Press.

Nabelek, I., and Hirsh, I. J. (1969): On the discrimination of frequency transitions. *Journal of the Acoustical Society of America* 45:1510–1519.

Plomp, R. (1966): *Experiments on Tone Perception*. Soesterberg, Netherlands, Institute for Perception.

Plomp, R., and Smoorenberg, G. F. (eds.): *Frequency Analysis and Periodicity Detection in Hearing*. Leiden, A. W. Sijthoff.

Pollack, I. (1968): Detection of rate of change of auditory frequency. *Journal of Experimental Psychology* 77:535–541.

Schouten, J. F. (1940): The perception of pitch. *Phillips Technical Review* 5:286–294.

Seashore, C. E. (1938): *Psychology of Music*. New York, McGraw-Hill Book Co.

Small, A. M., Jr. (1970): Periodicity pitch. *In* J. V. Tobias (ed.): *Foundations of Modern Auditory Theory*. Vol. 1. New York, Academic Press.

Stevens, S. S., and Davis, H. (1938): *Hearing: Its Psychology and Physiology*. New York, John Wiley & Sons.

Thurlow, W. R., and Hartman, T. F. (1959): The "missing fundamental" and related pitch effects. *Perceptual and Motor Skills* 9:315–324.

Tobias, J. V. (ed.) (1970): *Foundations of Modern Auditory Theory*. New York, Academic Press.

von Békésy, G. (1960): *Experiments in Hearing*. New York, McGraw-Hill Book Co.

von Békésy, G. (1963): Hearing theories and complex sounds. *Journal of the Acoustical Society of America* 35:588–601.

von Helmholtz, H. L. F. (1954): *On the Sensations of Tone*. (1st German Ed., 1863.) New York, Dover Publications.

Ward, W. D. (1963): Absolute pitch. *Sound* 2:14–21, 33–41.

Ward, W. D. (1970): Musical perception. *In* J. V. Tobias (ed.): *Foundations of Modern Auditory Theory*. Vol. 1. New York, Academic Press.

Wickelgren, W. A. (1969): Associative strength theory of recognition memory for pitch. *Journal of Mathematical Psychology* 6:13–61.

Winckel, F. (1967): *Music, Sound, and Sensation*. New York, Dover Publications.

Chapter Seven

LOUDNESS

SANFORD E. GERBER AND BENJAMIN B. BAUER

In general, loudness is the perceptual correlative of sound intensity. It is that perceived property of sounds which permits us to order them on a scale extending from very quiet to very loud. It is the case, however, that loudness does not depend entirely upon the intensity of the signal. Loudness also depends upon frequency and wave complexity, and therefore the word "loudness" cannot be used synonymously with such terms as intensity.

In this chapter, we first consider absolute loudness; that is, we talk about what it is that makes sounds audible at all and what are the limits of audibility. We then talk about relative loudness or the *difference limen* for loudness and consider briefly the subject of the recruitment of loudness. Thirdly, we turn our attention to the construction of a scale of loudness based upon the unit called the sone. And, finally, the chapter addresses the interesting topic of equal loudness, that is, the properties of signals of different spectra which cause them to sound as loud as one another.

It is important to stress again that loudness does not depend in total upon signal intensity or sound pressure. In fact, intensity can remain constant while loudness changes. It is also to be stressed that, while we can continuously vary the intensity level of a signal, loudness does not vary continuously but moves instead in discrete steps.

151

The study of loudness as a psychoacoustic phenomenon dated essentially from the earliest beginnings of modern psychoacoustics. The topic had been considered, for example, by the first giant of psychophysics, E. H. Weber (1795–1878), who had formulated what we now call Weber's law. Weber's law was not viewed as a law for some years until G. T. Fechner (1801–1887) had called it such. In fact, it was Fechner's refinement of Weber's observations which constituted perhaps the most significant early research on the subject of loudness. Weber had said that the just-noticeable difference in perceiving a stimulus bears a constant ratio to the stimulus. Weber's work had first been done on the sense of touch, but he later extended it to vision and audition. Fechner had been concerned with some motor problems when he recognized that an "absolute increase of intensity might depend upon the ratio of the increase of bodily force to the total force" (Boring, 1950). Later, Fechner recognized the generality of this observation, and it is to the more general statement that Boring applied the term Fechner's law. In any case, Fechner is justifiably called the "Father of Psychophysics," and he had formulated his notions of the just noticeable difference by 1851.

Among modern investigations of loudness, Littler (1965) credits Kingsbury (1927) with the earliest investigations. However, Sabine had written a paper called "Sense of Loudness" that was published originally in 1910, republished in 1923, and again in 1964.

ABSOLUTE LOUDNESS

There is an absolute threshold of loudness; that is to say, there are some tones which are just not loud enough to be heard. Such signals are generally said to be below the threshold of audibility. At the opposite extreme, some signals are so intense that the notion of loudness does not really apply, and we find ourselves speaking instead of such things as the threshold of feeling, the threshold of tickle, and the threshold of pain.

THE THRESHOLD OF AUDIBILITY

The threshold of audibility is specified in units of sound pressure or of sound pressure level and refers to the number of units required to elicit a response in a listener a specified number of times. As you learned in Chapter 5, we usually take threshold value to be the number, in physical units, to which an observer will respond exactly half the time. So, the threshold of audibility, then, is the number of decibels of sound pressure level which can be heard by a given observer half the time. When operating near the threshold of audibility, the percentage of time a response is evoked is related directly to the intensity level or sound pressure level of the signal.

Traditionally, there had been two ways to determine the threshold of audibility. One was to measure the *minimum audible pressure,* and the other to measure the *minimum audible field.* The traditional method for determining the minimum audible pressure was that employed and reported by Sivian and White (1933). The essential question to be answered in a minimum audible pressure experiment is: How small a sound pressure measured at or in the ear canal will lead to a threshold of audibility in a large number of normally hearing, healthy young persons? Sivian and White developed a procedure whereby a tiny probe microphone could be inserted into the ear canal of a listener and the ear could be covered by a tightly fitting earphone. In this way, when a signal was transduced by the earphone, the listener's response could be elicited simultaneous with the measurement of sound pressure in the ear canal. If we ask, then, how little sound pressure will elicit a response only half of the time, and if we raise this question at several different frequencies, we will derive the MAP contour, as shown in Figure 7–1. The first thing which should attract one's attention is that the MAP contour is by no means a horizontal line: the minimum audible pressure varies as a function of frequency. Referring to Figure 7–1, it may be seen that for a tone of, say, 100 Hz to be minimally audible requires about 40 decibels more sound pressure level than does a tone of 1000 Hz to be minimally audible. Similarly, the 1000 Hz tone requires some 20 decibels less sound pressure level than does a tone of 10,000 Hz to be minimally audible. What this indicates is that healthy, normally hearing, young persons are more sensitive to tones of medium frequencies than they are to tones at either very low or very high frequency. Moreover, except for the extremes of the frequency range, these listeners are more sensitive to high frequencies than they are to low ones. What we are saying, therefore, is that greater pressure is required to cause a low-frequency or high-frequency tone to be audible than is required for a tone of medium frequency to be audible. This turns out to

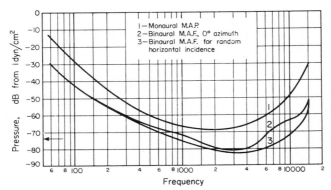

Figure 7–1 Threshold curves determined for minimum audible pressure (M.A.P.) and minimum audible field (M.A.F.). (From Littler, T. S.: The Physics of the Ear. Elmsford, N.Y., Pergamon, 1965.)

be biologically very useful: von Békésy (1960) pointed out that if we were more sensitive at low frequencies, our very footsteps would sound like· thunder to us, and if we were more sensitive to high frequencies, the blood rushing through the vessels in our ear would sound like driving rain. So there is a basic biological protective function of this curve of minimum audible pressure.

The other traditional measurement of the threshold of audibility is that of the minimum audible field. This, too, was measured by Sivian and White (1933). In a manner similar to that in which they measured the minimum audible pressure, they placed a probe microphone in the sound field, but removed both the listener and the earphone with which he was listening. Then they did essentially the same measurements that had been done with minimum audible pressure, which is to say, they applied the same signal levels to the transducer which led to the minimum audible pressures, plotted the amount of pressure in the sound field, and called these measurements the minimum audible field. The MAF is also shown on Figure 7–1, and (surprise!) the MAF curve does not overlay the MAP curve. In fact, the MAF curve lies somewhat below the MAP curve and varies not only as a function of frequency but also as a function of the angle of incidence of a sound wave striking both microphones and emanating from a loudspeaker in the field. Notice also that not only does the MAF lie below the MAP, but the curves are not parallel. Sivian and White thought the difference between MAP and MAF may have been because of diffraction of sound waves due to the fact that the listener's head is present in the sound field. This phenomenon, the "shadow effect," is discussed in the chapter on binaural hearing. The fact is, however, that no one has been able "to find any satisfactory solution to explain the total difference between the two thresholds" (Littler, 1965).

Many different studies have been made of both the minimum audible pressure and minimum audible field, and the MAF has consistently been found to lie below the MAP. The variation ranges from 5 dB to 13 dB and, in general, over the entire distribution of both curves, averages out to be about 6 dB. In fact, this has come to be known in the psychoacoustical literature as "the case of the missing 6 dB." Of course there is another explanation, which is that the minimum audible pressure is measured monotically under an earphone, whereas the minimum audible field is measured diotically in the sound field. The minimum audible field, then, is subject to the phenomenon of binaural summation, which would be expected to make the listener more sensitive to a signal of a given sound pressure. Nevertheless, the number of 6 dB remains a mystery and presumably those six decibels are forever missing. Even Stevens and Davis (1938) could not "account for all the discrepancies."

RANGE OF SENSITIVITY

In the section immediately preceding we learned about the lower limits of the sensitivity range of normally hearing persons. Of course, there must also be an upper limit. Some sounds are too loud; in fact, some of them are so much too loud as to become painful. As one might expect, it is difficult to do research on the threshold of pain and subjects do not readily volunteer. And, so, the threshold of pain is not firmly established, but it is generally thought to lie no higher than the 140 dB sound pressure level for most listeners. Furthermore, when we look at the ceiling of our sensitivity, we find that it does not vary as a function of frequency. That is, the amount of sound pressure sufficient to cause pain in a normally hearing person is about the same at any frequency. If the minimum audible pressure and the minimum audible field vary as a function of frequency and they constitute the floor of the area of hearing, but the ceiling does not vary with frequency, it is evident that the range of sensitivity is decidedly narrower at extreme frequencies than it is at middle frequencies. And this is well known to be the case.

The threshold of pain, again, is difficult to determine not only because

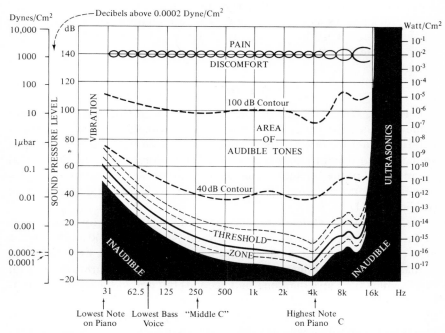

Figure 7–2 *The area of audible tones* was determined for a group of otologically normal men listening with both ears, facing the source, in a free acoustic field. The heavy lower contour represents their median hearing thresholds: the shaded zones show one and two standard deviations (σ) above and below it. Dips at 4000 and 12,000 Hz are due largely to resonance in the ear canal and diffraction patterns around the head. The area of audibility at low frequencies merges into vibration. On the high-frequency side lie the inaudible ultrasonics. The practical upper limit is the threshold for pain, at about 140 dB SPL. (From Davis, H., and Silverman, S. R.: Hearing and Deafness, 3rd ed. New York, Holt, Rinehart, and Winston, 1970.)

people do not readily volunteer for pain experiments, but also because what one person reports as painful another may report as only very uncomfortable. Nevertheless, high pressures give rise to tactile sensations in the auditory system instead of, or in addition to, auditory sensations. This "threshold of feeling" is generally thought to be in the neighborhood of 120 dB SPL and also does not vary significantly as a function of frequency. In general, the auditory mechanism has an upper limiting intensity of the order of 100 dB, and greater intensities elicit a sensation of discomfort.

Different loudness behaviors are exhibited at different points in the range of sensitivity. Since the top curves (whether of discomfort, feeling, or pain) are generally flat, it must be concluded that we do not show relative differential frequency sensitivity at very high levels. It is also the case at very, very low levels that we show rather little frequency sensitivity. Littler (1965) claimed that when a tone is barely audible, it does not have a tonal quality as do more intense sounds. Sounds close to the threshold of audibility lack a full quality of pitch. Figure 7–2 displays the distribution of the range of sensitivity as a function of frequency. It is also to be noted therefrom that as that range becomes extremely narrow, tonal quality disappears as well as intensity discrimination. In this figure, the curve labeled "Threshold of Hearing" is equal to the curve of the minimum audible pressure.

EFFECT OF DURATION

It turns out that while all the above is indeed true, the truth varies somewhat as a function of how much time is available to listen to the signal. If we want to compare the loudnesses of two tones which are of equal sound pressure and frequency, but of different durations, we will find that the intensity of the briefer one needs to be increased in order to maintain equality, as its duration becomes progressively less than 200 msec (Gulick, 1971).

Garner (1947) showed that the threshold of audibility for tones varies directly with duration when tone duration is less than 500 msec. In the next chapter, this phenomenon is discussed at length. The essential point is that our ability to detect a tonal signal at all varies with duration for brief signals (i.e., less than one-half second) but not with longer durations (i.e., longer than one-half second), as shown in Figure 7–3. Gulick (1971) claimed, for a 1000 Hz tone, loudness will decline over a period as long as two minutes and then will stabilize. Even so, although threshold will vary up to one-half second, perceived loudness increases up to durations of about a second (Littler, 1965). Also it matters whether the tone is continually present or whether it is only intermittently present. If the pulses are very brief, they just might not last long enough to achieve their full loudness. It takes about 200 msec for a tone to reach maximum level, and then the loudness begins to decline (von Békésy, 1967). Again, detailed

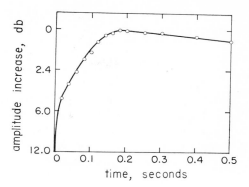

Figure 7–3 Increase of loudness of a tone as a function of stimulus duration. (From Von Békésy, G.: Sensory Inhibition. Princeton, N.J., Princeton University Press, 1967.)

discussion of the interactions between stimulus duration and perceived loudness is to be found in the next chapter.

BINAURAL SUMMATION

The topic of binaural summation is discussed at length in Chapter 9. In that chapter the reader will learn that the term "dichotic" refers to a condition when the ears are each receiving a different signal. The term "diotic" refers to the condition in which the same signal arrives at both ears, and "monotic" refers to a signal reaching one ear only. Dichotic signals are louder than either diotic or monotic signals.

Refer again to Figure 7–1 and also to the discussion to the effect that the MAF might be expected to be less than the MAP because two ears are used. Notice also that there is a difference in the two MAF curves shown as a function of the angle of incidence of the stimulus sound waves. It is simply the case that, for purposes of sensitivity, two ears are better than one. Not very much better; we would expect (by the physics of the situation) the threshold of audibility to be 6 dB better for two ears in a sound field than for one. And that is generally what was discovered. It is also the case that our sensitivity to loudness change is improved when listening with two ears. However, apparently because of summation between the two ears, if we present a tone of a fixed sound pressure level in one ear and a tone of a varying sound pressure level in the other, we will find that the intensity difference between the ears required to produce a perceptible change of loudness (by virtue of a localization response) is greater than if we have diotic or monotic serial presentation of tones (Rowland and Tobias, 1967).

RELATIVE LOUDNESS

What, then, about our ability to detect changes of loudness? Is this a uniform behavior, or is it in some way related to absolute loudness? And, how does it differ between normal and abnormal ears?

DIFFERENCE LIMENS

Recall that the term *difference limen* is synonymous with the term *just-noticeable difference*. In this section, we deal with the matter of the intensive difference limen or the just noticeable difference for intensity.

We find that the difference limen (henceforth symbolized DL) depends upon sensation levels. The term *sensation level* relates intensity to the threshold of audibility of a particular ear or listener. Sensation level is reported in decibels above threshold for that ear or listener. If we are dealing with pure tones or with bands of noise narrower than a "critical band," it is the case that loudness is proportional to the power of the signal. If, however, we are dealing with a band of noise wider than a critical band, loudness is found to increase with bandwidth. Furthermore, as the signal becomes louder, its DL also increases. Our ability to detect change of loudness varies as a function of loudness, so that the louder the signal is, the more its intensity must change before we can determine that it has changed. And isn't this again reminiscent of Fechner's law? In fact, loudness varies as the logarithm of intensity. Another way of stating this was "the ratio. . . of the increment to the level from which the increase was made remains quite constant" (Hirsh, 1952). Hirsh explains that "if we represent both loudness and the intensity of the sound on logarithmic scales, the loudness increases very rapidly at low intensities while at higher intensities the function decelerates, indicating a smaller logarithmic increment in loudness for each successive increment in intensity." Over the entire range, every 10 dB increase of sound intensity amounts to a two-fold change of loudness.

RECRUITMENT

For some people the loudness DL does not increase as loudness increases, or at least does not increase as much as it does for normal persons. This phenomenon is called the *recruitment* of loudness; it is an abnormal growth of loudness. Frequently, in those hearing impairments in which the site of pathology is in the cochlea, the patient will have a severely diminished dynamic range. That is to say, the range of sensitivity from his threshold of audibility to his threshold of discomfort is decidedly decreased. For this patient, sounds of moderate intensities are inaudible, but sounds of high intensities are at least as loud as they are for normally hearing persons.

Figure 7–4 illustrates recruitment quite clearly. It shows a normal ear and an impaired ear. The curve marked *A* represents the case when the two ears are equal — normal or otherwise. The curve marked *C* indicates the case when the impaired ear has no recruitment, while the curve marked *B* indicates an impaired ear with recruitment. Notice that curves *A* and *C* are parallel while curve *B* bends upward from a common point with *C* to a common point with *A*. This demonstrates clearly the abnormal growth of loudness.

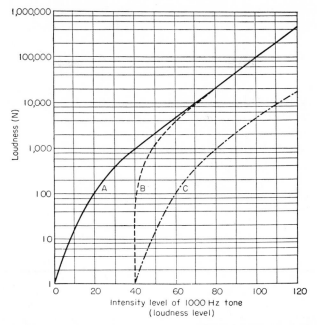

Figure 7-4 Theoretical functions relating loudness to Intensity Level for three cases: (A) normal hearing; (B) 40 dB hearing loss with recruitment; (C) 40 dB hearing loss with no recruitment. (From Hirsh, I. J.: The Measurement of Hearing. New York, McGraw-Hill, 1952.)

LOUDNESS SCALES

It is often desirable to know how much louder one sound is than another. And so, from this point of view, it is required to establish a scale of loudness. In order to do this, one has to ask people when a given sound is louder than another sound. In 1938, Stevens and Davis established two criteria for a scale of loudness which continue to be entirely relevant. The first criterion was that the numbers on the loudness scale must have "true numerical significance," which meant that if they were arithmetically manipulated, they would render results that would correspond to physical operations. The second criterion was that the scale should bear "a reasonable relation to the experience of the observer."

A scale of loudness can be developed quite directly by having a listener adjust the level of a sound until its loudness, in his judgment, doubles, triples, etc. The first question, however, has to do with double or triple of what? To this day, we follow the procedure of Stevens and Davis in which we assign the arbitrary number one to an intensity 40 dB above threshold; that is to say, given a tone of frequency 1000 Hz at 40 dB sensation level, we will arbitrarily state that it has a loudness of one *sone*. Now, in order for it to satisfy the requirement of numerical significance, it follows that a sound which is twice as loud (regardless of intensity) must be represented by two sones; and similarly 0.5 sone designates half as loud. Employing such a procedure renders the curve displayed in Figure 7–5.

First of all, one will notice in Figure 7–5 that, while there are different curves for different frequencies, all the curves but one are for very low frequencies. This is because it has been empirically determined that the curve for 1000 Hz is essentially accurate for all frequencies between 700 and 4000 Hz (Stevens and Davis, 1938) or perhaps even from 500 to 4000 Hz (Gulick, 1971). However, for lower frequencies, the loudness function becomes quite a bit steeper. Notice also that, with the exception of the very lowest frequencies, the curves for all frequencies come together at high intensity levels. Remember that we had pointed out previously that our ability to appreciate changes of either pitch or loudness diminishes severely at very high levels. In Figure 7–5, all the

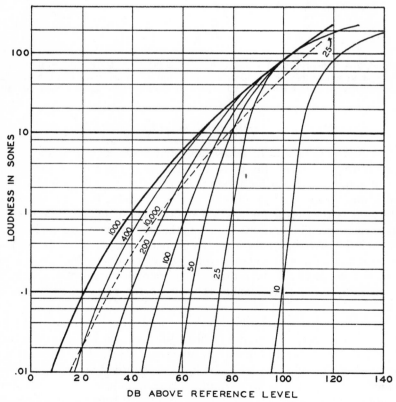

Figure 7–5 The loudness function. Showing how the perceived loudness of various tones depends upon the intensity of the stimulus. Frequency is the parameter. (From Stevens, S. S., and Davis, H.: Hearing. New York, John Wiley and Sons, Inc., 1938.)

curves meet at the 100 dB sensation level. Incidentally, notice also in that figure that there are no curves to the left of the curve for 1000 Hz.

A minor amount of caution is required in acquiring and interpreting these data. Characteristically, loudness functions are derived by a method of fractionation. This is the familiar method, again, in which we ask the listener to find twice the loudness, three times the loudness, etc. Remember the warning that sometimes methods which appear to be equal are not, and therefore do not derive identical answers. Littler (1965), for example, pointed out that "doubling a sound in loudness and then halving the resultant does not give the initial sound." In other words, using a tone with a loudness of one sone as the reference, ask the listener to double his loudness, and he will generate what we have decided to call two sones. If we now present a tone equivalent to two sones and ask him to adjust it half as loud, he does not generate the same sound pressure as the initial reference of 40 dB SL. Changing the reference changes the resultant.

If you look again at Figure 7–5, you will notice two things about the curves: first, they are not parallel, and second, they are not straight lines. We had indicated this phenomenon earlier in the section on the difference limen. Notice that the curve for low frequencies gets steeper as the frequencies get lower. A just detectable increase of sound intensity goes up both as the intensity goes up and as the frequency goes down.

EQUAL LOUDNESS

A matter which is at least as interesting as the problem of loudness itself has to do with the way in which to judge whether one sound is more or less loud than another sound. Remember, in the preceding discussion, loudness referred to the variation of perceived intensity at a given frequency. And we asked: how does loudness change with intensity for that frequency? When we come to the subject of equal loudness, we ask instead: how does loudness change as a function of frequency? To distinguish this phenomenon from loudness, Fletcher and Munson (1933) used the name *loudness level*. Today, two terms — equal loudness and loudness level — are used synonymously. Moreover, these terms refer to something quite specific, although some recent authors seem to have forgotten just how specific it is. Fletcher and Munson defined loudness level as "the equally loud reference tone . . . obtained by adjusting the intensity level of the reference tone until it sounds equally loud" to the sound being measured. Even more specifically, the reference tone was always a sinusoid of 1000 Hz. Therefore, it must be noted that "loudness level. . . tells us, not how loud a tone is, but rather how intense a 1000-cps tone must be in order to sound equally loud" (Hirsh, 1952).

The fact is that when making equal loudness measurements, one does not customarily behave in this manner. First of all, the notion of loudness level being dependent upon intensity level (re: 10^{-16} W/cm^2) implies listening in a free sound field, as would obtain in an anechoic chamber. In practice, however, loudness level measurements are made under earphones, and therefore, Stevens and Davis (1938) admonished that it makes much more sense to adjust the loudness not to the intensity level of the reference signal but rather to the sensation level of the reference signal. It is this procedure which is customarily followed.

The history of the measurement of equal loudness is, in fact, longer than that of loudness measurement. Littler (1965) claimed that the first equal-loudness contours were done by Kingsbury in 1927. However, Sabine, as early as 1910, had demonstrated the phenomenon of equal loudness for a series of organ pipes. There have been several standard studies of loudness levels to which we often return for our basis. These are the papers of Fletcher and Munson (1933), Churcher and King (1937), and Robinson and Dadson (1956). All of these classic papers have used the *phon* as their unit of measurement.

THE PHON

The phon is the unit of loudness level. The loudness level in phons of a tone of some frequency is equal to the intensity level of a 1000 Hz reference tone in decibels. In other words, applying a reference tone of 1000 Hz at 40 dB sensation level, we say that it has a loudness level of 40 phons. A tone of any other frequency judged to be equally loud to that reference is also said to have a loudness level of 40 phons. Remember that the same reference tone, 1000 Hz at 40 dB SL, was said to have had a loudness of one sone. There is an equation that demonstrates the relations between loudness and loudness levels or, better, the relation between the sone and the phon.

Figure 7–6 demonstrates the relationship between loudness in sones and the loudness level in phons, according to the following equation:

$$S = 2^{\frac{(P-40)}{10}} \qquad \text{or}$$

$$P = 40 + 10 \log_2 S.$$

What this means, according to Bauer and Torick (1966), is that loudness varies approximately as the 0.6 power of the ratios of the pressures of the comparison tones. Another way to put that is

$$\frac{S_1}{S_2} = \left(\frac{P_{c1}}{P_{c2}}\right)^{0.6}$$

The phon, unlike the sone, is a unit designated to indicate equality rather than to indicate a scale measure. In other words, equal phons rep-

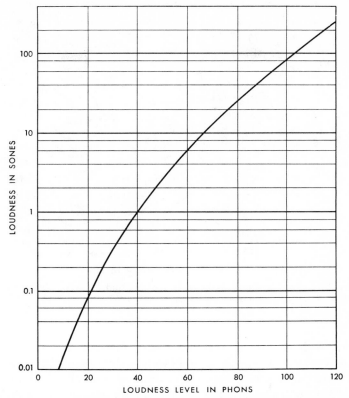

Figure 7–6 The loudness function, showing how perceived loudness (in sones) depends on the loudness level of the stimulus (in phons). (From Denes, P. B., and Pinson, E. N.: The Speech Chain. Bell Telephone Laboratories, 1963.)

resent equal loudnesses, but changes in a number of phons correspond only as the above equation with the scale of loudness measured in sones. The phon, then, is not a scalar.

FLETCHER AND MUNSON, AND OTHERS

Most people listening alternately to two tones of different frequency find it rather easy to decide which one is louder and to adjust the loudness of the other until their loudnesses are found to be equal. When making measurements of loudness level, one of these two frequencies is always a 1000 Hz tone of known sound pressure level. The well-known equal-loudness contours of Fletcher and Munson (1933) were obtained by such a process. Their contours are shown in Figure 7–7.

These measurements were made in an anechoic chamber with the listeners facing the source of sound. Obviously, not everyone has an absolutely free sound field, such as an anechoic chamber, so subsequent work

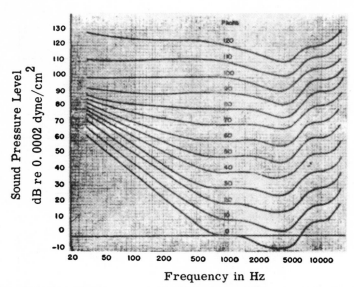

Figure 7–7   Equal-loudness contours of Fletcher and Munson. (After Bauer et al.: IEEE Trans. Audio Electroacoust., AU-15:177–182, 1967.)

was done with the aid of calibrated earphones, as mentioned earlier. While the Fletcher-Munson contours were widely accepted in the United States, there was some divergence of opinion. Therefore, Churcher and King (1937) published another set of equal-loudness contours, the set shown in Figure 7–8. It is to be noted that they vary almost not at all from the original curves of Fletcher and Munson. Some variation may be observed, however, in Figure 7–9, the equal-loudness contours of Robinson and Dadson (1956).

     There are some interesting generalizations which may be made from observation of all three sets of curves. First of all, they are obviously highly similar. Secondly, it is equally obvious that as the loudness level

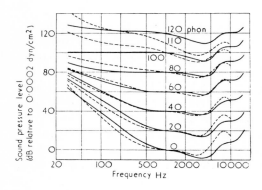

Figure 7–8   Equal-loudness contours of Churcher and King compared with Fletcher and Munson. (From Robinson, D. W., and Dadson, R. S. With permission from the National Physical Laboratory, Crown Copyright reserved. In Harris, J. D. (ed.): Forty Germinal Papers in Human Hearing. Groton, Conn., The Journal of Auditory Research, 1969, p. 194. Permission of the Controller of Her Brittanic Majesty's Stationery Office has been obtained.)

goes up, the variation of loudness level with frequency diminishes. That is to say, the upper curves are substantially flatter than the lower curves. If one notes the Robinson-Dadson contours, it may be seen that a contour for the MAF is shown there also. In one sense, the MAF (or the MAP) may be considered to be a zero phon contour. So this bottom equal-loudness contour represents, in a sense, a normal threshold of hearing. It shows that we are most sensitive in the area of 3000 Hz, least sensitive for very low frequencies, and intermediately sensitive for very high frequencies. But all the contours show that, as the sound pressure increases and the loudness level increases with it, our relative sensitivities with respect to frequency begin to diminish. Indeed, the curves do not become absolutely flat and the low point is still around 3000 Hz. But the ends of the several phon contours get ever closer together.

Two things matter. One has to do with whether we are adjusting the intensity level or the sensation level of the reference. The other has to do with whether we adjust the reference to be equally loud to the probe tone or the probe tone to be equally loud to the reference tone. Stevens and Davis (1936) adjusted the intensity level of the test frequency until it was equal to the reference tone, whereas Fletcher and Munson adjusted the intensity level of the reference tone until it was equal in loudness level to the test zone. This change matters, but only a little bit.

Stevens (1956) noted that when one tone is standard and the other is variable, listeners tend to set the variable one a little bit higher. But he

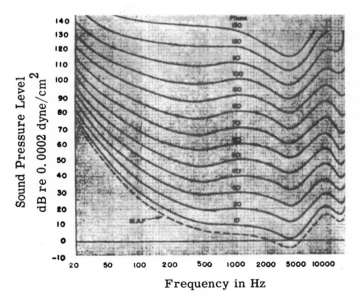

Frequency in Hz

Figure 7–9 Equal loudness contours of Robinson and Dadson. (After Robinson, D. W., and Dadson, R. S.: Br. J. Appl. Phys., 7:166, 1956. Copyright by The Institute of Physics. With permission.)

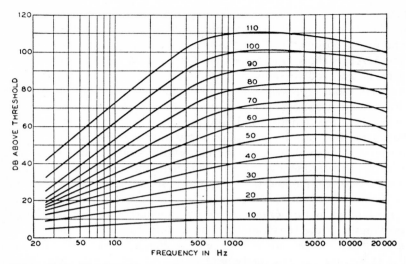

Figure 7–10 Equal-loudness contours plotted against sensation level (ordinate). All of the tones lying on each contour sound equal in loudness. The number (parameter) attached to a curve gives its loudness level. (From Stevens, S. S., and Davis, H.: Hearing. New York, John Wiley & Sons, Inc., 1938.)

also noted that the difference is smaller via loudspeaker (i.e., à la Fletcher and Munson) than when listening through earphones (i.e., à la Stevens and Davis). If we show equal-loudness contours plotted against sensation level, we get something which looks like an upside-down image of equal loudness contours plotted as a function of intensity level, such as the set of contours shown in Figure 7–10.

Figure 7–10 is very interesting because it so strongly illustrates the point made immediately above that our sensitivity diminishes as we get farther and farther above threshold. In this case, the lower curve represents the equal loudness of tones when they are adjusted to a 1000 Hz tone only 10 dB above threshold.

If our relative sensitivity diminishes as we get farther and farther from threshold, then the curves must come closer and closer together. And this is what may be seen exactly by looking at the very low frequencies. All of these curves, however, demonstrate equal loudness for tones. Of course, it is the case that we do not spend our auditory lives listening to sine waves, but rather to complex acoustic phenomena.

COMPLEX SIGNALS

If we do not go around listening to pure tones, do data from sinusoidal signals transfer meaningfully to data gathered when listening to complex signals? Stevens (1956) showed that equal loudness contours could be constructed with signals having bandwidths greater than 1 Hz and showed further that, if the bandwidth is not too wide, the contours agree rather well with pure-tone contours.

In attempting to measure the effect of bandwidth, Stevens found that it was easier to match a tone to a one-octave band than to a two-octave band even when either band contained that tone. Looking at narrower bandwidths, he found "excellent agreement" when comparing octave and third-octave calculations. This finding was confirmed by Milner (1969) for a 70-phon loudness level contour for one-third-octave bands and one-octave bandwidth. Expanding still further, Stevens (1961) found that it could be done for third-octave, half-octave and one-octave bandwidths. It is interesting that this holds at least up to a full octave for loudness level, but this phenomenon is not true for loudness (in sones).

Given the limitation on bandwidth, the spectrum matters little. That is to say, the loudness of fractional octave bands of pink noise is essentially the same as that of white noise. However, this does not apply to groups of sinusoids harmonically related. If one were to sound a complex tone made up of 10 harmonic components, one would find its loudness level contours to vary considerably from that of either a single sinusoid or a narrow band of noise. The loudness level of one-third octaves of pink noise, however, has been shown to be quite consistent with the original early data of Fletcher and Munson. For illustration, a 70-phon contour is shown in Figure 7–11. Gulick (1971) claimed that while this is not true of loudness, it is true of loudness level.

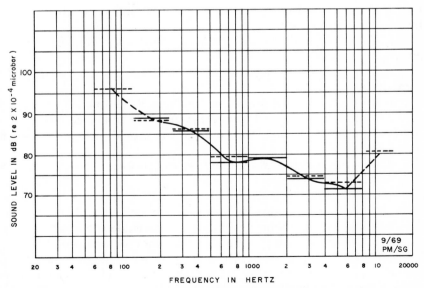

Figure 7–11 70-phon equal-loudness contour for one-third octave bands of pink noise. (After Gerber and Milner: J. Aud. Engineer. Soc., 19:656–659, 1971.)

Perhaps the most recent determinations of equal loudness have been those of Gerber and Milner (1971), who were concerned with the transitivity of loudness levels. Remember that in almost all experiments, all test tones were set to be equal in loudness to the reference tone of 1000 Hz. However, almost never were the test tones set to be equal in loudness to each other. It is not obvious *a priori* that they would be. On the other hand, Gerber and Milner have shown that transitivity of loudness level does obtain at 70 phons. They found that any octave band of pink noise of 70-phon loudness level was equal to any other octave band of pink noise at 70 phons. They predicted that this would hold for any spectrum of sound, whether the stimulus was white noise, pink noise, sinusoid, or some other spectral distribution. They predicted further that this would hold for other moderate loudness levels. On the other hand, since the loudness level contours for the extremes of loudness are of such different shape from each other and from those in the middle of the set of contours, it is possible that transitivity does not hold. This has not yet been demonstrated.

Bauer et al. (1967) have established the reliability of loudness level. They have shown that most listeners with practice will adjust the loudness level of two sounds within an average variation of only one decibel. Given that listeners perform reliably, is it then possible to predict loudness level?

LOUDNESS LEVEL PREDICTION

When psychoacousticians attempted to predict the loudness of multicomponent sounds from measured sound spectra, they employed the following line of reasoning:

1. Each component of the sound can be thought of as producing a given sensation of loudness S.

2. This loudness is calculable from the loudness level of the given component.

3. If one were to determine the loudness S due to each component acting alone, and if all these loudnesses were to be combined by means of some arithmetical scheme, the combination should yield the resultant total loudness.

Among the first to offer the above approach were Fletcher and Munson; however, their method is applicable only to pure tones. In 1951, Beranek et al. proposed a method for calculation of loudness of distributed-frequency noise following the same general idea. These authors divided the noise spectrum into bands approximately one octave wide (actually, 300 mels wide). Following this, they determined the sound pressure level in decibels for each band. Next, using the relation between loudness level and loudness, they found the loudness in sones contributed by each band. And finally, they added these individual values of loudness to obtain the total loudness in sones.

Other investigators, however, questioned the validity of direct addition of partial loudnesses of the individual bands. For example, the sum of the loudnesses in the separate bands of a broad spectrum could exceed the observed loudness of the total noise by a factor greater than two. Given N adjacent bands of equal loudness S, assume that the first one produces the full measure of loudness, i.e., S, but each added band contributes only a fraction F of S to the sum. Thus the total loudness S_1 of the N equally loud bands, according to Stevens (1961) is

$$S_1 = S + F(N - 1)S$$
$$= S + F(\Sigma S - S)$$
$$= S[1 + (N - 1)F]$$

where ΣS means the sum of the loudnesses of all the bands. If the bands are of unequal loudness, Stevens reasoned that the greatest contribution to total loudness will be by the loudest band S_m, all the others contributing the F fraction of their sum. Stevens conducted numerous experiments and concluded that, for octave bands of noise, the factor F was 0.27, but he rounded this to 0.30 because of better fit with subsequent experimental data. If the bands are one-third-octave wide, instead of one-octave, F turns out to be about 0.15.

Another method of loudness calculation has been proposed by Zwicker (1958), who added the further refinement of taking into account assumed differences in inhibition acting upward from lower to higher frequency bands as a function of the relative level of the bands.

While the methods of Stevens and Zwicker reportedly have served well for the calculation of the loudness of a variety of sounds, they have not been universally successful. For example, Corliss and Winzer (1965) employed these methods to calculate the loudness of footsteps, and pointed out a substantial disagreement between the calculated loudness and subjective measurements. The next question is, how about summation of bands of unequal loudness levels? Start with 70-phon octave bands of noise in groups of four adjacent bands. The lowest-frequency group spanned the range of 125 to 2000 Hz. The middle-frequency group extended from 250 to 4000 Hz; the high-frequency group covered 500 to 8000 Hz. If we compare the loudness of a group of bands with progressively diminishing levels toward the high-frequency end with a similar group in which the band level diminishes progressively toward the low-frequency end, what will be their relative loudness level?

The results are shown in Figure 7–12 from Bauer et al. (1967). The abscissa shows the incremental attenuation per band. The ordinate is the attenuation of the group to match a 70-phon band. It is seen that for two upper-frequency sets of bands, the direction of attenuation does not matter. The overall attenuation required to equalize the loudness of the sets against a 70-phon comparison tone follows the curve of 20 log the sum of normalized voltages, within 1 or 1.5 dB. With the set including the

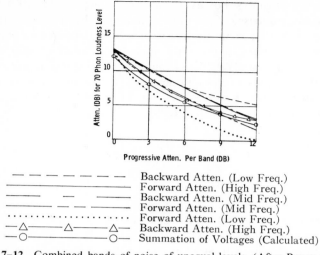

Progressive Atten. Per Band (DB)

— — — — — — —	Backward Atten. (Low Freq.)
———————————	Forward Atten. (High Freq.)
—————— — ————	Backward Atten. (Mid Freq.)
———— — — ————	Forward Atten. (Mid Freq.)
· · · · · · · · · · · · · · · · · · · ·	Forward Atten. (Low Freq.)
—△————△————△—	Backward Atten. (High Freq.)
—O——————————O—	Summation of Voltages (Calculated)

Figure 7–12 Combined bands of noise of unequal levels. (After Bauer and Torick: IEEE Trans. Audio Electroacoust., AU-14:141–151, 1966.)

lowest frequency, the direction of attenuation does make a difference. As expected, forward inhibition (or masking of low-level, high-frequency tones by high-level, low-frequency tones) is predominant. It is interesting to note that all equally loud four-octave band sets employed by Bauer et al. (1967) required that their level be attenuated 13 dB to be equally loud compared with a single octave band.

SUMMARY

In summary, then, we have shown that loudness is largely (but not entirely) the perceptual result of sound pressure level. Furthermore, we have demonstrated how different signals may be equated in loudness giving the phenomenon we call loudness level. And finally, we looked at the possibility of predicting loudness level and combining bands of different loudnesses. From now on, we hope, you will not confuse loudness with intensity; loudness is a property of persons, intensity is a property of signals.

REFERENCES

Bauer, B. B., and Torick, E. L. (1966): Researches in loudness measurement. *IEEE Transactions on Audio and Electroacoustics AU – 14*: 141–151.
Bauer, B. B., Torick, E. L., Rosenheck, A. J., and Allen, R. G. (1967): A loudness-level monitor for broadcasting. *IEEE Transactions on Audio and Electroacoustics AU – 15*:177–182.
Beranek, L. L., Marshall, J. L., Cudworth, A. L., and Peterson, A. P. G. (1951): Calcula-

tion and measurement of the loudness of sounds. *Journal of the Acoustical Society of America* 23:261–269.

Boring, E. G. (1950): *History of Experimental Psychology.* New York, Appleton-Century-Crofts.

Churcher, B. G., and King, A. J. (1937): The performance of noise meters in terms of the primary standard. *Journal of the Institute of Electrical Engineers* 81:57–90.

Corliss, E. L. R., and Winzer, G. E. (1965): Study of methods for estimating loudness. *Journal of the Acoustical Society of America* 38:424–428.

Fletcher, H., and Munson, W. A. (1933): Loudness, its definition, measurement, and calculation. *Journal of the Acoustical Society of America* 5:82–108.

Garner, W. R. (1947): Auditory thresholds of short tones as a function of repetition rates. *Journal of the Acoustical Society of America* 19:600–608.

Gerber, S. E., and Milner, P. (1971): The transitivity of loudness level. *Journal of the Audio Engineering Society* 19:656–659.

Gulick, W. L. (1971): *Hearing: Physiology and Psychophysics.* New York, Oxford University Press.

Hirsh, I. J. (1952): *The Measurement of Hearing.* New York, McGraw-Hill Book Co.

Kingsbury, B. A. (1927): A direct comparison of the loudness of pure tones. *Physical Review* 29:588–600.

Littler, T. S. (1965): *The Physics of the Ear.* New York, The Macmillan Co.

Milner, P. (1969): *Loudness Phenomenon in Hearing.* Stamford, Conn., CBS Laboratories, Report 9001–141.

Robinson, D. W., and Dadson, R. S. (1956): A redetermination of the equal loudness relations for pure tones. *British Journal of Applied Physics* 7:166–181.

Rowland, R. C., and Tobias, J. V. (1967): *Interaural Intensity Difference Limen.* Oklahoma City, Federal Aviation Administration, Office of Aviation Medicine, Report AM 67–10.

Sabine, W. C. (1910): Sense of loudness. *In Collected Papers on Acoustics.* Cambridge, Mass., Harvard University Press, 1923; New York, Dover Publications, 1964.

Sivian, L. J., and White, S. D. (1933): On minimum audible sound fields. *Journal of the Acoustical Society of America* 4:288–321.

Stevens, S. S. (1956): Calculation of the loudness of complex noise. *Journal of the Acoustical Society of America* 28:807–832.

Stevens, S. S. (1961): Procedure for calculating loudness, Mark VI. *Journal of the Acoustical Society of America* 33:1577–1585.

Stevens, S. S., and Davis, H. (1936): Psychophysiological acoustics: pitch and loudness. *Journal of the Acoustical Society of America* 8:1–13.

Stevens, S. S., and Davis, H. (1938): *Hearing, Its Psychology and Physiology.* New York, John Wiley & Sons.

von Békésy, G. (1960): *Experiments in Hearing* (translated and edited by E. G. Wever). New York, McGraw-Hill Book Co.

von Békésy, G. (1967): *Sensory Inhibition.* Princeton, N.J., Princeton University Press.

Zwicker, E., (1958): Über psychologische und methodische Grundlagen der Lautheit. *Acustica* 8:237–258.

Chapter Eight

AUDITORY TEMPORALITY

SANFORD E. GERBER

The phenomena of pitch and loudness have been well investigated indeed; they are appreciated by most psychoacousticians. We understand that acoustic signals are perceived by their frequency and by their amplitude. We also understand that acoustic signals exist in time. Psychoacousticians traditionally have spent less effort on the study of temporal phenomena in audition than they have on pitch and loudness phenomena. In a sense this seems peculiar because many studies have indicated that audition is the temporal modality. That is to say, the resolution of time by ear is far superior to its resolution by any other sense modality.

Several questions need to be asked about auditory time perception. One class of such questions has to do with the absolute perception of time: How long is long enough? How long must an acoustic event exist in time for it to be perceived as having occurred at all? This problem is cast under the heading of the *minimum audible duration*. A similar question has to do with the perception of silence: How far apart in time must two acoustic events be so that a listener considers them to be two rather than one? This is the *minimum temporal separation* (Hirsh, 1959). How long does an acoustic signal need to last for it to be not only sensed but identified? Similarly, how much separation does there need to be between two brief acoustic events for a listener to tell if they are the same or different and, if different, which came first? How well do we discriminate temporal order? Another class of questions is: How fast is too fast? How rapidly

172

can a series of acoustic events be presented and still be identified as a series of events rather than as one continuous event? This phenomenon is given the name of *auditory flutter*. Still another class of temporal questions: what about absolute time perception? Can we, for example, count the number of pulses occurring in a period of time? How good are we at this? This topic is the one of *temporal numerosity*. And finally, how sensitive are we to alterations in time? Pollack (1970) has called this auditory *"jitter."*

In 1956, Georg von Békésy pointed out that there are no theories of hearing, only theories of how the ear discriminates pitch. The following year Hallowell Davis suggested that attention should be given to temporal aspects since hearing has a time dimension. Why should we give more attention to temporal phenomena of audition? By the time the reader has completed this chapter, the answer to this question ought to be clear. In brief, the reason why temporal phenomena of audition require increased attention is that it seems that hearing *is* the temporal sense.

Consider the following. Imagine a group of people seated around a table with you at the head. One of those persons raises his hand and you are able to see him do so and you point at him. You have had no difficulty whatsoever in visually locating that person in the room. Let us assume, however, that the room were dark. If a person seated at the table were to ring a bell in the darkness, you would find it exceedingly difficult to point directly at the person making the sound. The object of this little experiment is to demonstrate that it is very easy to locate signals in visible space, but extremely difficult to locate signals in audible space. It is simply the case that vision exists largely for the purpose of telling us *where* things are. ". . . time is the dimension within which patterns are articulated for hearing in a manner analogous to the way in which space is the dimension for vision" (Hirsh, 1959).

If we interrupt a light a number of times per second, the number would have to be rather small for us to acquire the percept that the light was on continuously. The most familiar example of this is the ordinary fluorescent light. In this country, our urban homes are wired on 60 cycles alternating current; that is to say, the provision of electricity to our houses goes on and off 60 times every second. If the electricity is provided only 60 times every second, then that means that our lights must go on and off 60 times every second. Now look at the fluorescent light over your head. Do you notice that it is going on and off 60 times a second? Certainly not. Our eyes are unable to resolve visible temporal phenomena to that extent. A light going on and off 60 times per second appears to be on all the time. However, a noise which goes on and off 60 times per second sounds indeed like an interrupted noise to many people. For some people it would have to go on and off more often than that for them to acquire the percept that it is on all the time. This experiment demonstrates that our ears are more finely tuned than are our eyes to the extent of physical phenomena in time. Our ears are more sensitive than are our eyes to the temporal aspects of signals. It is for this reason that I say that the ear exists to tell us when things are; the eye exists to tell us where things are.

HOW LONG IS LONG ENOUGH?

How long must a stimulus extend in time for us to be aware of its existence? What is the minimum duration of a sound within which it is still audible? It turns out that the answer to this question is not simple, but is involved with the intensity of the sound. Simply stated, there is an interaction of duration and loudness so that briefer sounds may be heard if they are louder.

The response to light has a longer latency than the response to sound or to a touch on the skin. That is, our response time to visual stimuli is longer than it is to auditory or tactile stimuli. Since touch and hearing are very similar, we ought not be surprised to discover that the reaction time to either is about 140 msec, whereas the reaction time to light is about 180 msec. Again, this interacts with the intensity of the stimulus so that a weak sound or a strong light might bring slower or quicker responses. Furthermore, the response times compare with the signals most important to hear speech. So that, for example, consonant articulations in syllables occur at intervals which are similar to time periods of the neural pathways (Lehiste, 1970).

If you use a camera, you know that you must increase the size of the shutter opening as you decrease the exposure time. Or you must increase the exposure time if there is insufficient light. This is known as the Bunsen-Roscoe law to the effect that the intensity of the light multiplied by its duration determines its effect. The product of this multiplication is called the "quantity of light." The same equation applies to the threshold of hearing. At durations of about two or three milliseconds or less, an audible stimulus is clearly definable as a click. At longer durations, about 50 milliseconds, a stimulus is identifiable as a tone. As stimulus duration is decreased from 50 milliseconds, perception tends to be of a tone which is similar to a click in its sudden onset; and at still briefer durations (less than 10 msec), the perception is that of a click which has a pitch quality known as "click pitch" (Licklider, 1951). In general, "click pitch" refers to the perception of a click which seems to have a tone; whereas, "clicks with tonal pitch" refers to perceptions of tones which seem to begin and end with sharp clicks. For durations somewhat longer, sensations seem to increase in loudness for perhaps as long as 200 or 300 msec. For durations less than this value, it is still possible to balance time against intensity and get the same loudness for a constant product of intensity and time. One of the problems in hearing which does not exist in vision is that the presentation of repeated stimuli leads to fatigue. That is to say, the presentation of a single tone at fairly high levels decreases our sensitivity for a following tone. The more intense the first tone, the higher is the threshold for the following tone.

THE RELATION OF DURATION TO LOUDNESS

In the previous paragraphs we have suggested that our absolute perception of time is related to the loudness of the signals. This is, in effect, the same as the Bunsen-Roscoe law but applied to audition. It says in essence that the less time, the more energy is needed for a given percept. Clearly, there are some upper and lower limits to this. Stevens and Davis (1938) told us that "tones lasting less than half a second appear less loud than tones of the same amplitude whose duration is greater." To describe this, they mentioned an equation devised by Lifshitz:

> For pure tones of short duration, the law reduces to $It = K$, where I is the loudness level of sound (in decibels), t is time in seconds, and K is a constant. This equation states that, in order to maintain constant loudness, the loudness level must be increased by the same proportion that the time is decreased.

They said that Lifshitz was able to support this equation with data over times from 12 to 690 msec and levels from 34 to 84 dB within the range 50 to 4000 Hz. That covers a good portion of the audible range of brief tones. A similar observation was made by Hughes (1946) to the effect that threshold intensity is inversely proportional to duration.

It was observed by Plomp and Bouman (1959) that there must be some minimal stimulus intensity "which is not an effective stimulus for the ear." They devised a formula to give threshold intensity in decibels as a function of duration. Figure 8–1, taken from the paper of Plomp and Bouman, is a curve of the threshold of hearing at several different frequencies and several durations. The curve shows the average threshold of responses of their two listeners. It can be seen that, as a function of frequency, threshold of hearing versus duration varies from as little as about 2 dB to more than 36 dB. It can be seen (consonant to the above-mentioned comment of Stevens and Davis) that, for durations longer than about a half-second, there is rather little change with loudness. It is when the durations are less than a half-second that we see rather large effects of both loudness (i.e., sufficient to achieve threshold) and frequency. We can also see that low frequencies require greater intensity than high frequencies to achieve threshold at any given duration less than a half-second. This relationship between duration and frequency was discussed in Chapter 6. The observation which needs to be derived from this particular discussion is clear: the shorter the duration, the greater must be the intensity of the signal for it to be perceived at all. Therefore, the answer to the question "How long is long enough?" is involved in the question "How loud is loud enough?" and "long enough" can be as little as only one msec, providing that the frequency is medium-high and the intensity is great.

Stevens and Davis (1938) considered the qualitative differences among short noises having different waveforms: "Witness the qualitative differences between the sharp crack due to a spark and the dull boom of distant gunfire." They considered this to be a function of a time constant — a change of sound pressure as a function of time. Figure 8–2 shows how the loudness of an impulse varies with duration; it also shows the time constant T. It can be seen from this figure that as T increases, the loudness level also increases until T achieves a value of about 1 msec, beyond which the loudness level seems not to increase. This experiment (which Stevens and Davis reported was done by Steudel in 1933) makes essentially the same point as that made more recently by Plomp and

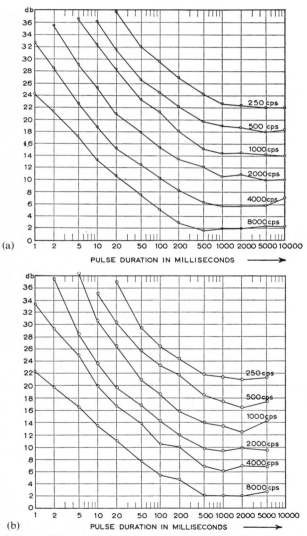

Figure 8–1 (*a*) Masked threshold as a function of the duration of the tone pulse for observer 1. (*b*) Masked threshold as a function of the duration of the tone pulse for observer 2. (After Plomp and Bouman: J. Acoust. Soc. Amer., 31:749, 1959.)

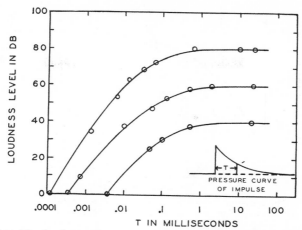

Figure 8-2   The loudness of an impulse varies with its duration. The impulse has a form as shown by the pressure curve and a time-constant, T, as shown by the abscissa. (From Stevens, S. S., and Davis, H.: Hearing. New York, John Wiley and Sons, Inc., 1938.)

Bouman. The number varies somewhat but that is probably a function of the wave form. Again, the answer to the question "How long is long enough?" is to be found in the neighborhood of 1 msec.

THE RELATION OF DURATION TO PITCH

It was suggested earlier in this chapter that tones of very brief duration seem to lack a pitch quality. Chapter 6 discussed the close relationship between the perception of pitch and temporal events. In particular, we discussed the important idea of periodicity pitch. In this much briefer section, we iterate some of the important interactions between time and pitch.

As we decrease the duration of tones down to the neighborhood of 2 or 3 msec, they tend to lose their pitches. At this duration, one's percept is tonelike, but the tone is very similar to a click in that it has a sudden onset; in fact, when the duration is less than 10 milliseconds, the percept is decidedly that of a click, but a click which has a pitch quality (Licklider, 1951).

Is this a matter of the absolute time or is it instead a matter of how many waves are taken from the tone? Stevens and Davis asked whether a single wave taken from a 1000-Hz tone would have a higher pitch than a single wave of a 500-Hz tone. Another way of phrasing this issue would be, do clicks have pitch? Clicks of duration in the neighborhood of 10 milliseconds appear to have pitches lower than similar clicks of longer duration. Figure 8-3 shows that the pitch of tones seems to fall with shortened durations. It also seems to be the case that there is a minimum time required to identify the pitch of a tone.

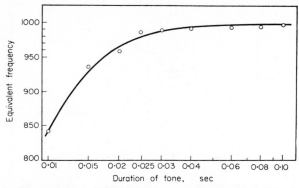

Figure 8–3 The variation of the pitch of a tone as a function of its duration. (From Littler, T. S.: The Physics of the Ear. Elmsford, N.Y., Pergamon, 1965.)

THE PROBLEM OF SUCCESSIVENESS

By how much must the onsets of two tones be separated in time in order for them to appear to be successive rather than simultaneous? The question was phrased very well by Hirsh (1959): "We wish to know how great a temporal interval must intervene between the onsets of two pure tones of different frequency in order for a listener to be able to report correctly which of the two tones came first." Stevens and Davis (1938) reported an experiment by Burck, Kotowski, and Lichte which showed that the just detectable temporal separation varied as a function of the average frequency, the "average" meaning the frequency midway between the two frequencies tested. Hirsh (1959) found no such result. He found that: "The ability of listeners to report correctly the order in which two tones of different frequency occurred ... did not vary as the difference in frequency between the tones was varied." It now appears that Hirsh may have been wrong. A recent experiment by Perrott and Williams (1971) required listeners to judge the interval between two tone pulses. They said that temporal resolution "was observed to decrease as the frequency disparity between the successive pulses increased." However, there is an important difference between the two experiments. Hirsh's listeners reported differences between onset times of two tones. Perrott and Williams' listeners reported gaps between the offset of one tone and the onset of a following tone. Perhaps these are two different experiments. In any case, the matter of successiveness does appear to be related to pitch. Recently, Divenyi (1973) has been investigating the perception of time gaps between tone bursts. His listeners hear a pair of bursts separated by a fixed interval, t_1, and then another pair separated by a variable interval, t_2. The listeners' task is to set t_2 equal to t_1. In general, listeners set t_2 shorter than t_1 for all stimuli in which the fourth tone burst is of a different frequency from the first three. The size of the temporal error is related to the frequency difference up to the third octave, but a marked change of the intensity of the fourth burst essentially eliminates the effect.

Accuracy does vary, however, as a function of the interval between onset times. This approaches the question, "Which came first?" and this question was investigated by Hirsh in 1966. He concerned himself with a number of possibilities. Not only was he interested in the temporal separation between two tones of different frequency, but he was also interested in the temporal intervals between high- and low-frequency noise, between tone and noise, and between a click and a tone. A prior question to Hirsh's experiment has to do with the separation time required for a listener to know that there are two stimuli rather than one. If two brief clicks are delivered to the same ear and if they are separated by an interval of less than 2 msec, they will be perceived as a single sound. Hirsh (1966) called this a measure of the "temporal grain" of the auditory system. If the interval between the clicks exceeds 2 msec, then the clicks will be perceived correctly as being two clicks. How much longer than 2 msec is required for the listener to report correctly which came first? Hirsh concluded that a 75 per cent correct response can be achieved only when the interval between two pure tones is as long as 20 msec. The same interval also seems to hold when the stimuli consist not of tones but of bands of noise of different pitch. Furthermore, this duration applies to the condition when the stimuli consist of a click and a noise, or a click and a tone. Hirsh's data are shown in Figure 8–4. It may be seen clearly in Figure 8–4 that the data points cluster quite closely to the line drawn. The point of this is that there is no consequential deviation as a function of the nature of the stimuli. Click stimuli, tonal stimuli, and narrow band stimuli in rela-

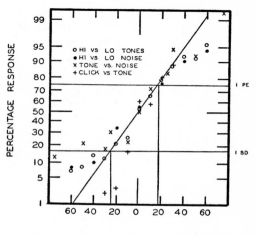

Figure 8–4 Probability of judgment concerning which of two sounds came first as a function of the temporal separation between sounds. Points corresponding to one probable error (75% judgment) and one standard deviation (16% judgment) are shown. (After Hirsh: J. Acoust. Soc. Amer., *31*:759, 1959.)

tion to each other tend to behave in about the same way. Hirsh concluded:

> Our experiments clearly indicate that two sounds that are separated just enough to be heard as two cannot be placed in correct order until the temporal separation is increased about tenfold . . . This greater temporal interval appears to be about ten times larger, or about 17 milliseconds, for the judgments to be 75 per cent correct.

In other words, the human ear requires about 17 milliseconds to tell which of two stimuli occurred first.* On the other hand, different series of the same two or three sounds can be discriminated even when the durations are too brief to permit identification of position (Warren, 1973). This is, in fact, a very important question in auditory perception. Hirsh used the example of the word "mist" versus the word "mitts." It is certainly important for the listener to know which came first, the *t* or the *s*. A musical example was employed by Stevens and Davis. They pointed out that an orchestra conductor might want to know which of two musicians began too early or too late. So the question of the minimum temporal separation is one of considerable practical value.

In summary, we have shown that if two acoustic stimuli are separated by less than 2 msec, the ear will not perceive them as two but only as one, as simultaneous rather than successive. If, on the other hand, the interval between two stimuli exceeds 2 msec, the ear will report them as being successive and not simultaneous, but cannot tell which came first until the separation is in the order of 17 msec or more. Beyond a separation of 17 msec, the ear can tell not only that there are two stimuli but which came first, and the nature of the stimuli is not relevant to this identification.

HOW FAST IS TOO FAST?

How rapidly can a series of acoustic events be presented and still be identified as a *series* of events rather than as one continuous event? What does this have to do with threshold of hearing? When we engage in clinical audiometry, we take it for granted that the stimulus is present for a relatively long period of time and that it is followed by a relatively long period of silence. What if, instead of these long durations, the stimulus were to go on and off rather rapidly? This question was raised by Garner in 1947. He obtained auditory thresholds for separated, short, sine waves that were repeated between one-quarter and 100 times per second. They, therefore, had tone durations between four seconds and 50 msec. We have already seen how the loudness, or the threshold, of a tone varies as a function of

---

*Scharf (1970), however, found longer separations to be required. His data on tones showed that not until about 50 msec will two tone bursts begin to be heard as separate sounds.

duration. How does the threshold of hearing vary if we have repeated brief stimuli rather than continuous stimuli? Garner reminded us that the total energy in the stimulus can be changed by varying either the repetition rate or the duration; however, the threshold of hearing is influenced solely by the duration. Garner found that decrements of duration produce "an equivalent shift in the threshold."

Noise stimuli are not subject to certain variations peculiar to pure-tone stimuli. If one interrupts pure tone stimuli periodically and rapidly, then one introduces an additional tone at a frequency equal to the rate of interruption — a modulating tone. In the kind of investigation done by Garner, there is the strong possibility that he had investigated the threshold of hearing for the modulating tone rather than for the tone being interrupted. Miller (1948) proposed the use of bursts of white noise. He pointed out, however, "A short burst of noise must be more intense in order to be equal in effectiveness to a longer noise." Thus the threshold of hearing is lowered by increasing the duration of the noise up to durations at least as long as one second. The use of noise has the advantage that "Noise interrupted at a steady rate has essentially the same spectrum over the range of frequencies transduced by the earphone as does continuous noise" (Miller and Taylor, 1948).

Given now that we will use noise rather than tones, and thereby avoid the introduction of modulating tones as well as the effects upon threshold: "How fast is too fast?" We pointed out that it matters how you phrase the question. The experiments to answer the question "How fast is too fast?" depend very heavily upon how you phrase it. Recently, for example, Zwislocki, commenting upon a paper by Scharf (1970), said: "... it is interesting that when you ask the subject a different question, his result changes very much." The reason for raising this issue at this point is that two different psychophysical methods have been employed to answer the question, "How fast is too fast?" Data obtained by a method of limits do not agree with those obtained from a paired-comparison method. If we present noise bursts interrupted at a slow rate (e.g., 30 per second) and increase the number of bursts per presentation, we eventually come to a rate at which a listener reports that he no longer experiences interruption. To this phenomenon is given the name *auditory flutter fusion*. The rate at which the perception of interrupted sound becomes a perception of continuous sound is called a flutter fusion threshold. Symmes, Chapman, and Halstead (1955) found that the fusion threshold varied between 45 and 120 bursts per second and averaged about 82 bursts per second. Gerber (1967) and Wolf and Gerber (in press) used a method of limits and found fusion data very similar to those reported by Mayer (1874) employing the same method: the fusion threshold is generally found between 45 and 55 bursts per second. Chistovich (1960) and Miller and Taylor (1948) employed a method of paired comparison and found very high fusion thresholds. Miller and Taylor reported the detection of interruptions at rates well above 1000 per second. Two conclusions need to be observed.

The first is that these are obviously different experiments. The second is that if we interrupt the sound at a rapid enough rate, we can detect interruptions at extremely high frequencies. There is, however, a very interesting distinction between the *detection* of interruption and the *identification* of interruption. If we ask a listener to detect the presence of interruption, to use the terminology of Miller and Taylor, we find that he does so at very rapid rates. If, on the other hand, we ask him to tell us when a sound which he already identified as being interrupted becomes no longer interrupted, then he does that at a much lower rate. Furthermore, if we present to the listener a stimulus which he identified as continuous and ask him to tell us when it becomes interrupted, we find still a different answer. Gerber (1967) also investigated the opposite of flutter fusion. To this phenomenon he gave the name "descending flutter threshold." In a descending method, the initial signal presentation was at 120 bursts per second and decreased in steps of three until the subject reported a sensation of flutter. For this experiment the average flutter threshold was found to be in the neighborhood of 100 bursts per second. The question "How fast is too fast?" depends very much upon whether the signal is speeding up or slowing down. If the signal is speeding up, the answer to the question is found in the neighborhood of 50 interruptions per second; if the signal is slowing down, however, the answer is found in the neighborhood of 100 interruptions per second; and if we ask the listener only to detect the presence of interruption, the answer is found well above 1000 interruptions per second. It might even be higher than that. Miller and Taylor suggested that for some listeners, "a qualitative difference between the interrupted noise and a steady noise can be detected" up to 2000 interruptions.

The data are consistent. The consistency was pointed out by Chistovich (1960) that ". . . the limiting distinguishable noise interruption rate reaches 1000 times per second, while the minimum distinguishable interval between pulses amounts to 1.0–1.5 milliseconds. . . ." Miller and Taylor's outside number of 2000 interruptions per second is supported by neurophysiological data. Goldstein and Kiang (1957) reported: "Synchronous neural activity has been recorded by gross electrodes from the auditory nerve in response to repeated impulsive stimuli at rates up to 2000/sec."

Now, Wolf and Gerber (in press) have shown higher fusion thresholds for male listeners than for female. Furthermore, they found that fusion threshold depends in part upon loudness.

CAN WE COUNT?

If we hear a series of discrete pulses, how accurately can we report the number of pulses? Cheatham and White (1954) gave to this phenomenon the name of *temporal numerosity,* while Woodworth and Schlosberg

(1954) gave the word *numerousness* "to that property of a collection of items which you discriminate, without counting, when you estimate the number of items." If one reviews the literature on this subject, he finds first that there isn't very much and, secondly, most of it deals with vision. There may be a good reason for this. Cheatham and White observed: "The task of reporting the number of sound pulses heard was found to be much more difficult than the reporting of perceived flashes in the visual counterpart of this study." Perhaps this is due to the fact that "auditory intervals are judged to be subjectively longer than comparable visual intervals" (Behar and Bevan, 1960). That is to say, maybe it's just harder to do.

There seems to be, however, a clear upper limit on our ability to report the number of stimuli in either modality. According to Cheatham and White (1954), there is a general tendency to *underestimate* the number of stimuli at any rate. Furthermore, the estimation of the number of stimuli decreases apparently in a linear fashion. And moreover, the variability increases when the number of stimuli exceeds five. For auditory stimuli, in fact, the subjective rate approaches a limit in the neighborhood of nine to 11 pulses per second, even though the number of stimuli may be as great as 10 to 30 pulses per second. That is to say, we seem to do fairly well in reporting the number of pulses heard when that number does not exceed five per second. From five up to about 10 per second, we tend to make more and more errors. And beyond about 10 per second, we are hesitant to estimate any more than 10 pulses even though the number of stimuli may increase up to as many as 30 per second.

Cheatham and White reported that temporal numerosity for auditory stimuli was less accurate than that for visible stimuli. That is, they found a great deal more variability among responses to acoustic stimuli than among responses to visible stimuli. This is in contrast to a conclusion by Pieron (1952), who claimed that auditory precision is maximum for temporal acuity. However, Pieron's data are consistent with those of Cheatham and White in that the ability to report distinguishable temporal stimuli decreases greatly in the neighborhood of 10 per second. Since Cheatham and White had investigated the visual counterpart of auditory temporal numerosity (1952), they were able to compare data from the two modalities. Based upon these comparisons, they concluded that peripheral mechanisms are not responsible for the limitations. To be sure, this implication is consistent with some we have suggested earlier — that the peripheral auditory mechanism is capable of tracking intermittent stimuli at rates greater than those possible in the auditory cortex.

TEMPORAL IRREGULARITIES

Our ability to detect irregularities in audible signals extending in time may be the strongest datum with respect to the very high temporal resolving power of the auditory system. If we listen to a train of pulses over a

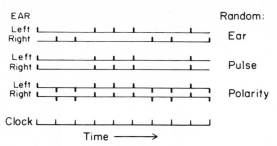

Figure 8-5 Schematic representation of non-jittered, non-repeated pulse patterns based upon a periodic clock (reference procedure) and three modifications from the reference procedure. (From Plomp, R., and Smoorenburg, G. F.: Frequency Analysis and Periodicity Detection in Hearing. Leiden, Sijthoff, 1970.)

period of time, the train having a fixed interpulse interval, we get a percept of pitch (cf. Chapter 6). If we introduce an irregularity in the interpulse interval (i.e., if we time-shift some pulses), we may elicit a percept of "jitter." If we look at Figure 8-5 (which is taken from Pollack, 1970), we can see three different kinds of jitter paradigm. In the upper pair of lines, we see pulses randomly assigned to each of the two ears, so that the pulse train in the right ear differs from that in the left. In the second pair of lines, the ears are both receiving the same series of randomly occurring pulses. The third pair of lines shows both ears receiving the same series of periodic pulses but with random polarity or phase inversion. If the pulse rate is high, then the addition of jitter to the pulse train leads to a change of pitch. At low pulse rates, the percept is rather one of an additional roughness. The issue is: how little jitter will lead to these perceptual changes? This is another question of auditory temporal resolving power.

The fact is, according to Pollack (1970), that one's jitter sensitivity is related to the pulse rate. When the interpulse intervals are long (i.e., low rates), the jitter threshold is about the same for all three procedures shown in Figure 8-5. At short interpulse intervals, all three versions are ineffective. When jitter is heard, the jitter threshold is found to be very sensitive. It amounts to about 0.1 per cent, which is not very interesting at low rates, but startling at high rates. It means, for example, that at a pulse rate of 10,000 pulses per second, we can hear jitters as small as 0.1 msec. Again, the temporal sensitivity of the human auditory system is shown to be very great.

CONCLUSIONS

In general, we have seen that the auditory system is capable of finer temporal resolutions than the visual system. Some of these resolutions are apparently mediated at relatively high-order neural centers and may apply equally to vision, audition, and other senses. We have seen further that the temporal resolving power of the auditory system is necessary for the perception of speech and of music. Both speech and music depend to a very large extent upon the auditory system's ability to discriminate serial acoustic phenomena. It is important to know which came first and when.

REFERENCES

Behar, I., and Bevan, W. (1960): Analysis of the prime psychophysical judgment. *Perceptual and Motor Skills 10*:82.

Cheatham, P. G., and White, C. T. (1952): Temporal numerosity: I. Perceived number as a function of flash number and rate. *Journal of Experimental Psychology 44*:447–451.

Cheatham, P. G., and White, C. T. (1954): Temporal numerosity: III. Auditory perception of number. *Journal of Experimental Psychology 47*:425–428.

Chistovich, L. A. (1960): Discrimination of the time interval between two short acoustic pulses. *Soviet Physics—Acoustics* (translation of *Akusticheskii Zhurnal*) *5*:493–497.

Davis, H. (1957): Biophysics and physiology of the inner ear. *Physiological Review 27*:1–49.

Divenyi, P. (1973): Discrimination of the silent gap in two-tone sequences of different frequencies. II. Dichotic case. Paper presented to the 85th meeting of the Acoustical Society of America, Boston.

Garner, W. R. (1947): Auditory thresholds of short tones as a function of repetition rates. *Journal of the Acoustical Society of America 19*:600–608.

Gerber, S. E. (1967): Flutter perception in normal listeners. *Journal of Speech and Hearing Research 10*:319–322.

Goldstein, M. H., and Kiang, N. (1957): Cortical responses to repeated clicks and bursts of noise. *Journal of the Acoustical Society of America 29*:773.

Hirsh, I. J. (1959): Auditory perception of temporal order. *Journal of the Acoustical Society of America 31*:759–767.

Hirsh, I. J. (1966): Auditory perception of speech. *In* E. C. Carterette (ed.): *Brain Function. Vol. III (Speech, Language, and Communication)*. Berkeley, University of California Press.

Hughes, J. W. (1946): The threshold of audition for short periods of stimulation. *Proceedings of the Royal Society B133*:486–490.

Lehiste, I. (1970): The quest for phonetic reality. *In* A. J. Bronstein, C. L. Shaver, and C. Stevens (eds.): *Essays in Honor of Claude M. Wise*. New York, Speech Association of America.

Licklider, J. C. R. (1951): Basic correlates of the auditory stimulus. *In* S. S. Stevens (ed.): *Handbook of Experimental Psychology*. New York, John Wiley & Sons.

Mayer, A. M. (1874): Researches in acoustics, Paper number 6. *American Journal of Science 108*:241–255.

Miller, G. A. (1948): The perception of short bursts of noise. *Journal of the Acoustical Society of America 20*:160–170.

Miller, G. A., and Taylor, W. G. (1948): The perception of repeated bursts of noise. *Journal of the Acoustical Society of America 20*:171–182.

Perrott, D. R., and Williams, K. N. (1971): Auditory temporal resolution: Gap detection as a function of interpulse frequency disparity. *Psychonomic Science 25*:73–74.

Pieron, H. (1952): *The Sensations: Their Functions, Processes, and Mechanisms* (translated by M. H. Pierenne and B. C. Abbott). New Haven, Yale University Press.

Plomp, R., and Bouman, M. A. (1959): Relations between hearing threshold and duration for tone pulses. *Journal of the Acoustical Society of America 31*:749–758.

Pollack, I. (1970): Jitter detection for repeated auditory pulse patterns. *In* R. Plomp and G. F. Smoorenburg (eds.): *Frequency Analysis and Periodicity Detection in Hearing*. Leiden, A. W. Sijthoff.

Scharf, B. (1970): Loudness and frequency sensitivity at short durations. *In* R. Plomp and

G. F. Smoorenburg (eds.): *Frequency Analysis and Periodicity Detection in Hearing.* Leiden, A. W. Sijthoff.

Stevens, S. S., and Davis, H. (1938): *Hearing, Its Psychology and Physiology.* New York, John Wiley & Sons.

Symmes, D., Chapman, L., and Halstead, W. (1955): The fusion of intermittent white noise. *Journal of the Acoustical Society of America* 27:470–473.

von Békésy, G. (1956): Current status of theories of hearing. *Science* 123:779–783.

Warren, R. M. (1973): Temporal order discrimination: Recognitions without identification by untrained subjects. *Journal of the Acoustical Society of America* 55:316 (abstract).

Wolf, K. E., and Gerber, S. E. (in press): Flutter fusion and intensity change.

Woodworth, R. S., and Schlosberg, H. (1954): *Experimental Psychology.* (Rev. Ed.) New York, Holt, Rinehart & Winston.

Chapter Nine

BINAURAL HEARING

HARRY LEVITT AND BARRY VOROBA

Binaural hearing refers to hearing with two ears. A monaural (monotic) listening situation involves the use of one ear only. Binaural listening utilizes both ears, but a distinction should be made between the terms "diotic" and "dichotic." In a *diotic* listening situation, the identical signal is applied to each ear of the listener. *Dichotic* listening also involves both ears, but different stimuli are applied to each ear. The terms *monophonic* and *stereophonic* are typically used to describe listening situations employing, respectively, one and two sound sources (e.g., loudspeakers) with the output of each sound source reaching both ears. Several phenomena are associated with binaural hearing, including binaural summation, binaural fusion, localization, masking level differences, enhanced intelligibility of speech, the precedence effect, binaural beats, and other forms of binaural interaction. These effects are of interest in themselves as perceptual phenomena and also because they provide considerable insight into the underlying hearing process, monaural or binaural. The purpose of this chapter is to provide an overview of the major effects of binaural hearing and how these effects throw light on the basic mechanisms of hearing.

THRESHOLD EFFECTS

BINAURAL SUMMATION

Binaural summation refers to the fact that the threshold of hearing for two ears is lower, i.e., more sensitive than the threshold in the better one of those same two ears. For example, if the threshold of hearing for a tone of a given frequency were, say, 10 dB SPL in one ear and 15 dB SPL in the other, then the binaural threshold would be expected to be 10 dB SPL or better. Binaural summation is greatest when the signals to the two ears are of equal sensation level. If the signal to each ear is just audible when heard monaurally, then when heard binaurally, the signal will be roughly 3 dB above the threshold of audibility.

The phenomenon of binaural summation is not limited to absolute thresholds or to simple signals. The speech reception threshold for two ears, for example, is better than that obtained for either ear, the improvement approaching 3 dB if the signals are of equal sensation level at the two ears. Similarly, the loudness of a binaural sound is greater than that of a monaural sound of equal intensity. If the level of the monaural stimulus is increased such that the binaural and monaural sounds are equally loud, the increase of intensity will vary from about 3 dB near threshold to roughly 6 dB at sensation levels of 30 dB or greater (Caussé and Chavasse, 1942). The sensitivity of the ear to changes of intensity or changes of frequency is also greater for binaural rather than monaural stimulation.

In general, it would appear that two ears are better than one. There is, however, a rather interesting example in which a binaural signal is less detectable than a monaural signal. Consider a low-frequency tone being presented to only one ear and a masking noise stimulus presented identically to both ears. The threshold for the tone in noise will be lower in this case than if both tone and noise were presented binaurally; i.e., the change from monotic to binaural presentation of the tone actually decreases the detectability of the tone. This effect turns out to be a special case of a *binaural masking level difference,* a topic considered in detail later in this chapter. In general, an interaural difference between signal and noise will enhance detectability; in the example cited above, the less detectable binaural mode of presentation involved stimuli that were identical at the two ears.

BINAURAL FUSION

In a normal listening situation, the signals reaching our ears are similar but not quite identical; yet we typically hear one sound. This phenomenon in which a single sound is heard for two separate inputs is known as *binaural fusion.* In the laboratory, a binaural fused image may be created by means of headphone listening. In the most basic case, two identical stimuli are applied, one to each ear, i.e., diotically. Under these conditions, a normal hearing listener almost always claims to hear a single, fused sound image within or near his head and close to or on the median plane (i.e., roughly in line with his nose).

INTERAURAL TIME DIFFERENCES

Early workers (Boring, 1942; von Békésy, 1930; von Hornbostel and Wertheimer, 1920) found that the introduction of an interaural time difference between signals reaching the two ears produced a shift in the perceived lateral position of the fused sound image. In one procedure (Teas, 1962) observers controlled the degree of interaural time difference between test pulses. They were asked to graph the perceived location of the sound image. Von Békésy (1930) used a stream of air directed at the subject's head as a pointing device for locating the lateral position of the sound image. Figure 9–1 displays the change of apparent lateral image position as a function of the time delay between input stimuli. The curves for suprathreshold stimuli rise rapidly at first, then flatten out at larger interaural delays. For delays greater than 2 to 3 msec, the image begins to break up and two percepts are heard—one at each ear.

For pulses, the split may occur with an interaural time delay of 2 to 3 msec, whereas for speech, a larger time delay reaching out to 15 msec can be tolerated.

For tones, an obvious split of the image does not occur, since tones are periodic and an interaural time delay equal to the period will bring the

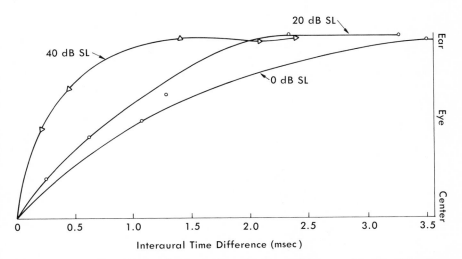

Figure 9–1   The change of apparent lateral image position as a function of the time delay between the input stimuli. (After Teas: J. Acoust. Soc. Amer., *34*:1460, 1962.)

tone back to its median plane position. The effect of systematically increasing interaural time delay in this case is to produce cyclic changes in apparent lateral position from the center of the head to one or the other extremity and back again. In the extreme condition, corresponding to a time delay of one-half period of the signal (which is the equivalent to 180° or π radians interaural phase difference), the auditory percept appears to differ from one individual to another. Some claim to hear a single, fused image emanating from all directions, while others claim to hear the image split into two parts, one at each ear.

The smallest detectable interaural time delay (the just-noticeable difference or jnd) varies with the type of signal employed. Jnd's as low as 10 microseconds have been reported when wide-band noise bursts or continuous speech were used as test stimuli (Tobias and Zerlin, 1959). For tones, the jnd of interaural time delay varies as a function of frequency. Zwislocki and Feldman (1956) observed a minimum jnd of the order of 30 to 50 microseconds at a frequency of 300 Hz, rising to about twice this value at higher frequencies. Similar data have been reported for narrow bands of noise.

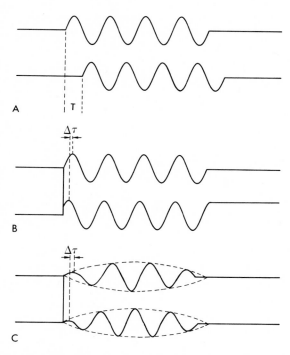

Figure 9–2 Tone bursts switched on (a) asynchronously, (b) synchronously with interaural time delay, (c) synchronously with time delay plus long rise and decay time.

An important consideration in experiments of interaural time delay is the manner in which the binaural signals are switched on and off. One approach is to have a sharp onset for the signals (see Fig. 9–2A). Another approach is to switch the signals synchronously but with an interaural time delay between the ongoing sequence (Fig. 9–2B). Transients in switching have a substantial effect on lateralization judgments, and the effect is likely to be most severe when there is a period of silence at one ear while there are switching transients at the other ear, as in Figure 9–2A. In this case, the judgment of apparent position may be critically dependent upon the switching transients. Switching transients also occur for the condition depicted by Figure 9–2B, but they occur in both ears simultaneously and should influence judgments of apparent position to a lesser extent. A preferred method of switching is to use synchronous switching as in Figure 9–2B, but with a relatively long rise time (greater than 25 msec) superimposed on the tone burst, as shown in Figure 9–2C. The long rise time substantially reduces the effects of switching transients which are further reduced by having both signals switched on synchronously. Unfortunately, published experimental data are contaminated by differences in experimental technique, and it is not always clear to what extent measured interaural jnd's reflect the interaural differences between the ongoing signals and interaural differences between switching transients.

INTERAURAL INTENSITY DIFFERENCES

Interaural intensity differences also produce change of the apparent lateral position of a fused sound image. In this case, there is a simple, monotonic relationship for all stimuli (including pure tones) between apparent lateral position and interaural intensity difference. The larger the interaural intensity difference, the greater the degree of laterality. In the limiting condition (i.e., extremely large interaural intensity difference), the signal will be well below threshold at one ear and heard only at the opposite ear. The jnd for interaural intensity difference is about 0.5 to 1.0 dB (Mills, 1960). The relative importance of interaural time and intensity differences upon apparent lateral position is very much a function of frequency. For low-frequency tones, both time and intensity differences are important. Interaural time differences become progressively less important with increasing frequency and do not have a measurable effect above approximately 1500 Hz.

Temporal and magnitude cues tend to compensate for each other's effects in a highly complex trading relationship. The compensation is incomplete, however, for the resulting fused sound image is more diffuse. Also, the range of interaural time and intensity differences that can be traded is necessarily limited; at large interaural differences, the adjusted interaural time delays are so great that the sound image splits into two parts, one at each ear. To add to the complexity, even for relatively small interaural time and intensity differences, there is not necessarily a unique trading relationship. Guttman, van Bergeijk, and David (1960), for example, found two separate trading relationships with tonal stimuli.

Additional factors which appear to shift lateral image position include head turning and jaw clenching, rotation or acceleration of the subject's head, interaction with visual stimuli, unilateral masking, unilateral fatigue, and the spectral content of the stimulus itself.

NONIDENTICAL STIMULI

Binaural fusion can occur also when nonidentical stimuli are used as long as the signal *envelopes* are the same. Figure 9–3 depicts two sine waves of differing frequency but identical envelopes (i.e., the gradual change of the amplitudes of the two sine waves is the same). Large differences between signals reaching the two ears need not cause a breakdown in fusion, provided the signals have a common envelope and the envelope frequency itself does not exceed 1500 Hz. This effect has been demonstrated in a number of experiments using such disparate stimuli as identically modulated sine waves of different frequency, the oscillatory responses of two different resonant circuits pulsed in synchronism, and also simultaneous bursts of uncorrelated noise.

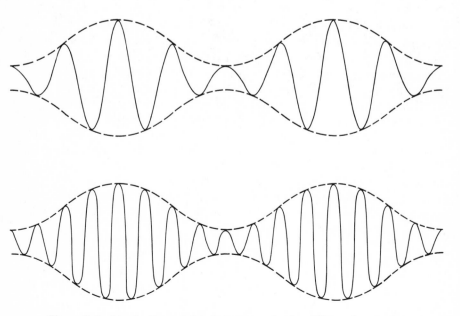

Figure 9–3 Identically modulated sine waves having different frequencies.

Binaural fusion has also been used with differentially filtered clicks by presenting the low-frequency components to one ear and the high frequencies to the other ear. Yet another means of creating a fused image is to present subjects with a speech signal that alternates from ear to ear. With a switching period roughly less than 100 msec, listeners report hearing a fused sound image. For slower switching rates, they observed one lateral image that fluctuated from side to side.

LOCALIZATION

STEREOPHONIC EFFECTS

The illusion of a single sound image may also occur to listeners under free-space listening conditions. The common example is the stereophonic effect which is produced when the stimuli emanate from two or more sources, e.g., loudspeakers in a free sound field. Localization is a term commonly used to describe the directional effect of a stereophonic sound image; whereas, lateralization refers to the image occurring with headphones. The reason for the different terminology is that the binaural fused image under headphone listening is internalized, i.e., it is heard either in or near the head. By far the most prominent coordinate of this internally fused image is its apparent lateral position. In the case of listening in free space, the sound is heard externally and in this case all three spatial coordinates are needed to specify the location of an external sound image.

The mechanism underlying the difference between internal and external sound images is not clear. Several investigators have suggested that in an everyday, non-free sound field, the constant tiny movements of the human head provide additional cues to form and locate an external sound image (see, e.g., Franssen, 1960). A 1940 experiment by deBoer (reported by Franssen) provided data which support this hypothesis. Microphones were mounted at ear level upon an artificial head and the amplified output fed dichotically through headphones to a listener. If the dummy head was placed upon a fixed object such as a table, an internal sound image was perceived. If, however, the dummy head was attached atop the subject's own head, an external sound image was reported.

The signals reaching the listener's ears are more complex under stereophonic listening than under dichotic. As shown in Figure 9–4, for the basic two-loudspeaker situation without reflections off walls or other surfaces, there are two signals reaching each ear. The signal reaching the left ear is the sum of the signals from the left channel over the path AD and the signal from the right channel over the path CD. The time delay and attenuation resulting from traveling the path AD may be represented as T (in msec) and I (in decibels), respectively; and the delay and attenuation resulting from traveling the path CD are $T + \Delta T$ and $I + \Delta I$, respectively.

ΔT is an additional time delay and ΔI is an additional attenuation,

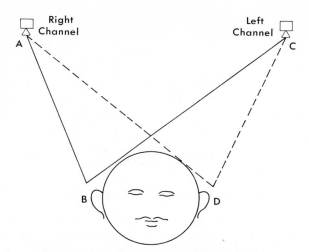

Figure 9-4   A stereophonic listening situation.

both incurred by traveling the greater distance AD. The signal reaching the right ear similarly consists of two components, a signal from the right channel and a delayed, slightly attenuated signal from the left channel.

A simple view of the situation is that either loudspeaker alone would produce a binaural sound image with values of interaural time and intensity differences that would place the sound image at or near the loudspeaker. When the two loudspeakers produce identical stimuli simultaneously, the combination of the two sets of signals balances each other out, resulting in the equivalent of one signal and its "echo" at each ear. The resulting sound image appears to emanate midway between the speakers. If an *interchannel* time or intensity difference is introduced, the balance will be disturbed and the image localized at some other point in space. Quantitative measures of the degree of accuracy with which a listener can localize a sound have been obtained. For free sound field listening conditions, the average error of azimuth made by a subject listening to sinusoidal sounds is about 20° for frequencies within the range 2000 to 5000 Hz. Localization improves to errors of about 5° for complex stimuli such as clicks and noise bands, presumably because of the presence of a wide range of intensity and time information within the stimulus. It should be noted, however, that jnd's and changes of position for stereophonic sound images require four to five times as much temporal or intensity disparity between the channels producing the stimuli as do similar effects for interaural images produced with headphones.

HEAD SHADOW

Additional temporal and magnitude localization cues may arise from the reflective properties and tiny movements of the human head. Sound waves may be reflected from or pass around an object, depending upon the relationship between the obstacle's dimensions and the frequency of the incident wave, as shown in Figure 9–5. Sounds with small wavelengths that encounter large objects will cast a shadow (Fig. 9–5a), while those signals with wavelengths that are large compared with the size of the obstacle will readily pass around the object (Fig. 9–5b).

An object the size of a human head will cast a substantial sound shadow above 2000 Hz. Interaural intensity differences between subjects' ears have been reported to be as large as 10 dB for a 4000-Hz tone presented in a sound field.

The value of this magnitude difference varies in a complex fashion as a function of both the frequency and azimuth of the arriving stimulus. Interaural intensity and time of arrival (phase) differences reach a maximum

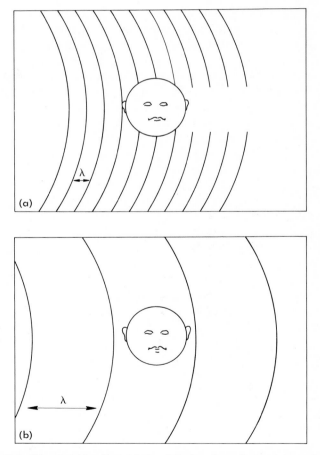

Figure 9–5 The obstacle effect: (a) sound shadow formed when λ is small compared to size of obstacle, (b) no shadow when λ is relatively big.

when the incident sound wave has a 90° azimuth (0° being the front of the head). This maximum time difference is slightly less than 1 msec for a headsized object. For frequencies above 1000 Hz, intensity rather than temporal differences would appear to play an important role in localization (as with lateralization). Because of the diffractive and reflective properties of the external ear, it is even possible to make very crude localizations of sounds using only one ear.

A related phenomenon important to localization of sounds is the precedence effect (Wallach, Newman, and Rosenzweig, 1949). The effect may be demonstrated by first creating a fused sound image with identical dichotic stimuli, followed very shortly afterwards by yet another pair of signals differing from the first set by small interaural time or intensity disparities (Fig. 9–6). Subjects report hearing a single image with an apparent position corresponding to the *initial* stimulus pair. Precedence will take place when two conditions are met:

1. The second pair of dichotic stimuli should not lag the first by more than a few milliseconds. Critical values range from one or two to over 40 milliseconds, depending upon the nature of the test stimuli.

2. The second stimulus pair should not exceed the first by more than 15 dB in level.

In the real world, we rely upon those stimuli arriving first at our ears for the determination of the direction of a sound source. Without this effect, one would be confused as to a sound's location even in moderately reverberant surroundings, such as a classroom or office.

Precedence and lateralization effects are most apparent when the test stimuli employed are impulsive. It seems that the auditory system makes use of, and is highly sensitive to, the wide range of frequency components within transient cues. When a binaural signal is presented which contains conflicting lateralization information, then the cues contained in the initial or transient portion of the waveform will dominate. It has been estimated that the effect of a brief transient cue may persist for several hundred milliseconds after its occurrence.

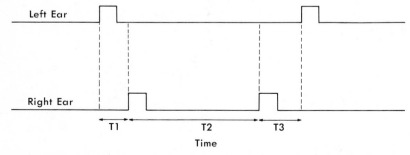

Figure 9–6 The precedence effect. Listeners perceive the fused sound image associated with the initial stimulus pair.

BINAURAL MASKING LEVEL DIFFERENCES

The binaural hearing mechanism assists the listener with more than localization of external sound sources. In highly reverberant surroundings, binaural listening facilitates the rejection of unwanted echoes that interfere with the desired acoustic signals. Similarly, the intelligibility of speech in noise (or more generally, the auditory detection of signals in noise) is improved substantially under dichotic rather than monotic listening. This improvement of a subject's detection performance for a signal within noise as a consequence of dichotic rather than monotic listening has been investigated by numerous researchers since Licklider (1948) and Hirsh (1948) first reported the effect. The phenomenon may be better understood by reference to Table 9–1 and through the following series of experiments.

At first, both a low-frequency tone and a narrow band of noise (with the same center frequency as the test tone) are presented to one of a listener's headphones. The magnitude of the test tone is adjusted until it is barely detectable against the background of the noise (the $S_m N_m$ condition, Fig. 9–7(a). The introduction of the identical noise waveform to the opposite ear yields a dramatic improvement in the detectability of the tone (the $S_m N_o$ condition, Fig. 9–7(b). Next, add the test tone to the opposite ear as well and the detectability drops markedly again (the $S_o N_o$ condition, Fig. 9–7(c). A greater improvement can be obtained by reversing the phase of the noise waveform between the two ears; the tone being applied binaurally in phase (the $S_0 N_\pi$ condition, Fig. 9–7(d). The largest improvements in detectability have been obtained binaurally out of

TABLE 9–1   *MLD Nomenclature*

SYMBOL	*BINAURAL PHASE RELATIONSHIP*
S_m	Signal monaural, no signal presented to opposite ear.
S_o	Signal in phase at the two ears.
S_π	Signal at one ear 180° (π radians) out of phase with the signal at the opposite ear.
N_m	Noise monaural, delivered to one ear only.
N_o	Identical noise presented to each ear.
N_π	Noise waveform at one ear is 180° out-of-phase with noise waveform at the other ear.
N_u	Uncorrelated noise (i.e. arising from two statistically identical but separate sources) at the two ears.
N_τ	The noise waveform at one ear is time delayed with respect to the noise waveform in the opposite ear.

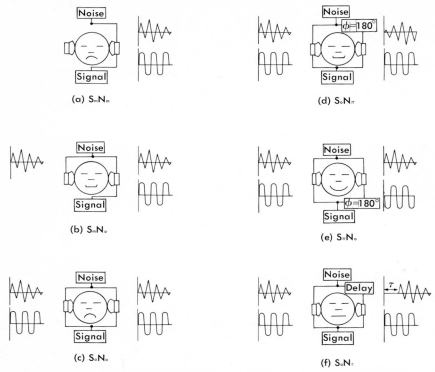

Figure 9–7   (a) The SmNm listening condition (both signal and noise delivered monaurally). The tone is barely detectable.

(b) The SmNo listening condition (signal monaural, noise in phase at both ears). The tone is clearly detectable.

(c) The SoNo listening condition (signals binaurally in phase, noise binaurally in phase). The signal is again barely detectable.

(d) The SoN$_\pi$ listening condition (signals binaurally in phase, noise 180° or π radians binaurally out of phase). The signal is highly detectable.

(e) The S$_\pi$No listening condition. This is the most detectable condition.

(f) The SoN$_\tau$ listening condition (signals binaurally in phase, noise delay to one ear). The signal detectability varies with the interaural delay.

phase, keeping the noise binaurally in phase (the $S_\pi N_0$ condition, Fig. 9–7e). A gain in detectability on the order of 15 dB has been reported for this condition (Green and Henning, 1969).

The detectability differences among these separate listening conditions has been variously labeled binaural release from masking, binaural unmasking, binaural analysis, binaural masking level differences (BMLD), and masking level differences (MLD). Masking level differences are typically specified in terms of the signal level in dB for detectability for the experimental condition relative to the signal level for the $S_0 N_0$ condition. As the signal frequency is raised, the MLD values decrease from 15 dB at 250 Hz to a fairly uniform value of 3 dB for frequencies above 2000 Hz. Masking level differences presumably depend upon the processing of phase (time) information, and the lack of improvement in MLD values above 2000 Hz may be linked to the ear's apparent insensitivity to temporal cues above 2000 Hz. In fact, it is quite surprising that a phase effect can play such a marked role at these high frequencies. Most effects involving temporal processing (e.g., binaural beats, periodicity pitch, localization, etc.) have been observed at lower frequencies.

Research into MLDs for frequencies below 250 Hz has yielded conflicting data. Hirsh (1948c) obtained a peak MLD value of 14 dB around 250 Hz, decreasing to about 3 or 4 dB at both 100 Hz and 5 kHz. Durlach (1972) and Webster (1951) found that MLD values below 200 Hz remain constant at about 14 dB (see Fig. 9–8). An adequate explanation for these disparate findings has not yet been found, although procedural differences among the studies may be an important factor. It should be noted, for example, that in Webster's experiment, the intensity of the tone was kept constant, while the noise level was adjusted to mask the tone. Other experimenters have typically held the noise level fixed and adjusted the magnitude of the tone.

Another factor influencing the MLD results is the level of the noise. It has been reported that MLD values increase as the spectrum level* of the noise increases (Hirsh, 1948). Figure 9–9 displays the change of the MLD for the conditions $S_\pi N_o - S_o N_o$ as the spectrum level of white noise increases. For a test tone of 200 Hz, the MLD values range from about 4 dB at 9 dB spectrum level to about 14 dB at a more intense spectrum level

---

*The term "spectrum level" refers to the power per unit bandwidth of the noise.

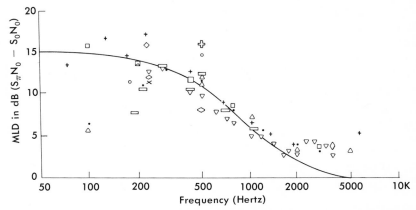

Figure 9–8   The change in MLD values as a function of tone frequency. The data points represent the diverse results of many studies. (After Durlach in Tobias: Foundations of Modern Auditory Theory, Vol. II. New York, Academic Press, 1972.)

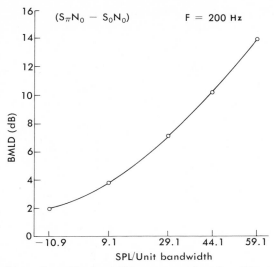

Figure 9–9   Binaural masking level differences as a function of the spectrum level of a white noise background. (After Hirsh: J. Acoust. Soc. Amer., 20:536, 1948.)

of 59 dB. It has been suggested that these particular masking level differences may be linked to the variability of neural firings under different conditions of signal magnitude (Green and Henning, 1969).

One of the variables influencing binaural release from masking is the degree of correlation between the noise signals reaching the two ears.* If two separate noise signals are used, one to each ear, having the same statistical characteristics (e.g., as produced by separate but identical noise generators), then the detectability of a binaurally in-phase tone in this background of uncorrelated noise will be about 3 dB greater than that of the S_mN_m case (Robinson and Jeffress, 1963).

Another way of producing decorrelated noise is to introduce a substantial time delay between the noise waveforms delivered to each ear. This condition is shown in Figure 9–7(f). The subject listens to the identical sinusoid in each ear and a narrow band noise in each ear. In one ear, however, the noise waveform is delayed by some time, $\Delta\tau$. The correlation between two narrow-band noise waveforms follows a cyclic pattern with a gradual decrease in peak heights as $\Delta\tau$ increases (Fig. 9–10). The variation in MLD values due to the interaural time delay of the noise waveform is displayed in Figure 9–11A. The relationship is cyclic in nature with successive maxima and minima occurring, respectively, at the half- and full-period times for the particular narrow-band signal employed.† At

---

*By correlation is meant the degree of similarity in the structure of the waveforms. Correlation may be expressed mathematically as the normalized product of two waveforms integrated over the total time the waveforms are observed.

†The narrower the band of the noise, the closer it approximates a modulated sine wave varying slowly in amplitude and frequency.

very large interaural delays, there is negligible correlation between the noise waveforms reaching the two ears, and a steady MLD of 3 dB is reached.

A number of models have been proposed to account for MLD data; by far the most comprehensive is the Equalization-Cancellation model of Durlach (1972). According to this model, the detection mechanism manipulates the stimuli waveforms at each ear so as to equalize the noise at the two ears. The equalized signals are then subtracted so as to eliminate the noise. This model would yield perfect detectability were it not for the presence of small errors in the temporal and amplitude processing of the signals. Estimates of the magnitude of these errors that would yield a good fit to published MLD data show a relative amplitude variance of $(0.25)^2$ and a time-jitter variance of $(105 \ \mu sec)^2$.

Masking level differences for speech stimuli have also been studied. It is important to distinguish between binaural release from masking for the *detection* of speech (MLD), and the release from masking at a specified level of speech intelligibility. For the latter case, the term "binaural intelligibility difference" (ILD)* has been suggested (Levitt and Rabiner, 1967a). The data on the binaural enhancement of speech in noise are quite disparate. ILDs as low as 3 dB and as high as 12 dB have been reported. The magnitude of the ILD, however, appears to depend on the intelligibility level, a greater ILD being observed for low levels of intelligibility. It has been determined that the low-frequency region of the

---

*The nomenclature BMLD and BILD was originally used in the Levitt and Rabiner paper, but has been shortened to MLD and ILD in order to be consistent with nomenclature used in this chapter and elsewhere.

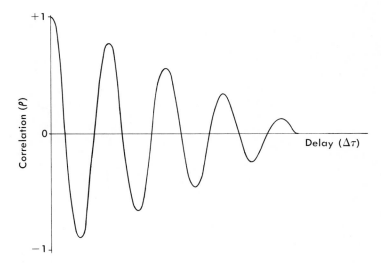

Figure 9–10   The change in correlation for two narrow band noise waveforms as a function of the interaural delay between waveforms.

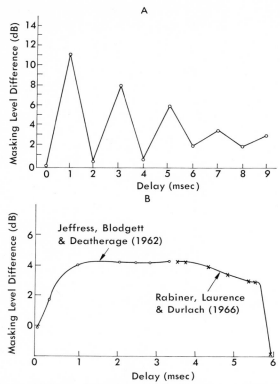

Figure 9–11 A, MLD vs. τ in background of positively correlated noise. (After Langford and Jeffress: 1964). B, Binaural masking level differences as a function of the interaural
time delay between noise waveforms at each ear. (After Jeffress et al., 1957; Langford and
Jeffress, 1964; Jeffress et al., 1962; Rabiner et al., 1966.)

speech signal (around 300 Hz) is of primary importance in release from
masking (MLD), while both high and low portions of the speech spectrum play a significant role in binaural gain in intelligibility (ILD), although the lower frequencies are relatively more important. Levitt and
Rabiner (1967b) have provided a simple numerical procedure for predicting the ILD and MLD values for speech which indicates that ILD values
become progressively larger as one moves from high intelligibility levels
to low intelligibility levels, until zero intelligibility is reached. At this
point, speech is just detectable but no longer intelligible, and a maximum
improvement, equal to the MLD, is achieved. The MLD for speech may
be thought of as a limiting case of the ILD.

OTHER BINAURAL EFFECTS

When two pure tones of differing frequency are presented dichotically, the presence of a single tone that fluctuates in magnitude is often

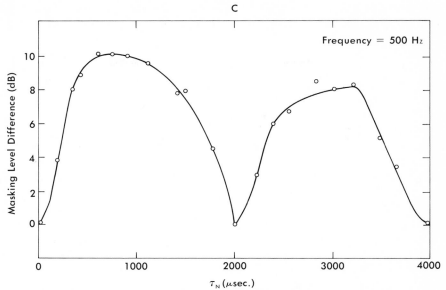

Figure 9–11 *Continued.* C, MLD vs. interaural time delay between the noise waveforms.

reported. This phenomenon, called binaural beats, should be distinguished from objective beats perceived by either or both ears due to the interaction of the tones outside the head. Early studies (Lane, 1925; Rayleigh, 1907) reported the occurrence of binaural beats only when frequencies below 1000 Hz were employed. Subsequent research (Wever, 1949) provided data which extend this frequency limit and suggests that the effect is linked to the complex synchrony of neural firings.

Almost every psychoacoustical effect appears to be enhanced when binaural rather than monaural listening is utilized. As discussed earlier, for example, the auditory threshold for binaural listening is from 3 to 6 dB better than for monaural conditions and, too, the perceived loudness of a sound is greater for the binaural case (cf. Chapter 7). In addition, improvements in just noticeable differences for frequency have been noted as well as the reduction of both listening fatigue and the so-called critical band of hearing which relates to the ears' ability to filter out noise or other stimuli not in the immediate frequency region of the target signal. Substantial improvements have also been observed in the binaural intelligibility of speech under reverberant conditions even when there are no interaural differences.

RIGHT EAR ADVANTAGE

Licklider, in his classic 1948 study on binaural release from masking for speech, found that if noise was presented to both ears and speech to only one ear, then the intelligibility scores for the right ear were superior to those for the left ear. A right-ear advantage was also observed by Broadbent (1958) in an experiment involving competing dichotic stimuli. In this experiment, pairs of digits were presented simultaneously, one to each ear. After three such pairs, the listener was required to repeat the digits he heard. The listeners reported all the digits heard in one ear before reporting the digits heard in the opposite ear.

Kimura (1961a, b; 1964) studied the effect in greater detail using both speech and nonspeech stimuli. She found a right ear advantage for speech and a left ear advantage for nonspeech stimuli, such as a melody. She attributed the effect to the prepotency of the contralateral neural pathway from the right ear to the language-dominant left hemisphere of the brain. Kimura's observations have since been confirmed by a number of researchers, the thrust of much current research being on the extent of the differences between different types of speech sounds (Gerber and Goldman, 1971; Studdert-Kennedy and Shankweiler, 1970, and references cited therein). In practical terms, the magnitude of the right ear advantage for speech is small and has only been measured under rather special dichotic listening conditions with competing stimuli at each ear. As an investigative tool, experiments of this type have provided important new insights into the basic mechanisms of auditory perception.

SUMMARY

Several important characteristics of the ear may be learned from the wealth of data obtained through experiments on binaural hearing. Generally, the remarkable sensitivity of the auditory system is even greater under binaural (as opposed to monaural) listening. The threshold of audibility is lower for binaural signals, as is differential sensitivity for intensity and frequency. Also, binaural stimuli are substantially louder than monaural stimuli of equal intensity. Even more remarkable is the precision displayed by the binaural system in the processing of temporal information, as in the lateralization and localization of sounds. Whereas the time scale of an individual nerve firing is measured in milliseconds, just-noticeable differences in interaural time delays as small as 10 microseconds have been obtained. Clearly, a good deal of statistical averaging of neural events must be taking place in order to achieve such precision.

The ear would also appear to be highly nonlinear with respect to localization phenomena. The precedence, stereophonic, and other localization effects clearly display the ear's reliance upon initial rather than ongoing cues. Similarly, with high frequency signals, the signal envelope dominates localization and fusion effects, indicating some form of nonlinear detection process. Temporal processing also appears to play a substantial role in most binaural effects. Apart from fusion, lateralization, and localization effects, the phenomenon of binaural release from masking illustrates dramatically the importance of phase or temporal cues. In this case, improvements in detectability approaching a 100-fold reduction in signal power (i.e., 20 dB) have been reported.

Since a listener can pay attention to one or the other ear, much of the research on attention mechanisms has involved the auditory system (rather than visual, or other sensory systems), leading to some important findings regarding a human listener's ability to tune in to one of several simultaneous messages. In particular, the intelligibility of speech in noise is enhanced considerably under binaural conditions, provided there are interaural differences between the speech and interfering noise. Experiments of this type have also shown a marked asymmetry between the ears in that speech appears to be processed more readily in the right ear and nonspeech stimuli more readily in the left ear. These findings support neurophysiological data on the prepotency of the contralateral pathway from the right ear to the language-dominant left hemisphere. Thus, two ears may be better than one, but they are not identical.

Of all the effects that have been reported in binaural hearing, perhaps the most remarkable is that of binaural fusion. Despite the many differences between the signals reaching the two ears (including reflections) and despite the rapid changes in these differences that are continually occurring as a result of head movements and other changes, we perceive a single, stable auditory image of the world around us.

REFERENCES

Boring, E. G. (1942): *Sensation and Perception in the History of Experimental Psychology.* New York, D. Appleton-Century Co.
Broadbent, D. E. (1958): *Perception and Communication.* Oxford, Pergamon Press.
Caussé, R., and Chavasse, P. (1942): L'écoute binauriculaire et monauriculaire pour la perception des intensités supraliminaries. *Compte Rendu Société Biologique* (Paris) *136*: 405.
deBoer, K. (1940): *Stereofonische Geluidsweergave.* Dissertation, Delft (cited by Franssen, q.v.).
Durlach, N. I. (1972): Binaural signal detection: equalization and cancellation theory. *In* J. V. Tobias (ed.): *Foundations of Modern Auditory Theory.* Vol. II. New York, Academic Press.
Franssen, N. V. (1960): *Some Considerations on the Mechanism of Directional Hearing.* Thesis, Technische Hogeschool, Delft.
Gerber, S. E., and Goldman, P. (1971): Ear preference for dichotically presented verbal stimuli as a function of report strategies. *Journal of the Acoustical Society of America 32*:1329–1336.
Green, D. M., and Henning, G. R. (1969): Audition. *Annual Review of Psychology 20*: 105–128.
Guttman, N., van Bergeijk, W. A., and David, E. E., Jr. (1960): Monaural temporal masking investigated by binaural interaction. *Journal of the Acoustical Society of America 32*: 1329–1336.
Hirsh, I. J. (1948): The influence of interaural phase on interaural summation and inhibition. *Journal of the Acoustical Society of America 20*:536–544.
Kimura, D. (1961a): Some effects of temporal lobe damage on auditory perception. *Canadian Journal of Psychology 15*:156–165.
Kimura, D. (1961b): Cerebral dominance and the perception of verbal stimuli. *Canadian Journal of Psychology 15*:166–171.

Kimura, D. (1964): Left-right differences in the perception of melodies. *Quarterly Journal of Experimental Psychology 16*:355–358.

Lane, C. E. (1925): Binaural beats. *Physical Review 26*:401–412.

Levitt, H., and Rabiner, L. R. (1967a): Binaural release from masking for speech and gain in intelligibility. *Journal of the Acoustical Society of America 42*:601–608.

Levitt, H., and Rabiner, L. R. (1967b): Predicting binaural gain in intelligibility and release from masking for speech. *Journal of the Acoustical Society of America 42*:820–829.

Licklider, J. C. R. (1948): The influence of interaural phase relations upon the masking of speech by white noise. *Journal of the Acoustical Society of America 20*:150–159.

Mills, A. W. (1960): Lateralization of high frequency tones. *Journal of the Acoustical Society of America 32*:132–134.

Rayleigh, Lord (1907): On our perception of sound direction. *Philosophical Magazine 13*: 214–232.

Robinson, D. E., and Jeffress, L. A. (1963): Effect of varying the interaural noise correlation on the detectability of tonal signals, *Journal of the Acoustical Society of America 35*:1947–1952.

Studdert-Kennedy, M., and Shankweiler, D. (1970): Hemispheric specialization for speech perception. *Journal of the Acoustical Society of America 48*:579–594.

Teas, D. C. (1962): Lateralization of acoustic transients. *Journal of the Acoustical Society of America 34*:1460–1465.

Tobias, J. V., and Zerlin, S. (1959): Lateralization threshold as a function of stimulus duration. *Journal of the Acoustical Society of America 31*:1591–1594.

von Békésy, G. (1930): Zur Theorie des Hörens; Über die Richtungshören bei einer Zeitdifferenz oder Lautstärkenungleichheit der beiderseitigen Schalleinwirkungen. *Physikalische Zeitschrift 31*:824–835, 857–868; also: Chapter 8 in von Békésy, G. (1960): *Experiments in Hearing* (translated and edited by E. G. Wever). New York, McGraw-Hill Book Co.

von Hornbostel, E. M. and Wertheimer, M. (1920): Über die Wahrnehmung der Schallrichtung. *Sitzung Berlin Akademie der Wissenschaft 15*:388–396.

Wallach, H., Newman, E. B., and Rosenzweig, M. R. (1949): The precedence effect in sound localization. *American Journal of Psychology 62*:315–336.

Webster, F. A. (1951): The influence of interaural phase on masked thresholds: I. The role of interaural time deviation. *Journal of the Acoustical Society of America 23*:452–462.

Wever, E. G. (1949): *Theory of Hearing.* New York, John Wiley & Sons.

Zwislocki, J., and Feldman, A. S. (1956): Just noticeable difference in dichotic phase. *Journal of the Acoustical Society of America 28*:860–864.

Part Four

ACOUSTICS
OF SPEECH

There is, after all, one major point in being able to hear — to be able to communicate with others. Therefore, the hearing of speech is paramount. In Part Four, we are concerned with speech as an acoustic phenomenon, with speech sounds as acoustic events, and with a very special process called speech perception. In this part, we see that speech differs from other audible sounds in a number of particular ways. We learn about acoustic models of speech, ways to analyze speech, and even ways to synthesize it. Finally, in the last chapter of the book, we examine speech perception and find that it is actually different from other kinds of perception. Part Four, in many ways, is more difficult than the first three parts — necessarily — since this most important of topics is the most specialized. So, like dessert, we have saved the best for last; but, like dessert, it isn't satisfying unless you approach it by the proper route.

Chapter Ten

THE ACOUSTICS OF SPEECH

Hisashi Wakita

Treated from the viewpoint of acoustics, a speech event is a vibration of air in a complex mode changing rapidly with time. Let us briefly observe how a voiced sound becomes a vibratory event. Vibration of air is caused by the closing and opening motion of the vocal cords sending out a train of air puffs into the vocal cavity through the glottis. The vibration of air produced at the glottis is deformed in various ways while proceeding toward the lips according to the different configurations of the vocal tract, thus radiating different sounds from the lips. In the case of voiceless sounds, a turbulent flow of air is created by making a constriction within the vocal tract but without involving any vibratory motion of the glottis. The sound radiated from the mouth is then transmitted through the air, and when it reaches the ear of a listener, it causes vibration which is physiologically processed by the auditory organs and finally perceived as sound. Thus, vibration plays an important role in the production and perception of speech. The acoustics of speech is a science which makes

209

clear this intricate mechanism of the vibration event so that we can get better understanding of speech production and perception processes.

Although the history of speech research dates back to the eighteenth century, in the past 20 years highly advanced mathematical and engineering techniques have been introduced into the study of speech and many remarkable accomplishments have been achieved. Study is being rigorously continued by many researchers all over the world. The purpose of this chapter is to provide the reader with the basic scientific concepts involved so that he can more fully appreciate the work in this field.

WAVEFORMS

Normally, you cannot see the vibratory motion of air with your own eyes. As you learned in Chapter 3, however, it is possible to convert the variation of air pressure into a variation of electrical voltage by means of an electroacoustic transducer, and we can see a replica of the variation of air pressure in terms of the variation of electrical voltage. As an example, a portion of an utterance, "Thieves who rob friends deserve jail," is shown in Figure 10–1. This was recorded at a fixed point about 15 inches from the mouth of the speaker and shows a period of only approximately 500 msec. Thus we can visualize the variation of air pressure in terms of the variation of electrical voltage which is evidently the entity of a speech sound. Suppose the utterance shown in Figure 10–1 were a portion of

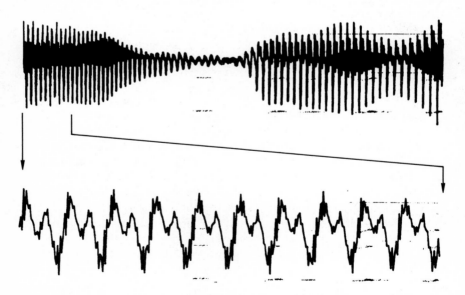

Figure 10–1 A portion of the waveform of the utterance, "Thieves who rob friends deserve jail." (a) The waveform for a portion "----ieves who ro----" (about 500 msec). (b) Expanded waveform of the first 50 msec of the waveform in (a) above.

what your close friend spoke to you through a curtain. You would probably be able to identify the voice as your friend's, not to mention that you understand what is said. Sometimes you will be able to guess your friend's emotional state. Consequently, it is certain that the waveform as shown in Figure 10-1 bears the information or a part of the information on what is spoken, who spoke it, and sometimes in what emotional state it was spoken. Truly, the waveform as shown in Figure 10-1 is the only available physical entity of speech sounds; although, under certain circumstances, such factors as facial expression, lip movements, etc. will also give supplementary information to listeners. Thus, our investigation starts from observing the waveforms of speech sounds and trying to look for those elements that bear such information.

FILTERS

Sometimes it is desirable to alter the spectral envelope or eliminate some of the frequency components artificially. Systems having this function are called *filters*. Three types of filters are often used: a low-pass filter (LPF), a high-pass filter (HPF), and a band-pass filter (BPF). If a signal as shown in Figure 10-2(a) is passed through each of these filters, the output

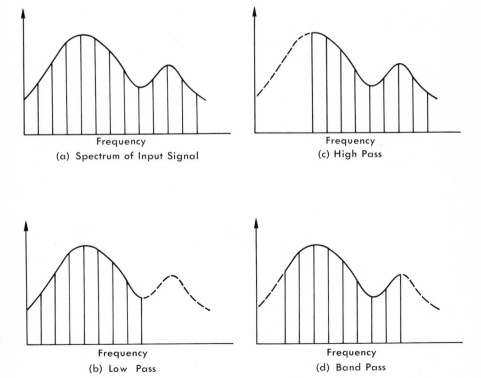

Figure 10-2 Output spectra from three filters for the same input.

spectra can be illustrated as shown in Figures 10–2(b), (c), and (d). The frequency components shown by the broken lines are eliminated by the filters. This effect of a filter system on the input spectrum is called the *frequency characteristic* of the system or the *transfer function* of the system. These terms are used quite often for electroacoustic transducers and electrical devices such as microphones, loudspeakers, and amplifiers. Usually, it is desired in these devices that the frequency components of an input signal are not altered while the signal is transmitted through them.

RESONATORS

There is another kind of system, called a *resonator*, which emphasizes particular frequency components of a signal. Its frequency characteristic is as shown in Figure 10–3. The frequency characteristic of a resonator is usually specified by the frequency of the maximum amplitude which is called the center frequency or the resonance frequency. The bandwidth of a resonance is defined as the frequency range where the amplitude of the frequency component is 3 dB below the amplitude of the center frequency or, in other words, the frequency range around the center frequency where 50 per cent of the power is included. If you use an impulse as an input to a resonator, the constant spectrum of the input is deformed by the frequency characteristics of the resonator, and the output spectrum would look exactly as shown in Figure 10–3; the output waveform will be a damped sinusoid. The output signal of a system when an impulse is applied as an input is usually called an impulse response. Thus, the impulse response of a resonance system is a damped sinusoid. As you will see later, the resonance system plays an important role in building a speech synthesizer as well as in understanding the speech production system.

SPEECH PRODUCTION MODEL AND ACOUSTIC FEATURES

Based on the various acoustic concepts you learned in the previous sections, let us try to make a simple model of speech production. The

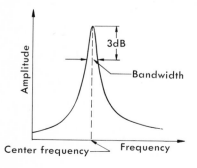

Figure 10–3 Frequency characteristics of a resonator.

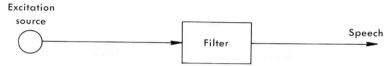

Figure 10-4 Speech production model.

simplest model for producing the voiced sounds such as vowels is given in Figure 10–4. The glottal wave caused by the vibration of the vocal cords is expressed by the excitation source, and the vocal tract is regarded as a kind of acoustic filter. The frequency characteristics of this filter are varied by changing the positions of the vocal organs such as the tongue, the jaw, the lips, and so on, thus generating different sounds as output. By virtue of the vibration of the vocal cords, a train of air puffs is sent out into the vocal tract. While the train of air puffs travels through the vocal tract, the amplitudes of some of the frequency components are reduced and others are emphasized in a complex manner, depending on the vocal tract configuration. Let's look at a simple example shown in Figure 10–5. The input, (a), shows the glottal wave which is roughly triangular shaped, and (b) shows the output of the filter. It is to be noted how a relatively simple input waveform is changed into a complicated waveform by the vocal tract filter. Let's take a look at this event in terms of the changes of the power spectral envelope. Figure 10–6(a) shows the spectral envelope of the excitation source and 6(b) shows the output spectral envelope of the

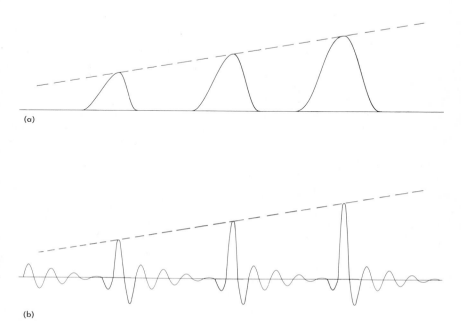

Figure 10–5 Waveforms of the filter input and output. (a) Waveform of excitation source. (b) Waveform of sound output.

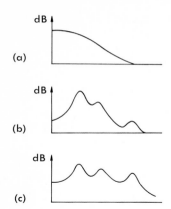

(a)

(b)

(c)

Figure 10–6 Frequency characteristics. (a) Excitation source, (b) output, (c) filter.

excitation source changed by the frequency characteristics of the vocal tract filter. To see the frequency characteristics of the vocal tract filter more clearly, characteristics of the excitation source can be subtracted from the output spectral envelope if the amplitude is expressed in decibels. The frequency characteristics of the vocal tract filter thus obtained are shown in 6(c).

EXCITATION

You might be surprised if you were told that even such a simple model of speech production can explain most of the important properties of voiced sounds. Then, what are their properties and how can we describe them? Observe the waveforms in Figure 10–5: you will notice that the peaks in the excitation waveform are still preserved in the output waveform. These peaks tell us the number of repetitions of air puffs per second in the excitation source, which is called the fundamental frequency of the voice and is directly related to the pitch of the sound. When the fundamental frequency is increased, the pitch goes higher (cf. Chapter 6). Usually, the average fundamental frequency of male voices is around 125 Hz, and that of female voices around 230 Hz. Another significant feature about the excitation waveform, as indicated by the dotted lines in Figure 10–5, is the amplitude of the peaks. They are well reflected in the output waveform. Thus, the amplitude of the excitation source determines the power of speech and, hence, the loudness of the sound. These two quantities, the fundamental frequency and the amplitude, are considered to be the most important properties pertaining to the excitation source.

FORMANTS

As is clear from the frequency characteristics of the filter in Figure 10–6(c), its significant property is the conspicuous peaks. The center frequency of each peak is called the *formant* frequency. From lower to higher they are called the first, the second, the third formant frequencies and so on. As mentioned in the previous section, each peak can be described by its center frequency and bandwidth. Thus, the frequency characteristics of the filter (i.e., the vocal tract) can be described by formant frequencies and bandwidths. As described later, each sound is characterized by the locations of the formant frequencies. Thus, formant frequency is known to be the most important acoustic property of a speech sound. Usually, the first three formant frequencies are dominant and they are usually below 3500 Hz.

For the production of consonants, a noise source is considered to be at the place of the consonantal constriction where turbulent noise is generated — plus a glottal excitation source if the consonant is voiced. For the production of nasal sounds, a nasal filter corresponding to the nasal tract is branched from the vocal tract filter. However, it is very difficult to separate the frequency characteristics of the nasal tract. Acoustically, all the consonants are described by their frequency spectral characteristics. More specific models of speech production are described later. Before proceeding to them, let us examine various methods for finding the properties of speech sounds discussed in this section.

SPEECH ANALYSIS

In order to examine the acoustic properties pertaining to a particular sound, it is necessary to know how to obtain those properties in an efficient way. This has long been a primary topic for speech researchers. In the early days, a technique of photographically recording speech waves was used to examine the fundamental frequency of the speech sound, and laborious calculations of Fourier transforms were tried by the use of a hand calculator in order to obtain the frequency spectrum of a sound. With the development of electronic techniques, various machines were developed to analyze speech. The sound spectrograph, among others, played (and is still playing) an important role in speech analysis (Potter, Kopp, and Green, 1947). A great deal of speech information has been obtained with this machine by many researchers. Since the development of digital computers, especially in the last 10 years, highly sophisticated techniques have been applied to speech analysis, allowing us fast and accurate computation. Digital computer techniques are especially suitable for processing large amounts of speech data. In the following sections, the sound spectrograph and some digital computer methods of speech analysis are described.

THE SOUND SPECTROGRAPH

The sound spectrograph, developed in 1947 (Potter, Kopp, and Green), provides various data on speech sounds, such as formant struc-

ture, voicing, friction, stress, and fundamental frequency. Figure 10–7
shows a schematic diagram of one type of sound spectrograph. By setting
the microphone switch in the record position, a speech sample is recorded
on a magnetic disc which is rotating with a certain speed (generally it
takes about 2.4 seconds for one rotation). Then, the switch (SW1) is
changed to "analyze" from "record" and another switch (SW2) is set in
the spectrogram position with the filter selection in "wideband." An electrically sensitive paper is fixed to a drum which rotates on the same shaft
as the magnetic disc. The reproduced signal is sent to the analyzing band-
pass filter, the output of which appears through the marking amplifier on a
stylus which is in contact with the paper fixed on the drum. The output
current of the band-pass filter is in proportion to the energy of the original
speech signal contained in the same frequency range as the band-pass
filter. Electrical current from the stylus burns the paper in proportion to
the current magnitude, and leaves a mark with a density roughly proportional to the logarithm of the current magnitude. With the first rotation of
the magnetic disc, the reproduced signal is passed through a band-pass
filter with a frequency range of 0 to 300 Hz, and the stylus leaves a burned
mark on the bottom part of the paper. At the end of the first rotation of the
disc, the frequency range of the band-pass filter is shifted 20 Hz upward
and the stylus is also moved slightly upward. By the second rotation of the
magnetic disc, energy of the signal within 20 to 320 Hz is taken out by the
filter and the burned mark is produced on the paper. In this fashion, for
each playback of the disc, the frequency range of the band-pass filter and
the position of the stylus are shifted, thus producing a time-intensity-
frequency plot of the signal on the paper. An example of a spectrogram
made with a wide-band filter is shown in the upper part of Figure 10–8.

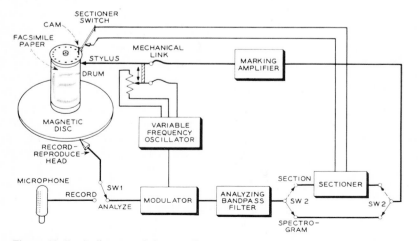

Figure 10–7 A diagram of the sound spectrograph. (From Flanagan, J. L.: Speech
Analysis, Synthesis, and Perception, 2nd ed. New York, Springer-Verlag, 1972.)

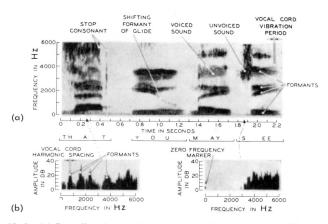

(a)

(b)

Figure 10–8   (a) Broadband sound spectrogram of the utterance "That you may see." (b) Amplitude *vs.* frequency plots (amplitude sections) taken in the vowel portion of "that" and in the fricative portion of "see." (From Flanagan, J. L.: Speech Analysis, Synthesis, and Perception, 2nd ed. New York, Springer-Verlag, 1972.)

The horizontal scale shows time, the vertical scale shows frequency, and the amplitude of the spectrum is shown by the darkness of the pattern. Since formant frequencies are peaks in the frequency spectrum, they appear as darker marks in the spectrogram. Besides formant structure of the sound, you can see the duration of sounds, voiced and unvoiced portions, etc. If you are accustomed to the spectrogram, you can read the main features of the utterance as indicated in the diagram.

If you select the narrow-band filter, the fundamental frequency and its harmonics are emphasized in the pattern, and you can measure the fundamental frequency accurately, for example, by measuring the frequency of the tenth harmonic and dividing by 10. An example of a narrow-band spectrogram is shown in Figure 10–9.

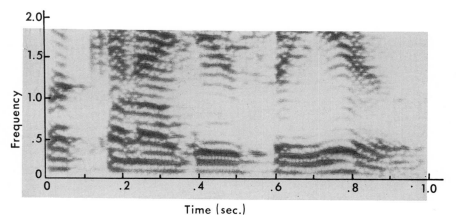

Figure 10–9   Narrow-band spectrogram of the utterance, "What can I do for you?" by a male speaker.

A frequency vs. amplitude diagram at any instant can also be obtained by properly setting the switch (SW2) in the "section" position. Examples.are shown in the lower diagrams of Figure 10–8. Since the section has an intensity range of approximately 45 dB, instead of only 12 dB as in the wide-band spectrogram, it is quite useful for examining amplitude spectra over a greater intensity range.

FORMANT ANALYSIS

As mentioned before, formant frequencies specify the frequency characteristics of the vocal tract which characterize each sound. Thus, it is indispensable to know the formant structure of sounds in order to examine their acoustic properties. The sound spectrograph is still a widely used tool to do this. However, a recent development in computer techniques has made possible automatic tracking of formant frequency, thus making possible fast and accurate analysis of a large amount of data. The most efficient and promising computer methods, among others, would be the cepstrum method and the linear prediction method, both of which are based on highly sophisticated mathematical procedures, so they are not yet fully exploited by speech researchers.

In the cepstrum method (Fig. 10–10), the Fourier transform is applied to a certain length of a speech wave by the use of a computer program which obtains the frequency spectrum of the sound. If we take the Fourier transform of the logarithm of this frequency spectrum, we obtain a different kind of spectrum called *cepstrum*. The vocal cords' excitation appears in the high-time portion of the cepstrum as rapidly varying peri-

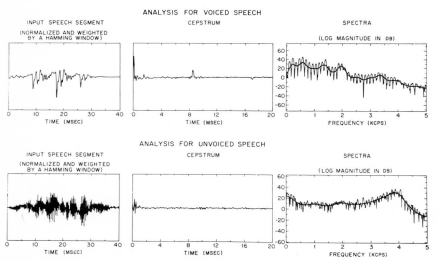

Figure 10–10 Spectrum and cepstrum analysis of voiced and unvoiced speech sounds. (From Flanagan, J. L.: Speech Analysis, Synthesis, and Perception, 2nd ed. New York, Springer-Verlag, 1972.)

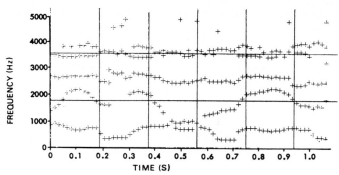

Figure 10–11 Digital inverse filter analysis of phrase: "I am now a man." (After Markel: IEEE Trans. Aud. Electroacoust., AU-*20*:137, 1972.)

odic components, whereas the vocal tract transmission function appears in the low-time portion of it as slowly varying components having the formant information. Thus, we can separate the vocal transmission function from the vocal tract excitation. If we take the low-time portion of the cepstrum and apply the Fourier transform to it again, we obtain a smooth spectrum showing clear formant peaks. You may feel as if you were watching the feat of a magician while reading the idea of the cepstrum method; truly it is a magic of mathematics. In Figure 10–10, examples of cepstrum analysis of voiced and unvoiced sounds are shown. You can see how the formant information is separated from the fundamental frequency information in the cepstrum shown at the middle of the top row. The smoothed spectra are shown by the solid lines in the right-hand figures for voiced and voiceless sounds.

The linear prediction method is another magic of mathematics. In this method, the present amplitude of a speech sound is predicted by the past amplitude values of the sound. Unknown variables, called prediction coefficients, are determined in such a way that the difference between the predicted and the actual values is minimized to a certain criterion. The prediction coefficients thus obtained are mathematically related to the formant frequencies which can be computed in a very efficient manner. The linear prediction method is considered very reliable and accurate for obtaining formant frequencies of voiced, non-nasalized sounds, and the mathematical procedure is quite suitable for computer processing. An example of the result obtained on the utterance, "I am now a man," is shown in Figure 10–11. This method, however, has a disadvantage for nasal sound analysis since it neglects the anti-resonance due to the nasal cavity which affects formant frequencies.

Although there are various other methods, each of them has its own merits and demerits. It is very important for us as users to select the most appropriate method, depending upon the purpose of our study, and to know the advantages and disadvantages of the method we choose. For example, if you have a large amount of data to analyze, you might think of using digital computer techniques, whereas the sound spectrograph will be a handy tool for relatively small amounts of data.

FUNDAMENTAL FREQUENCY ANALYSIS

One of the earliest methods of obtaining the fundamental frequency was a phonophotographic technique in which a replica of the speech vibration was recorded on photographic paper. As mentioned before, the air vibration caused by the vocal cords' vibration is preserved in the sound wave. The peaks of the triangular-shaped glottal wave are normally clear in the sound wave. The fundamental frequency can be figured out by measuring the time difference between two successive peaks in the sound wave and then computing the reciprocal of it. However, this procedure is extremely time-consuming. The development of the sound spectrograph saved much labor in measuring fundamental frequency. The narrow-band spectrogram gives us the harmonic structure of the voiced sounds. However, even the sound spectrograph is not suitable for processing a large amount of data, for example, for examining the statistical properties of fundamental frequencies of various speakers. A recent development in electronics provided us a machine called a pitch meter which allowed us real-time analysis. It would be a handy tool, depending upon the purpose of your study. If your study requires more accuracy, the machine may not be satisfactory to you. A relatively reliable and efficient method would be the use of the digital computer. There are several methods developed for computer processing. A simple one is the autocorrelation method which is, so to speak, a computerized "peak-picking" method which extracts the periodicity of the sound wave by knowing peak locations in its autocorrelation function.

A disadvantage of this method is the interaction between the source excitation and the first formant frequency, thus, sometimes giving a false result. Experience tells, however, that such a case is not encountered frequently, and it serves our purposes quite well. If you want to avoid such a disadvantage, the cepstrum method would satisfy you, since the periodic component is completely separated from the vocal tract characteristics in the cepstrum as exemplified in Figure 10–10. The linear prediction method is also a valuable tool for fundamental frequency analysis as well as formant analysis. The prediction error, after eliminating the combined characteristics of the glottal wave shape, the vocal tract, and the radiation, still preserves the information on source periodicity. Thus, we can extract this information from the prediction error by such a method as autocorrelation.

Formant frequencies are necessary to know the acoustic attributes of each sound. Fundamental voice frequency, together with other acoustic properties such as voice intensity level and phonetic duration, gives information on the prosodic variation of the voice such as stress, intonation, individual voice characteristics, and emotional characteristics. Since the amplitude of the glottal wave is known to be proportional to voice intensity level, it is easily measured by an electronic device or computed by a digital computer. However, there is no reliable way of automatically measuring sound duration; the sound spectrograph is most widely used for this purpose.

Formant bandwidth is another acoustic quantity needed to specify the shape of the spectral envelope of a sound. Normally, formant bandwidth is obtained as the combined effects of the glottal wave, the vocal tract, and the radiation at the mouth. It is difficult to know the contribution of the vocal tract to formant bandwidths due to interactions with the glottal wave and the radiation.

SPEECH SYNTHESIS

In the previous sections, we studied the acoustic properties of speech sounds and how they can be extracted; but we don't know yet whether or not these extracted properties are truly valid. One way of testing is to reconstruct the original speech sounds based on these acoustic properties. We can also learn more about how speech is produced in the human vocal tract by "speech synthesis."

Besides the basic study of speech sounds, speech synthesis has many practical applications, such as computer terminals which provide such information as airline and hotel reservations, selective stock market quotations, medical data, etc. Since speech synthesis is of such importance, practically as well as basically, it has been studied in detail in the past two decades, although interest in the matter started at least as far back as the late eighteenth century (cf., e.g., von Kempelen, 1791). There are various ways to synthesize speech, depending upon the vocal tract model chosen. In this section, we study several methods of synthesizing speech so that we can understand more about the acoustic process of speech production.

TERMINAL ANALOG MODEL

As mentioned before, the simplest model of speech production is to regard the vocal tract as a filter which is excited by the glottal source. A speech synthesizer based on this simple model is called a *terminal analog* synthesizer. Since the conspicuous peaks in the frequency characteristics of the vocal tract are due to its resonances, the filter in this model consists of several resonant circuits connected in series or in parallel.

A typical example of a terminal analog synthesizer is shown in Figure 10–12. Let us examine how it works, first by considering the synthesis of voiced sounds. For synthesis of vowels, fundamental frequency (F_0) is produced by the pulse generator, and then formed into a triangular-shaped glottal wave by the pulse-forming circuit. The amplitude A_0 of the glottal

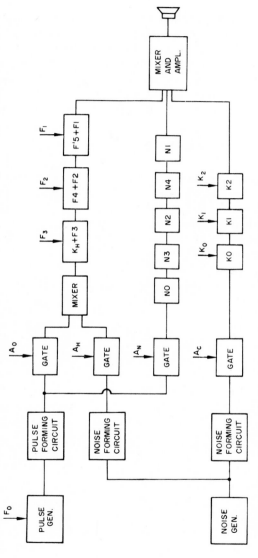

Figure 10-12   Terminal analog speech synthesizer. (From Hanley and Peters, in Travis, L. E. (ed.): Handbook of Speech Pathology and Audiology, p. 115. Copyright © 1971 by Meredith Corporation. Reproduced by permission of Appleton-Century-Crofts, Educational Division, Meredith Corporation.)

wave is also controlled. For vowels, only gate 1 is open, and the circuit in the top row corresponding to the vocal tract is excited. This circuit consists of six series-connected resonant circuits in which each resonance frequency corresponds to each formant frequency. The first three formants, F_1, F_2, and F_3, are variable, whereas F_4 and F_5 are constant. K_H is for the connection of higher formant frequencies and is fixed. By properly setting the variables for the values obtained from analysis, one can generate vowel sounds to see if the analysis was or was not valid by listening. For generation of voiced consonants, the same circuit is used. For some voiced consonants, noise and pulses are mixed to excite the vocal tract circuit. Four resonant circuits (N_1 through N_4) and an anti-resonant circuit (N_0) in the middle row correspond to the nasal cavity and are used for generation of nasal sounds. All the resonant frequencies are fixed in the nasal model. Two other resonant circuits (K_1 and K_2) and another anti-resonance (K_0) are used for synthesizing voiceless consonants with three frequencies and the noise amplitude as variables.

A particular synthesizer, called ÖVE II, was developed by Fant (1960). The control data were given by patterns handwritten on a plastic film with inductive ink, and were then converted into the electrical signal to excite the synthesizer. Some other types of terminal analog synthesizers are connected to digital computers, and the control signals are sent to the synthesizer via the computer.

ACOUSTIC TUBE MODEL

In another type of speech synthesizer, the vocal tract is regarded as a non-uniform acoustic tube. We have not yet studied sound-wave behavior in an acoustic tube, so we begin considering it for a uniform tube. It is known that two waves exist in the tube: one, the incident wave, advancing in a given direction; and the other, the reflected wave, advancing in the opposite direction. A traveling sound wave has both pressure and velocity; since they are related to each other, we consider the velocity wave for the sake of convenience. If the pressure wave varies sinusoidally, so does the velocity wave (cf. Chapter 2). Suppose one end of the tube is closed, and the tube is excited sinusoidally at the other end. Since the wave cannot move at the closed end wall, the velocity there must always be zero. In Figure 10–13, at the left, the velocity of the incident wave (solid line) and the reflected wave (dotted line) are illustrated in successive times. The total velocity is illustrated at the right. It should be noted that the velocity at the end wall is always zero. Keeping this state, if the other end of the tube is closed, then the velocity there must also be zero. Thus, only those velocity waves that become zero at both ends can exist. For a tube of length L, the first three such waves are illustrated in Figure 10–14. You can easily understand that the wavelength of such waves is determined by the length of the tube.

Since wavelength is determined by the length of the tube, waves of

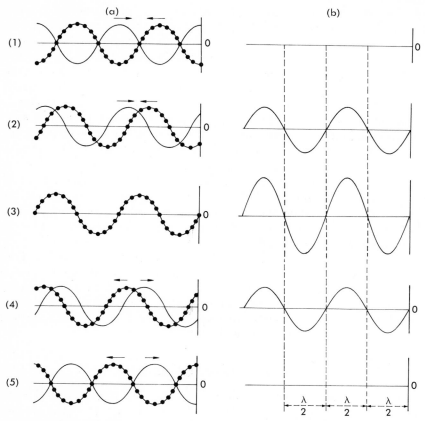

Figure 10–13 Velocity waves at the closed end. (a) Incident and reflected velocity waves. (b) Velocity wave.

other frequencies (i.e., other wavelengths) die out quickly, while waves of this particular length, or frequency, remain for a long time. A tube like this is a *resonator,* and the frequency of the wave remaining for a long time is called a *resonant frequency* or a *resonance.* The lowest resonant frequency is the fundamental frequency, and the rest are called harmonics (i.e., whole-number multiples of the fundamental). In the above example, the fundamental frequency is $c/2L$, where c is sound velocity. All the higher harmonics are integer multiples of the fundamental frequency. For instance, assuming a sound velocity of 34,000 cm, the resonant frequencies of a tube of 17 cm are 1000 Hz, 2000 Hz, 3000 Hz, and so on. It should be noted that the fundamental frequency of a resonator is different from the fundamental frequency of speech sounds. The former corresponds to the first formant, while the latter corresponds to the pitch.

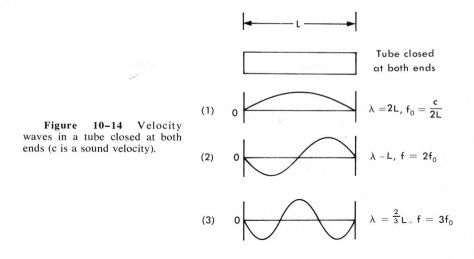

Figure 10–14 Velocity waves in a tube closed at both ends (c is a sound velocity).

If a uniform tube is open at one end and closed at the other end, the velocity at the open end is known to become maximum. The first three waves in such a tube are illustrated in Figure 10–15. Thus, the tube has different resonance frequencies which are also determined by the length of the tube L. The fundamental frequency is $c/4L$, and all the higher harmonics are odd multiples of the fundamental frequency. For instance, the resonance frequencies for a tube of 17 cm are 500 Hz, 1500 Hz, 2500 Hz, 3500 Hz, and so on. When we consider the vocal tract as an acoustic tube, the resonant frequencies correspond to the formant frequencies, but they are not in harmonic relation anymore because of a complex non-uniform shape. We can understand from this model that a short vocal tract has higher resonant frequencies, i.e., higher formant frequencies which are characteristic of the female and child voices.

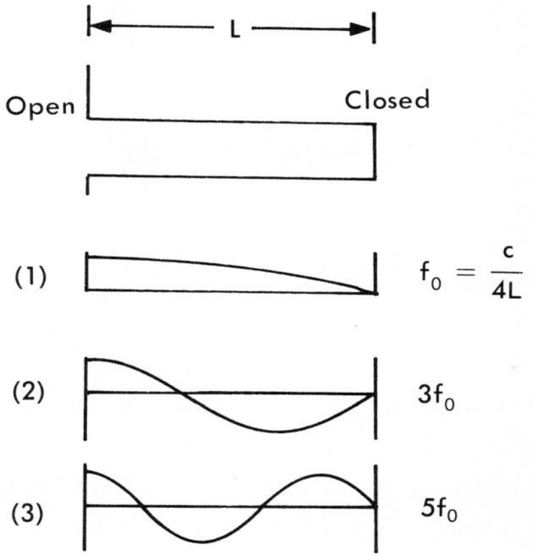

Figure 10–15 Waves in a tube open at one end and closed at the other end (c is a sound velocity).

Let us return to the speech synthesis model based on the non-uniform acoustic tube. The shape of the vocal tract is represented by the cross-sectional area along its length. Since the vocal tract shape is too complicated to be expressed by a continuous mathematical function, it is usually approximated by a concatenation of cylindrical sections of equal length. This model is more closely related to the physiological process of speech production than a terminal analog synthesizer in the sense that the variables for this model are the cross-sectional area for each cylindrical section. In a terminal analog synthesizer, the individual resonance frequencies of the vocal tract were represented by single resonant circuits which were connected in series or in parallel. Instead of controlling the shape of the vocal tract, resonant frequencies (formants) and bandwidths were controlled. Thus, the two models are intrinsically identical.

In practical synthesis based on the acoustic tube model, however, it is not easy to obtain the data for real configurations of the vocal tract. To obtain the vocal tract shape, a mid-sagittal x-ray photograph was used with palatography or a plaster cast of the mouth as a supplementary tool. However, x-ray technique is not suitable to obtain necessary and sufficient data, since the derivation of the tract shape is a laborious task and there is a safe dosage limitation of x-rays. There are some studies on indirectly deriving the vocal tract shape for the voiced non-nasal sounds, based on acoustic measurements or directly from the speech waves.

ARTICULATORY MODEL

In another type of speech synthesis which is most closely related to the physiological process of speech production, efforts are concentrated on the description of movements of speech articulators such as tongue, jaw, lips, etc. For this purpose, various techniques and mathematical models have been tried to obtain the movements of those articulators. However, in the actual synthesis of speech, the result of the measurement must be interpreted in terms of the cross-sectional area along the vocal tract. Easy transformation from the movements of articulators to the vocal tract area function has not yet successfully worked out.

ACOUSTIC PROPERTIES OF SPEECH SOUNDS

In previous sections, we studied the general acoustic aspects of speech production. Now we investigate more detailed acoustic properties pertaining to American English sounds. We can acoustically categorize speech waveforms according to the type of excitation source. Among voiced sounds, when only the laryngeal source is employed to produce a sound, the resultant waveform will usually have a quasi-periodic component in it. Vowel sounds, for example, have quasi-periodic waveforms. Some voiced sounds have double-periodic waveforms produced by the recurrent vocal mechanism: the waveforms for alternate periods correspond more closely than those for successive periods. Some other voiced sounds have irregular-periodic waveforms which are produced by the recurrent vocal mechanism and which vary in an irregular manner for successive periods.

In contrast to the voiced sounds, a quasi-random waveform results when a turbulent noise source is active during the production of a sound. Such sounds as the voiceless fricatives and sibilants, and the whispered sounds, have quasi-random waveforms. A speech burst is another wave type resulting from a noise excitation which has the form of an impulse produced by release of a closure in the vocal tract, such as in the production of stop articulations. Since an impulse results in an oscillatory response, the resulting waveform usually consists of the superposition of a complex oscillatory waveform upon a quasi-random waveform caused by turbulent airflow during the release.

When no excitation source is active, the acoustic speech waveform is defined as quiescent, and all values of instantaneous amplitude are approximately zero. A quiescent speech wave is produced during a voiceless interval, for example, when the occlusion of a voiceless plosive takes place.

WAVE TYPES

Peterson and Shoup (1966) defined the various types of waveforms described above as the basic speech wave types to describe a speech sound. In Figure 10–16, oscilloscope tracings of the basic speech wave types are shown. Some sounds are characterized by a composite form of more than one type of basic speech wave. The combined speech wave types do not always result in a simple superposition, but often result in a modulated waveform. Such a case, for example, can be seen during the production of a voiced sibilant in which the air flow against the edge of the teeth normally is periodically reduced or interrupted by the closure of the true vocal folds.

SPECTRA

Acoustic properties which appear in the waveforms are often not fully satisfactory to describe the various speech sounds. More often we seek equivalent acoustic properties in the frequency spectra of speech sounds. Acoustic parameters, such as formant frequencies, formant bandwidths, formant amplitudes, and fundamental frequency, are obtained and used as quantitative specifications of the acoustic speech wave. To obtain these parameters, various techniques are used, as mentioned in previous sections. Quite extensive studies have been made, especially by the use of the spectrograph, although the use of the digital computer has become popular. In the following sections, we study some

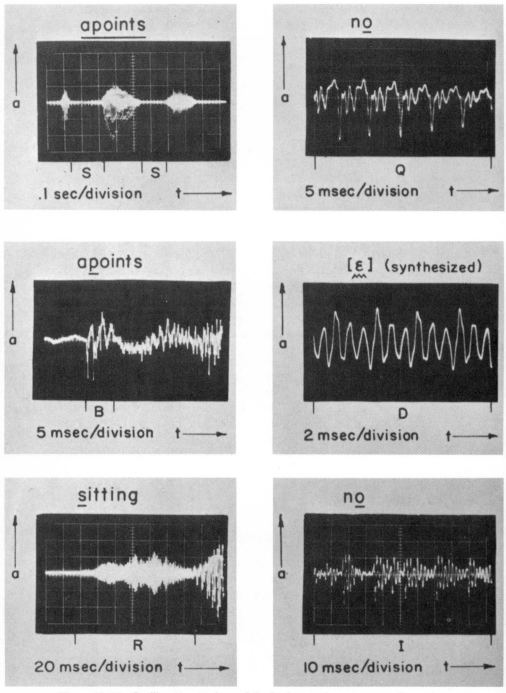

Figure 10–16 Oscilloscope tracings of the basic speech wave types: S = quiescent; B = burst; R = quasi-random; Q = quasi-periodic; D = double-periodic; I = irregular-periodic. (After Peterson and Shoup: J. Speech Hear. Res., 9:68, 1966.)

of the data obtained for different sounds, such as vowel, sonorant, fricative, sibilant, stop, and nasal manners of articulation.

VOWELS

The vowel sounds are produced by exciting the vocal tract with a
train of air puffs caused by vocal cord vibration. The vocal tract is con-
figured such that the pharynx and mouth form a transmission path for the
laryngeal excitation. The schematic configurations to show the position of
the tongue for each of the eight vowel sounds /i, e, ε, a, ɔ, o, u/ are shown
in Figure 10–17. If you consider these different configurations in terms of
the non-uniform acoustic tube model, you can easily imagine how the
cross-sectional area changes along the vocal tract for each vowel, thus
causing different resonant frequencies for the different vowels. For an
isolated sustained vowel utterance, the resulting waveform at the lips consists mainly of a quasi-periodic type of wave.

The study of vowel sounds has a history as far back as the first half of
the eighteenth century. Since then, vowel sounds have been studied in
various ways. However, the number of subjects to be analyzed was rather
limited before the invention of the spectrograph. Peterson and Barney
(1952) made extensive spectrographic measurements of the fundamental
voice frequency and the formant frequencies of vowel utterances spoken
by 76 different speakers. Averages of fundamental and formant frequencies and formant amplitudes for vowel sounds are shown in Table 10–1.
The 76 speakers included 33 men, 28 women, and 15 children. The
vowels were uttered in the context of "hVd," such as heed, hid, head, and
so on. As can be seen from Table 10–1, in general, children's formants are
highest in frequency, women's are intermediate, and men's are lowest in
frequency. More specifically, the first formants for children are about half

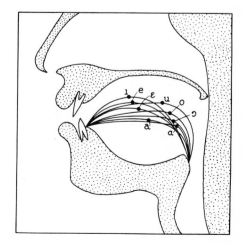

Figure 10–17 Tongue positions for
eight vowel configurations. (From Wise,
C. M.: Applied Phonetics. Englewood
Cliffs, N.J., Prentice-Hall, 1957.)

TABLE 10-1 *Averages of Fundamental and Formant Frequencies and Formant Amplitudes of Vowels by 76 Speakers*

		i	I	ɛ	æ	ɑ	ɔ	U	u	ʌ	ɝ
Fundamental Frequencies (Hz)	M	136	135	130	127	124	129	137	141	130	133
	W	235	232	223	210	212	216	232	231	221	218
	Ch	272	269	260	251	256	263	276	274	261	261
Formant Frequencies (Hz) F_1	M	270	390	530	660	730	570	440	300	640	490
	W	310	430	610	860	850	590	470	370	760	500
	Ch	370	530	690	1010	1030	680	560	430	850	560
F_2	M	2290	1990	1840	1720	1090	840	1020	870	1190	1350
	W	2790	2480	2330	2050	1220	920	1160	950	1400	1640
	Ch	3200	2730	2610	2320	1370	1060	1410	1170	1590	1820
F_3	M	3010	2550	2480	2410	2440	2410	2240	2240	2390	1690
	W	3310	3070	2990	2850	2810	2710	2680	2670	2780	1960
	Ch	3730	3600	3570	3320	3170	3180	3310	3260	3360	2160
Formant Amplitudes (dB)	L_1	-4	-3	-2	-1	-1	0	-1	-3	-1	-5
	L_2	-24	-23	-17	-12	-5	-7	-12	-19	-10	-15
	L_3	-28	-27	-24	-22	-28	-34	-34	-43	-27	-20

(After Peterson and Barney: J. Acoust. Soc. Amer., 24:183, 1952.)

an octave higher than those of men, and the second and third formants are also appreciably higher. These differences are due mainly to differences of vocal tract length among men, women, and children; women and children have shorter vocal tracts than men. From a uniform tube model you can easily understand that a tube of shorter length has higher resonant frequencies. An interesting fact to be noted is that vowel sounds cannot be defined by the absolute values of formant frequencies. All three types of speakers are capable of producing the same highly intelligible vowel with different formant frequency structures. This fact led to the hypothesis that the relative values of the formant frequencies determine the phonetic value of vowel sounds. Although various attempts have been tried so far to prove this hypothesis, there seems to be no satisfactory result yet obtained. A distribution of vowels by 76 speakers on the F_1–F_2 plane is shown in Figure 10–18. It is known that the first and second formants are most significant for the definition of the vowels. The third formant is considered to contribute increased exactness of phonetic quality, although it does not necessarily contribute to separate those areas that overlap each other.

Although less important to the definition of the phonetic quality of the vowels, the formant bandwidth (corresponding to the formant ampli-

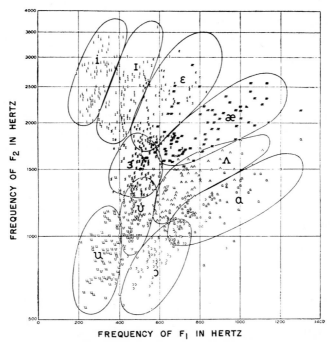

Figure 10–18   Frequency of second formant versus frequency of first formant for 10 vowels by 76 speakers. (After Peterson and Barney: J. Acoust. Soc. Amer., *24*:176, 1952.)

TABLE 10–2   *Average Half-Power Bandwidths of Three Vowel Formants (Hz)*

	Year	Number of Voices	Vowels	First Formant	Second Formant	Third Formant
Steinberg	1934	1	7	83	118	...
Lewis	1936	1	5	39	51	80
Lewis and Tuthill	1940	6	2	45	50	93
Tarnóczy	1943	?	4 to 9	110	190	260
Bogert	1953	33	10	130	150	185
van den Berg	1955	1	11	54	66	89
House and Stevens	1958	3	8	54	65	70
New spectrogram measurements	1961	20	10	50	64	115
30 pps measurements	1961	2	12	47	75	106

(After Dunn: J. Acoust. Soc. Amer., *33*:1737, 1961.)

tude) has been measured in various ways. The formant bandwidth gives us information for estimating the loss of sound energy involved in speech production. Such information is very useful, for instance, in the synthesis of high-quality speech. However, due to the difficulty of accurately measuring formant bandwidth, the results are not consistent among many studies. Table 10–2 shows the average bandwidths of three vowel formants measured by different people and by different measuring techniques. In general, the formant bandwidth tends to become large as the formant frequency increases.

So far we have looked at the acoustic properties of the steady-state portion of vowels. They get complicated in connected speech in which articulators are in continuous movement. The formant frequencies take different patterns depending on context, such as consonant-vowel (CV), consonant-vowel-consonant (CVC), etc. It happens quite often in CVC contexts that formant frequencies moving toward the steady-state values of the vowel from the initial consonant begin to move toward the final consonant before they reach the steady-state values of the vowel. The vowel sounds in this context are closely related to perception, and much remains to be studied. Some studies are being done with the aid of synthetic techiques in which we can vary any speech parameter in an arbitrary manner.

CONSONANTS

It is more difficult to describe the acoustic properties of consonants, owing to their short durations, less steady state, context dependency, and interspeaker variation, among other factors.

Although there has been a number of studies on acoustic properties of consonants, no sufficiently consistent acoustic properties have been obtained yet for many of the consonants. In this section, we review some of the acoustical analyses of consonants.

Fricatives and Sibilants

For the production of voiceless fricatives and sibilants, a frictional airflow is caused by constriction in the vocal tract, and the resulting waveform becomes quasi-random. In the production of voiced fricatives and sibilants, the laryngeal voice source is active as well as the friction source, thus resulting in waveforms consisting of both quasi-random and quasi-periodic wave types. It is observed in general that the /s/ and /ʃ/ have the highest relative intensity and the /f/ and /θ/ have the lowest, while /h/ is medium.

In the frequency domain, these sounds have energy components in a wide range of frequencies, normally up to as high as 10 kHz. However, due to large interspeaker variation, it is difficult to extract characteristics of each sound from the spectrum envelope to describe each phonetic value precisely. The energy contained in certain frequency bands has been found to be useful in discriminating these sounds. It is not clear, however, whether the fact is relevant to determination of the phonetic value of these sounds. Examples of frequency spectra for some of these sounds are shown in Figure 10–19.

From theoretical considerations, it is anticipated that the vocal tract configurations for these sounds produce formant frequencies and that the existence of a friction source at the constriction tends to produce anti-resonances. Although some synthetic speech studies of voiceless fricatives based on this theoretical consideration have given good identification and spectral matching, we will have to wait for more extensive study of fricatives and sibilants.

In perceptual studies, it was found that /s/ and /ʃ/ are identified more correctly by their steady-state portions, while the transitional portion is rather more important for the identification of /f/ and /θ/.

Stops

English stops are all plosives which are characterized by an acoustic burst resulting from a sudden release of a closure in the vocal tract.

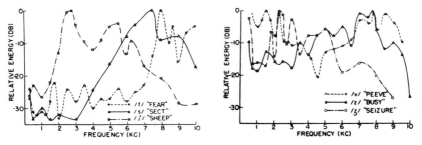

Figure 10–19 Spectra of some fricative consonants. (After Hughes and Halle: J. Acoust. Soc. Amer., *28*:306, 1956.)

Voiced or voiceless plosives are differentiated, depending on whether or not the laryngeal source is active during the period of closure. In distinguishing the voiceless /p/, /t/, /k/ from the voiced /b/, /d/, /g/, it is observed that in the production of voiceless plosives, more pressure is built up behind the closure than in the production of voiced plosives, thus resulting in higher intensity bursts, often followed by aspiration (which is not present in the voiced plosives).

It is known that stop consonants normally consist of three perceptually important portions: silence, burst, and transition. These are due to the complex movements of articulators involved in the production of stops. The rapid change in the spectrum is normally followed by a fairly long period of "silence," during which only the voicing component (below 300 Hz) exists. When a stop is preceded or followed by a vowel, the movement of the vocal tract configuration to and/or from the closure characterizes the formant transitions.

Some spectral properties of stop bursts have been observed. The bilabial stops, /p/ and /b/, have a primary concentration of energy between 500 Hz and 1500 Hz. The alveolar stops, /t/ and /d/, have a flat spectrum in which frequency components above 4000 Hz sometimes predominate, plus an energy concentration in the region of 500 Hz. The palatal or velar stops, /k/ and /g/, have strong energy concentrations between 1500 Hz and 4000 Hz. It is also known that the voiced stops have a strong low-frequency component due to the active laryngeal source and have less strong high-frequency components than the voiceless stops.

When a stop is preceded or followed by a vowel, the transitional portion of the CV or VC utterance characterizes the formant structure of the sound. The transition of the second formant is known to be especially characteristic. For example, the first and second formant transitions of /b/, /d/, and /g/ when followed by the vowel /a/ are shown in Figure 10–20. The second formant of /ba/ starts from a very low frequency and increases sharply toward the second formant of /a/. The second formant of

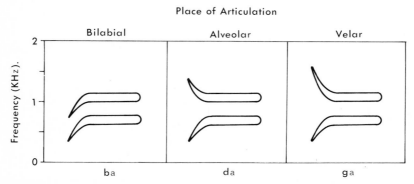

Place of Articulation

Bilabial   Alveolar   Velar

ba   da   ga

Figure 10–20 The transition of the first and the second formant frequencies of voiced stops followed by the vowel /a/.

/da/ starts from a frequency slightly higher than the second formant of /a/, whereas the second formant of /ga/ starts from a much higher frequency than the second formant of /a/. However, when these transitions are in the VCV context, they are affected by coarticulation with the initial vowel.

Perceptually, all three elements in a stop — silence, burst, and transition — can be cues for the identification of the stop. The silence especially is known to be a necessary cue for the perception of stops. For example, if the silence is filled by any type of sound except voicing, a stop is not perceived. The burst or the transition, plus the silence, are necessary for the identification of stops. The transitions of the second and third formants have especially significant influences on the perception of stops.

Sonorants

The sonorant consonants of English — /w/, /j/, /r/, and /l/ — are often called "semi-vowels" since they have formant structures similar to those of vowels. Waveforms of these consonants are quasi-periodic. Acoustic properties of the sonorants are known only qualitatively since the formant structures of these sounds are often influenced by the preceding or the succeeding sound, or according to position within an utterance.

Generally speaking, /w/ is similar to the vowel /u/, but has a lower first formant. For /j/, which is similar to /i/, the first formant is lower than that of /i/. For /r/ and /l/, the first and second formant frequencies are located fairly close to each other, and the third formant is relatively low in frequency.

Perceptually, the transition between a sonorant and the adjacent sound is also important. In this case, the duration of the transition is more influential than the rate of transition.

Nasals

Nasal consonants are normally characterized by opening the velum (thus making a passage to the nasal tract) and making an oral closure. The sound is radiated chiefly from the nostrils. The waveform is quasi-periodic, but its intensity is normally lower than that of vowels, mainly due to greater attenuation in the nasal tract and the small openings at the nostrils.

Theoretically, it is difficult to analyze the production of the nasal sounds, but we can get some gross features of them by schematizing the vocal tract and nasal tract configurations. Figure 10–21 shows one example of such schematization. In this case, the closed oral cavity acts as a side branch of the pharyngeal-nasal passage. It is known that a side branch causes anti-resonances which appear as dips in the output spectrum envelope. If we assume a uniform side branch of length L_m, then the frequency of the first anti-resonance is known to be $c/4L_m$ where c is sound velocity. All the other anti-resonance frequencies are odd multiples of the first one. If we assume a side branch of 7 cm and a sound

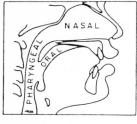

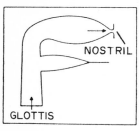

Figure 10–21   The upper figure is a tracing from a radiograph showing a midsagittal section of the vocal and nasal tracts during production of the nasal consonant /n/. The structure of the articulatory system is schematized in the lower figure as a joined three-tube model. (After Fujimura: J. Acoust. Soc. Amer., *34*:1865, 1962.)

velocity of 34,000 cm/sec (which roughly corresponds to the production of /m/), then the first anti-resonance frequency falls at approximately 1200 Hz. From this simple model, it is anticipated that the anti-resonance frequency of /ŋ/ is higher than that of /n/ and that of /m/, since the lengths of the side branches for /m/, /n/, and /ŋ/ become shorter in this order.

Figure 10–22 shows an example of a measured spectrum for the nasal consonant /m/ in real speech. In this example, the first anti-resonance appears to be reflected by the relatively broad dip in the spectrum. In a study by Fujimura (1962), anti-resonances for /m/ were observed between 750 Hz and 1250 Hz, those for /n/ were observed between 1450 Hz and 2200 Hz, and those for /ŋ/ above 3000 Hz. Based on observation of the nasal spectra, together with other synthetic speech experiments, it is generally considered that the nasals /m/, /n/, and /ŋ/ are characterized by low, medium, and high anti-resonances, respectively. The formants in the immediate vicinity of anti-resonance are influenced appreciably, whereas other formants are relatively intact. On the average, bandwidths of formants observed in nasal murmurs were comparable to, or greater than, those observed in vowels.

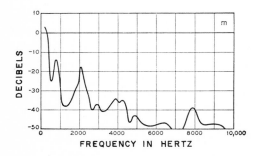

Figure 10–22 Measured spectrum for the nasal consonant /m/ in real speech. (From Flanagan, J. L.: Speech Analysis, Synthesis, and Perception, 1st ed. New York, Academic Press, Inc., 1965.)

Perceptual studies, however, have shown that highly intelligible nasals can be synthesized without anti-resonance, and thus, that the anti-resonance may not be essential for the perception of nasals. In the study of the perception of some nasal-vowel and vowel-nasal sounds, it has been found that perception was more influenced by the transitions than by the steady state.

PROSODY

We have observed the acoustic properties of vowels, sonorants, fricatives and sibilants, stops, and nasals. Suppose we can generate the acoustic waveform of any phone type with a certain duration and pitch from the acoustic properties representing the exact phonetic value of the phone. Then, by combining those waveforms corresponding to the individual sounds which make a sentence, we will get an utterance which can convey the minimum information pertaining to the sentence. However, as speech, it will sound quite unnatural. To make it sound more natural, we have to give it *prosodic variation*. What, then, are the acoustic correlates of prosody?

Suppose the sentence utterance is /ɪt ɪz faɪn/ (It is fine). First, we have to give an appropriate duration to each phone, connect phones with proper transitions, and then give proper fundamental voice frequency variation and voice intensity level variation such that they represent the intonation of the utterance as an affirmative sentence. If you want to stress the word "fine," you have to increase the fundamental voice frequency and voice intensity, and the duration of /aɪ/ will be, then, slightly lengthened. Thus, the important acoustic correlates of the prosodies which give some linguistic concepts are fundamental voice frequency, voice intensity level, and phone duration. All three parameters are correlated with each other, and it is a very difficult task to find the prosodic rules governing speech production in terms of acoustic parameters. Progress has been made in this area by the use of the synthesis-by-rule technique, and efforts have been made to unravel the intricate rules of human speech production. Yet, human speech is not limited to this stage. Besides prosodies giving linguistic concepts, such non-linguistic concepts as individual voice characteristics and emotional characteristics of the voice should also be understood.

REFERENCES

Fant, C. G. M. (1960): *Acoustic Theory of Speech Production.* The Hague, Mouton & Co.
Fujimura, O. (1962): Analysis of nasal consonants. *Journal of the Acoustical Society of America* 34:1865–1875.
Peterson, G. E., and Barney, H. L. (1952): Control methods used in a study of the vowels. *Journal of the Acoustical Society of America* 24:175–184.
Peterson, G. E., and Shoup, J. E. (1966): The elements of an acoustic phonetic theory. *Journal of Speech and Hearing Research* 9:68–99.
Potter, R. K., Kopp, G. A., and Green, H. C. (1947): *Visible Speech.* New York, D. van Nostrand Company.
von Kempelen, W. (1791): *Mechanismus der Menschlichen Sprache Nebst der Beschreibung Seiner Sprechenden Maschine.* Vienna, J. V. Degen.

Chapter Eleven

THE INTELLIGIBILITY OF SPEECH

Sanford E. Gerber

The Power of Speech Sounds
The Frequencies of Speech
The Temporal Aspect of Speech
The Power-Intelligibility
   Relationships

INTELLIGIBILITY
SUMMARY
REFERENCES

Since the ear is rather well-suited to the perception of speech, and since speech perception is really the main purpose of human hearing, it is important to know the acoustic characteristics of speech. The subject of acoustic phonetics is one on which we have a great deal of data, as shown in the previous chapter. In fact, present researchers are engaged in highly sophisticated and esoteric projects in basic research and clever technical projects in applied research.

Since speech is an acoustic event, we can describe it in terms of its frequency characteristics, its intensity characteristics, and its temporal characteristics. However, speech is an extremely complex phenomenon, and the critical nature of speech rests in those relationships which are most difficult to observe and describe. For example, it is difficult to describe acoustically the transition from one vocal sound to another; and this may be the most critical thing which occurs in the perception of speech. In any case, the marriage of speech and hearing is a good one. The acoustic characteristics of speech are among those to which the ear is most sensitive. In this section, we examine the characteristics of power, frequency, duration, and their various interactions and we also view some interesting problems in the intelligibility of speech.

238

THE POWER OF SPEECH SOUNDS

The power of the sounds of spoken English was measured nearly 50 years ago (Sacia and Beck, 1926). This measurement was sufficiently accurate and valid that the same values are used today. In Table 11–1 is a presentation of the power values in relative quantities as they are found in normal conversation. The reception of speech power is in terms of loudness, so it is well to know the *relative* powers of the sounds and the range within which they lie. For some sounds, we do not have information. The Table shows relative powers: the weakest sound, /θ/, was given a value of one; the most powerful, /ɔ/, 680. In other words, the loudest sound in our language is the vowel /ɔ/, as in f*a*ll, and it is 680 times as powerful as the weakest sound, the consonant /θ/, as in *th*ing; or /ɔ/ exceeds /θ/ by 28 dB.

The speech sounds of English cover a considerable range, but a range which is easy to hear. If one were to compare the power values with the area of hearing, it would be seen that speech sounds lie grossly within the middle ground of audibility. They are, in general, well above the threshold of audibility and far below the threshold of feeling. This means that they would be completely audible for the average listener and would not be distorted under normal conditions.

TABLE 11–1   *Relative Phonetic Powers of the Fundamental Speech Sounds* *

VOWELS		LIQUIDS, GLIDES, AND NASALS		CONSONANTS	
Sound	Relative Power	Sound	Relative Power	Sound	Relative Power
ɔ as in t*a*lk	680	r as in *r*ain	210	ʃ as in *sh*ot	80
a t*o*p	600	l *l*et	100	tʃ *ch*ief	42
ʌ t*o*n	510	w *w*et	?	dʒ *j*ot	23
æ t*a*p	490	j *y*et	?	ʒ a*z*ure	20
ou t*o*ne	470	ŋ ri*ng*	73	z *z*ip	16
U t*oo*k	460	m *m*e	52	s *s*it	16
eI t*a*pe	370	n *n*o	36	t *t*ap	15
ɛ t*e*n	350			g *g*et	15
u t*oo*l	310			k *c*at	13
I t*i*p	260			v *v*at	12
i t*ea*m	220			ð *th*at	11
				b *b*at	7
				d *d*ot	
				p *p*at	6
				f *ph*one	5
				θ *th*in	1

*Data from Fletcher, 1953.

THE FREQUENCIES OF SPEECH

In consideration of speech frequencies, one is primarily interested in a determination of energy distribution over frequency. If one has measured the power of a given phoneme, he was limited by the frequency response of his apparatus. Within the characteristics of the measuring system, it may be found that certain frequencies contain more power than others, and some frequencies may contain virtually no power. Moreover, there is a different energy-frequency distribution for each speech sound and for each speaker. An interesting thing is that we can all recognize the sounds of our language, regardless of who is speaking it. While the speech sounds are greatly influenced by the speaker, they must have sufficient characteristics of their own in order to be recognized independent of voice. In Figure 11–1 is shown the effect of a given voice upon the production of a vowel sound. The characteristics of the vocal resonance greatly modify the original waveform of the vowel; nevertheless, it must retain sufficient acoustic information to still be recognizable to the ear.

The drawings in Figure 11–1 represent a general case; however, while the laryngeal tone and the vocal resonance are different for every speaker, the vowel is consistently identifiable. The drawings represent what is known as a *line spectrum* in which the position of each line represents frequency, and height represents amplitude at that frequency. It

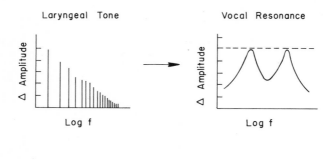

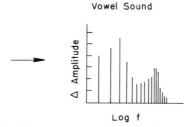

Figure 11–1   The effect of a given voice upon the production of a vowel sound.

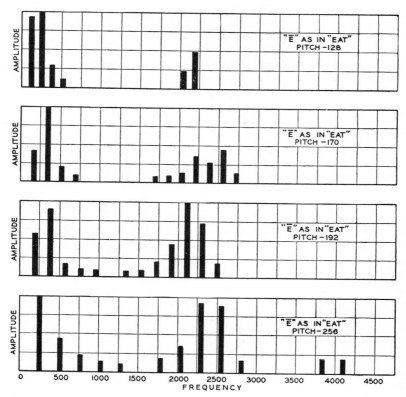

Figure 11–2   Line spectra of /i/. (From Speech and Hearing in Communication by Harvey Fletcher, © 1953. Reprinted by permission of D. Van Nostrand Company.)

may be seen that the frequency dimension is derived largely from laryngeal tone, and the amplitude dimension from vocal resonance. It is reasonable that for each and every phonetic event there must be some minimum number of spectral details which is sufficient to distinguish a given sound from all others. If one were to examine spectrograms of a variety of sounds, it would be obvious that they are very similar within or among speakers. Having this information, it is possible to draw simplified spectrograms unique for each word of a given vocabulary.

The particular frequencies which are represented in spectrograms are derived within the limitations of the apparatus. It is apparent, though, that even within these limitations there is enough information to specify a sound. A typical frequency range of a device for this purpose would be from 85 to 8000 Hz; this device, the speech spectrograph, was described in the previous chapter. The "formants" (concentrations of energy) seen in a line spectrogram must be within that range. This range has been found to be satisfactory in most applications. The fundamental frequency of the voice is rarely as low as 85 Hz. The average fundamental frequency for men is about 125 Hz, and for women it is about 212 Hz. So the measuring instrument certainly extends low enough for all but the rarest cases. The adequacy of the upper limit has been demonstrated empirically; that is, one doesn't find significant formants as high as 8000 Hz.

If we were to disregard the fundamental of the voice, apparently we can plot line spectra for various vowel sounds relatively independent of voice (see Fig. 11–2). The spectra are not entirely independent, however, since they do change somewhat with changes of the fundamental. Figure 11–2 represents line spectra for the same vowel /i/ (as in *eat*) with four different fundamentals. The upper diagram is for a fundamental of 128 Hz, and the bottom diagram is for a fundamental of 256 Hz.

Observation of the line spectra discloses significant features of the vowel /i/. There are certain common occurrences of energy at some frequencies. Detailed analyses of this vowel have revealed certain characteristic frequencies (i.e., formants), and they may be seen on the simple diagrams of Fig 11–2. They are in the areas below 500 Hz and around 2000 to 3000 Hz. If one were to examine line spectra for the diphthong /eɪ/ (as in *tape*), the 3000 Hz concentration would again be found. But for /eɪ/, the low-frequency characteristic is closer to 650 Hz. Even greater divergence obtains for /i/ or /eɪ/, as compared to /u/ (as in *pool*), where the high-frequency concentration is about 4000 Hz and the low about 1000 Hz. These concentrations will vary slightly among speakers, but seem to be sufficiently characteristic to distinguish among vowels. Characteristic

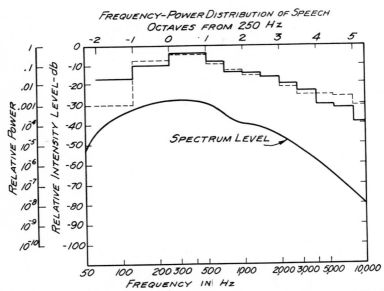

Figure 11–3 Frequency-power distribution of speech. (From Speech and Hearing in Communication by Harvey Fletcher, © 1953. Reprinted by permission of D. Van Nostrand Company.)

frequency concentrations have been determined for all vowels and most consonants. The total situation is summarized in Figure 11–3, which shows the relative power of speech in half-octave bands from 500 Hz up. Below 500 Hz, the device measures in one-octave bands. Measurements were made at a distance of 30 cm from the talker's lips. The chart in Figure 11–3 has as its upper level the average power for speech as a whole.

THE TEMPORAL ASPECT OF SPEECH

The frequency and power attributes of speech occur in time. When one considers temporal aspects of speech, the problem is seen to be twofold. The individual speech sounds present unique durational characteristics, and running speech presents rate characteristics. The matter of the rate of conversational speech is rather easy to observe; it is a simple counting problem. The average speaking rate for native speakers of American English is 165 words per minute. Trained listeners have judged fewer than 140 words per minute as too slow, and more than 185 words per minute as too fast (Hanley and Thurman, 1970).

The relative durations of the fundamental speech sounds do not have as wide a range as the relative powers of those sounds. The longest sound in English is the diphthong /aɪ/ (as in fly), which is four times as long as the shortest sound, the consonant /g/. In absolute terms, /aɪ/ is around 200 msec and /g/ is around 50 msec.

One of the nicer "matches" between speech and hearing is found in the temporal domain. Remember that the auditory modality has excellent temporal resolution, better than either the visual or tactual modalities. And speech is a serial signal, i.e., it is distributed in time. It is true that, in the production of speech, we coarticulate; that is, any given speech sound is modified by its phonetic environment. On the other hand, we perceive speech in discrete elements which are sometimes called phonemes. A phoneme is a speech sound which makes a difference; for example, "take" and "cake" differ by only one phoneme. Phonemes follow each other in speaking like the boxcars of a freight train. The sense of hearing deals with these speech events as they occur, that is, serially. Therefore, it is possible to talk about speech sound intelligibility as well as word intelligibility or even sentence intelligibility.

Again, although we produce speech continuously, we perceive it discretely. We do identify separate, discrete, independent elements of the speech signal. The matter of the perception of speech is the topic of the following chapter. The point to be made here is that speech perception is a discrete process. For example, given a sufficient quantity or duration of phonetic elements, a listener will make whole (i.e., categorical) judgments. Various speech sound segments can lead to different perceptual categories (cf., e.g., Gerber, 1971).

How do we measure the rate characteristics of conversational speech? We have already reported "too fast" and "too slow" rates of speaking in terms of words-per-minute (wpm). This can sometimes be a misleading unit. First of all, we don't speak in words; spaces between words are a property of writing, not of speaking. We don't pause between words. Secondly, all words are not of the same length either in absolute duration or in number of syllables. Obviously, polysyllabic words require more time than do monosyllabic words. So, perhaps we should make measurements in syllables per minute rather than in words per minute. The average rate of speaking American English is 440 syllables per minute.

Rather than inquiring about words or syllables per minute, it might be interesting to ask about the rate at which we say something. Verplanck (1958) has written about the notion of statements per minute in an experiment in which he was investigating the operant control of opinions. One of his principal findings was that reinforcement produced no significant change of the rate of making statements, and that the extinction level was (at the median) 5.2 statements per minute. Of course, one might debate about what constitutes a statement and how one can tell when one statement ends and another begins; nevertheless, this kind of figure may be more useful than either words or syllables per minute if we are interested in the rate at which language (rather than speech) is produced.

THE POWER-INTELLIGIBILITY RELATIONSHIPS

The relationship between vowels and consonants is an interesting one. We have seen that the vowels are more powerful than the consonants, and they last longer than the consonants. We have also seen that they are generally lower in frequency than consonants. One might consider these excesses as advantages, but the most critical measure of speech is its intelligibility. In Table 11-2 is a comparison of power and intelligibility in terms of frequency. It may be seen that the low frequencies (< 500 Hz) contain 60 per cent of speech power, but provide only five per cent of the intelligibility. The reverse is true for high frequencies — five per cent power and 60 per cent intelligibility.

The effect of this power-intelligibility relationship may be demon-

TABLE 11-2   *Per Cent Speech Power and Per Cent Intelligibility*

FREQUENCY RANGE (Hz)	PER CENT SPEECH POWER	PER CENT INTELLIGIBILITY
62–125	5 ⎱	1 ⎱
125–250	13 ⎬ 60	1 ⎬ 5
250–500	42 ⎰ ⎱ 95	3 ⎰
500–1000	35 ⎰	35 ⎱
1000–2000	3 ⎱	35 ⎬
2000–4000	1 ⎬ 5	13 ⎬ 60 ⎰ 95
4000–8000	1 ⎰	12 ⎰

strated in the laboratory. If one employs a compression device which reduces peak powers, the effect is to reduce the total contribution of vowels. It may be shown that considerable compression has virtually no effect on intelligibility. The percentages seen in Table 11-2 may be taken as suggestive of the relative contribution of vowels and consonants to intelligibility.

INTELLIGIBILITY

What are the properties of the intelligibility of speech? It is necessary for us to show here what is meant by intelligibility and what factors affect it. The American Standard Method for the Measurement of Monosyllabic Word Intelligibility (1960), in a footnote, distinguishes rather carefully between intelligibility and articulation. That standard points out that intelligibility is a property of meaningful parts of speech: words, phrases, sentences, etc. Articulation, on the other hand, refers to the repeatability or correct receipt of parts of speech which are not meaningful, for example, nonsense syllables or "logotomes." Traditionally, in speech research or in speech perception research, the terms intelligibility and articulation have often been used synonymously; they are not synonyms.

Hirsh (1952) defined intelligibility as the percentage of words correctly repeated or written down in any given test list. One might also consider the intelligibility of longer strings of speech such as phrases or sentences. The relation between intelligibility for words and intelligibility for sentences is discussed later. As a general rule of thumb, the intelligibility for sentences or for continuous discourse is about 15 per cent higher than the intelligibility for isolated words.

Many things influence the intelligibility of speech. Among them are the number of words to be intelligible, the bandwidth of the system through which the speech is heard, and the rate at which the speech is presented to the listener. Of course, one must always assume that his listener is familiar with the words in the list; that is to say, they are not words in a foreign language or words of a special or technical nature which he might not understand no matter how clearly transmitted. A similar concern, and one which was expressed in the literature by Lehiste and Peterson (1959), has to do with the recency of the words. Archaic words are, in effect, foreign words. For example, one word list which is commonly used for intelligibility testing was produced originally in 1944 (Egan). This list is still in common use, but it contains some words which are no longer in common use and which, for that reason alone, are not intelligible to the contemporary listener. One such word is "vamp." The word "vamp" has long since fallen into a condition of lesser use, and when many contemporary listeners hear "vamp," they respond with "ramp." This is not due to any failure of intelligibility, but rather to a failure of vocabulary. Upon hearing a word like "vamp," they reject it and substitute for it a word which is familiar.

PB Tests. It was Harvey Fletcher (1953) who did most of the pioneering work on what he called "articulation." He reserved the word "intelligibility" for sentences. If one were to examine Fletcher's 1953 book, *Speech and Hearing in Communication,* one would find many measurements of intelligibility (called articulation) which revealed several of the factors which influence it. It was not until some years later that more specifically *linguistic* attention was paid to the measurement of intelligibility. It was Egan (1944, 1948) who produced the phonetically balanced (PB) word lists. Egan argued, with considerably good reason, that if a list of words is to be a reasonable test of the content of the language for purposes of intelligibility, the elements in the list should reflect the properties of the language. To this quality he gave the name "phonetically balanced." There are 50 words in each phonetically balanced word list. Each list was intended to represent, thereby, the distribution of the sounds of spoken American English as it existed at that time. Actually, no word list does represent exactly the balance of speech sounds in American English, nor are the lists equivalent in balance to each other. There are two versions of the phonetically balanced word lists in common use. The first is the Harvard PB-50 word lists prepared by Dr. Egan during his tenure at the Harvard Psychoacoustic Laboratory during the early and mid-1940's (Fig. 11–4). A new list of phonetically balanced words was produced by Hirsh, who had been a colleague of Egan's at Harvard, and had gone to the Central Institute for the Deaf in St. Louis. There he produced CID Auditory Test W-22 (Hirsh, 1952). The W-22 word lists are identical in intent to the PB-50 word lists, but there was an attempt to rebalance them with respect to the content of the language and also an attempt to produce better quality recording. These recordings are still available. The differences in vocabulary between the PB-50's and the W-22's are very few in number (cf., Fig. 11–5). Still, both the PB-50 and W-22 sets of word lists intend to represent the distribution of speech sounds in the language and were intended for use in investigations of intelligibility.

An intelligibility test score is expressed in per cent correct responses when the test words are spoken either in isolation or in a carrier phrase. An example of a carrier phrase containing the test word would be, "You will write ____ now." Sometimes the test word comes at the end of the carrier phrase, as for example in, "Word Number Three is ____."

CNC Tests. The consonant-nucleus-consonant (CNC) word lists of Peterson and Lehiste (1962) are in many ways superior to the phonetically balanced word lists. Although CNC scores correlate very highly with PB scores, they have been updated by removing words which are no longer familiar. Also, unlike the PB lists, the CNC lists contain no consonant clusters. The purpose and organization of CNC lists are identical to those of the PB lists (see Fig. 11–6). The American Standard Method for the Measurement of Monosyllabic Word Intelligibility (1960), however, requires the use of the PB word lists. It further requires that if one does not use the PB lists, it is necessary to show the conversion from his scores

PB-50 List 3

1 why	26 size
2 turf	27 wedge
3 gnaw	28 deck
4 drop	29 hurl
5 jam	30 wharf
6 flush	31 leave
7 rouse	32 crave
8 neck	33 vow
9 sob	34 law
10 trip	35 stag
11 dill	36 oak
12 thrash	37 nest
13 dig	38 sit
14 rate	39 crime
15 far	40 muck
16 check	41 fame
17 air	42 take
18 bead	43 who
19 sped	44 toil
20 cast	45 path
21 class	46 pulse
22 lush	47 fig
23 shout	48 barb
24 bald	49 please
25 cape	50 ache

PB-50 List 4

1 float	26 new
2 sage	27 rut
3 cloak	28 neat
4 race	29 dodge
5 tick	30 sketch
6 touch	31 merge
7 hot	32 bath
8 pod	33 court
9 frown	34 oils
10 rack	35 shin
11 bus	36 peck
12 blonde	37 beast
13 pert	38 heed
14 shed	39 eel
15 kite	40 move
16 raw	41 earn
17 hiss	42 budge
18 fin	43 sour
19 scab	44 rave
20 how	45 bee
21 strap	46 bush
22 slap	47 test
23 pinch	48 hatch
24 or	49 course
25 starve	50 dupe

Figure 11–4 Some PB-50 word lists.

C.I.D. Auditory Test W–22 (PB Word Lists)

List 1A

1. an	26. you (ewe)
2. yard	27. as
3. carve	28. wet
4. us	29. chew
5. day	30. see (sea)
6. toe	31. deaf
7. felt	32. them
8. stove	33. give
9. hunt	34. true
10. ran	35. isle (aisle)
11. knees	36. or (oar)
12. not (knot)	37. law
13. mew	38. me
14. low	39. none (nun)
15. owl	40. jam
16. it	41. poor
17. she	42. him
18. high	43. skin
19. there (their)	44. east
20. earn (urn)	45. thing
21. twins	46. dad
22. could	47. up
23. what	48. bells
24. bathe	49. wire
25. ace	50. ache

List 2A

1. yore (your)	26. and
2. bin (been)	27. young
3. way (weigh)	28. cars
4. chest	29. tree
5. then	30. dumb
6. ease	31. that
7. smart	32. die (dye)
8. gave	33. show
9. pew	34. hurt
10. ice	35. own
11. odd	36. key
12. knee	37. oak
13. move	38. new (knew)
14. new	39. live (verb)
15. jaw	40. off
16. one (won)	41. ill
17. hit	42. rooms
18. send	43. ham
19. else	44. star
20. tare (tear)	45. eat
21. does	46. thin
22. too (two, to)	47. flat
23. cap	48. will
24. with	49. by (buy)
25. air (heir)	50. ail (ale)

Figure 11–5   Some W-22 word lists.

CNC Words
(Arrangement No. 1)

List 3A

fade	shock
rage	wail
man	cash
what	can
mirth	work
pack	wig
rice	shake
sung	foot
gull	war
noise	hoof
nice	give
net	size
him	said
toss	bug
well	purge
dose	life
dip	rat
long	rig
head	soon
shine	bar
toll	joke
numb	mill
pool	keen
keg	birch
till	for

List 4A

chin	chum
lake	mop
bush	rouge
bone	chief
more	gas
hire	house
with	keep
shut	peace
deal	perch
void	when
gap	faith
hut	vote
mate	right
date	pause
shake	leave
job	phone
take	lone
youth	room
thumb	tower
sheep	jail
reed	pike
pod	kid
yam	tone
bell	rage
dab	lap

Figure 11–6   Some CNC word lists.

to those which would have been derived had PB word lists been used. Since the correlation between the CNC lists and PB lists is very nearly 1.00, it is always possible to substitute CNC lists for PB lists.

Fairbanks' Rhyme Test.   The Rhyme Test of Fairbanks (1958) purports to measure intelligibility in much the same manner as the PB or CNC lists but with increased efficiency and economy. It is a multiple-choice test in which the listener is asked to select the stimulus word from six printed response choices. The choices are words which rhyme, so that the test stimulus is really only the initial consonant; however, it appears that Rhyme Test scores correlate highly with PB scores. The Rhyme Test has gotten increased use, owing to its high correlation with PB and to the relatively short time required to obtain a reliable score. There is another form of the Rhyme Test which is appropriately called The Modified Rhyme Test (House et al., 1963). The Modified Rhyme Test is identical in purpose and form to Fairbanks' original Rhyme Test, but contains words which vary only in the final consonant or only in the initial consonant. It is important to bear in mind, however, that the Rhyme Test does not claim any balance with respect to conversational American English. Moreover, the Rhyme Test does not claim that its several lists are of equal intelligibility. There is, however, a subform of the Rhyme Test which can be used when phonemic balance is desirable. Fairbanks, in his original 1958 paper on the subject, indicated which words would need to be selected from which of the Rhyme Test lists for achieving phonemic balance.

There are five Rhyme Test lists in the original version, each of which contains 50 words. In administering a Rhyme Test, the experimenter does not require the listener to write down or repeat his responses, as would be the case using PB or CNC word lists. Instead, the listener has before him an answer sheet (Fig. 11–7). On the answer sheet there are six choices for each stimulus, all of which rhyme, and the listener's task is simply to cross out the word which he believes he heard in the box containing six words. For example, one of the test words in the Rhyme Test lists is "hot." For that stimulus word, the listener might see in front of him a box containing the six words: "got," "hot," "lot," "not," "pot," and "rot." If he correctly identifies the word as being "hot," then that is the word he crosses out in that list. For the next list of 50 words, the listener will have before him the identical answer sheet. But this time the stimulus word might be "got." Now, from the same ensemble of six words, he is to cross out "got." Of course, he does not have his previous response before him to use as a guide. The reader can easily determine, then, that not only is the Rhyme Test simple to administer, but it also can be scored with great speed and convenience. This overall ease of administration has been what has often dictated the choice of the Rhyme Test for the evaluation of the intelligibility of speech. For comparison, Figure 11–8 is an answer sheet for a Modified Rhyme Test.

Free Conversation Tests.   Even before the development of the PB

Name _____
Form _____
Birthdate _____
Today's date _____

A		B		C		D		E	
got lot pot	hot not rot	fire mire tire	hire sire wire	den men ten	hen pen yen	din pin tin	gin sin win	fail nail sail	mail rail tail
day lay say	may pay way	bale male sale	gale pale tale	bark hark mark	dark lark park	bust gust must	dust just rust	fight might right	light night sight
cop hop pop	fop mop top	bent rent tent	dent sent went	boil foil soil	coil royal toil	fine mine pine	line nine wine	born horn torn	corn morn worn
feel keel reel	heel peel seal	boon loon noon	coon moon soon	big fig pig	dig jig wig	link pink sink	mink rink wink	cod hod rod	god nod sod
cake make take	lake rake wake	kick nick sick	lick pick tick	cage page sage	gage rage wage	bold gold sold	cold hold told	cock hock mock	dock lock rock
jaw paw saw	law raw yaw	came fame name	dame game same	cast last past	fast mast vast	bit hit sit	fit lit wit	bump jump lump	dump hump pump
bile mile tile	file pile vile	bide ride tide	hide side wide	gain main rain	lain pain vain	bed fed red	dead led wed	date fate late	gate hate rate
beat heat neat	feat meat seat	dip lip rip	hip nip tip	best rest vest	nest test west	bend mend send	lend rend tend	bell fell tell	dell sell well
book hook nook	cook look took	bore more tore	lore sore wore	bun gun run	fun nun sun	bid hid lid	did kid rid	bet let set	get met yet
bill fill till	dill kill will	bang gang rang	fang hang sang	deal meal seal	heal peal zeal	back lack rack	jack pack sack	buck luck suck	duck muck tuck

Figure 11-7 Rhyme test.

Name_____ Date_____ Test No._____

Form_____ Score_____

1	lick pick tick wick sick kick	14	sad sass sag sat sap sack	27	sung sup sun sud sum sub	40	cave cane came cape cake case
2	seat meat beat heat neat feat	15	sip sing sick sin sill sit	28	red wed shed bed led fed	41	game tame name fame same came
3	pus pup pun puff puck pub	16	sold told hold cold gold fold	29	hot got not tot lot pot	42	oil foil toil boil soil coil
4	look hook cook book took shook	17	buck but bun bus buff bug	30	dud dub dun dug dung duck	43	fin fit fig fizz fill fib
5	tip lip rip dip sip hip	18	lake lace lame lane lay late	31	pip pit pick pig pill pin	44	cut cub cuff cuss cud cup
6	rate rave raze race ray rake	19	gun run nun fun sun bun	32	seem seethe seep seen seed seek	45	feel eel reel heel peel keel
7	bang rang sang gang hang fang	20	rust dust just must bust gust	33	day say way may gay pay	46	dark lark bark park mark hark
8	hill till bill fill kill will	21	pan path pad pass pat pack	34	rest best test nest vest west	47	heap heat heave hear heath heal
9	mat man mad mass math map	22	dim dig dill did din dip	35	pane pay pave pale pace page	48	men then hen ten pen den
10	tale pale male bale gale sale	23	wit fit kit bit sit hit	36	bat bad back bath ban bass	49	raw paw law saw thaw jaw
11	sake sale save same safe sane	24	din tin pin sin win fin	37	cop top mop pop shop hop	50	bead beat bean beach beam beak
12	peat peak peace peas peal peach	25	teal teach team tease teak tear	38	fig pig rig dig wig big		
13	king kit kill kin kid kick	26	tent bent went sent rent dent	39	tap tack tang tab tan tam		

Figure 11–8 Modified Rhyme Test answer sheet.

lists, it was recognized that intelligibility may not be the only parameter of a transmission system which should be measured. As early as 1937, Grinsted described a method of testing "Immediate Appreciation." Basically, he conceived that transmission is satisfactory when two persons can converse without misunderstanding or strain. The development of the Immediate Appreciation Test was for the purpose of quantizing this principle. A transmission is judged to be satisfactory by the degree to which there is no misunderstanding or strain. While the Immediate Appreciation method has had considerable use by both the British and Australian telephone administrations, it has been recognized that scores so derived are difficult to quantize. In the effort to make the results of these kinds of tests more meaningful, the British Post Office along with other agencies of the British Government has developed the Free Conversation Opinions Test (Buck, 1959). Free Conversation Opinions Tests consist of having untrained subjects converse with each other over a transmission system and collecting their opinions of its performance by reference to a prearranged scale. The scale used has five levels varying from "complete relaxation possible" down to "no meaning understood." This test has been in use for a number of years but has had little use outside of England.

External Influences.   The preceding has demonstrated that there are various means whereby intelligibility may be measured. These means are roughly equivalent to each other. More importantly, all of the various tests are subject to the same external influences. The most directly obvious of these influences is simply the intensity or sound pressure level of the speech signal. Certainly, one of the questions which needs to be asked is: Can the listener hear the speech at all? Hirsh (1952) defined: "Having found the intensity (of speech) at which the observer reports that he hears something 50 per cent of the time, we shall have measured a *threshold of detectability*." The threshold of detectability, of course, is not very useful for the measurement of communications systems. One must assume that if the listener is operating at or below the threshold of detectability, the intelligibility is far below acceptable levels.

Pierce and David (1958) commented that "Intelligibility is the prime requisite for a communication system." That is to say, a message which is not intelligible cannot possibly be comprehensible. As Hirsh defined the threshold of detectability as that intensity level at which the listener reports he hears something 50 per cent of the time, so also he defined the threshold of intelligibility as *"the intensity of the speech* at which an observer can *repeat 50 per cent of the speech* that is presented." Again, all of us assume that we have an essentially high-quality transmission system and the vocabulary is familiar to the listener. This so-called threshold of intelligibility corresponds to what is also called the speech reception threshold, the threshold of intelligibility for spondaic words. It is defined thereby as the intensity level at which a listener can correctly repeat half of the spondees on a word list. A spondee, or spondaic word, is a bisyllable in which both syllables are stressed. Examples of spondees are: "baseball," "northwest," and "hothouse." Such words were employed by the Central Institute for the Deaf to make CID Auditory Tests W1 and W2. For a thorough discussion of the W1 and W2 word list, the reader is referred to any good textbook on clinical audiology, such as that by O'Neill and Oyer (1966). The name properly given to the 50 per cent score on the W1 or W2 lists is "the speech reception threshold." Figure 11–9 is a W2 list, and one may see that all the words are spondees but wonder why they should be. It is a property of speech perception that the longer the element, the more intelligible it is. Therefore, bisyllables, spondaic or otherwise, are inherently more intelligible than monosyllables. To assure this distinction in practice, then, one speaks of the speech reception threshold for spondees and the threshold of intelligibility for monosyllables. The term "speech discrimination" is employed when one has measured the intelligibility of monosyllables at some specified level above the speech reception threshold for that ear.

Frequency.   Clearly, then, the intensity of the signal is in some sense a parameter of intelligibility. It simply must be loud enough to be heard at all before it can be expected to be intelligible. An additional question was raised by Hirsh (1952): "At a given intensity, how intelligible is a given sample of speech?" The answer to that question depends upon the influence of many other acoustic and electroacoustic factors. First among these is the frequency bandwidth of the transmission system. When we speak of speech as being heard "in the clear," we mean face-to-face conversation at a distance of one meter. Speech transmitted over such a condition has an extremely broad bandwidth, extending from sometimes as low as 80 Hz perhaps to as high as 10,000 Hz. The low figure is chosen to represent the fundamental frequency of the most bass of male voices. On the average, superior male speakers employ a fundamental frequency in the neighborhood of 125 Hz. The upper figure of 10,000 Hz represents the uppermost frequencies found in some of the voiceless fricatives of speech such as /s/. It is our everyday experience that a range of frequencies from 80 to 10,000 Hz is not necessary for total intelligibility of speech. Our everyday experience is the ordinary telephone. The American telephone provides nearly 100 per cent intelligibility with a bandwidth of about 3000 Hz (200 to 3200). Does this mean, then, that the bandwidth of the transmission system has no effect on intelligibility? Of course, it does not.

What, then, are the exchanges of intelligibility for frequency? Miller, in 1951, reported the exchange of intelligibility for high-pass and for low-pass filters. If all the frequencies of speech below 3000 Hz were heard, there would be virtually no effect on intelligibility. Similarly, virtually no harm would be done by limiting the frequencies of speech to those found above 300 Hz. Figure 11–10 shows the exchange of cut-off frequency and per cent word intelligibility. It can be seen in that figure that the amount of intelligibility is the same above and below 1800 Hz. That is, if one heard only those frequencies found below 1800 Hz, the intelligibility of the

Word Lists for CID Auditory Test W-2

List A

Attenuation relative to level of first group		Attenuation relative to level of first group	
0	1. greyhound 2. schoolboy 3. inkwell	−18	19. baseball 20. stairway 21. cowboy
−3	4. whitewash 5. pancake 6. mousetrap	−21	22. iceberg 23. northwest 24. railroad
−6	7. eardrum 8. headlight 9. birthday	−24	25. playground 26. airplane 27. woodwork
−9	10. duckpond 11. sidewalk 12. hotdog	−27	28. oatmeal 29. toothbrush 30. farewell
−12	13. padlock 14. mushroom 15. hardware	−30	31. grandson 32. drawbridge 33. doormat
−15	16. workshop 17. horseshoe 18. armchair	−33	34. hothouse 35. daybreak 36. sunset

Figure 11–9   W-2 word list.

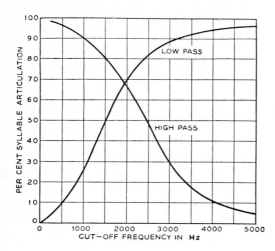

Figure 11-10 Intelligibility as a function of the cutoff frequency of a low-pass or a high-pass filter for speech of constant intensity. (From Pierce, J. R., and David, E. E.: Man's World of Sound. Garden City, N.Y., Doubleday, 1958.)

speech would be exactly the same amount as if he had heard only those frequencies found above 1800 Hz. You will also notice, however, that the amount of intelligibility at 1800 Hz is somewhat less than 70 per cent, a figure which leaves something to be desired. Clearly, however, the differential effects of high-pass and low-pass filtering are distinct. If we look, for example, at 1000 Hz in the figure, we can see that if we heard all the frequencies above 1000 Hz, monosyllabic word intelligibility would be found at about the 90 per cent level. On the other hand, if our hearing were limited to those frequencies found below 1000 Hz, our intelligibility score would drop to something below 30 per cent. This suggests that the higher frequencies are more important than the lower ones for speech intelligibility. Examination of the spectra for individual speech sounds will reveal that these high frequencies are found mainly in the consonants. That is to say, the vowel sounds of speech consist primarily of lower-frequency sounds, say, below 1000 Hz.

One might also want to say that the consonants contribute more to intelligibility than do the vowels. This is true, in fact, and can be demonstrated in writing as well as in speech. If one were to hear only the vowels of speech, or if one were to read only the vowels written in a word, one would find that word extremely difficult to decipher. Try the following example:_o_o__y__e. Now, if one were to read or to hear such an utterance, one would find it totally unintelligible. Let us try the following example, however: m_t_rc_cl_. One would have rather little difficulty determining that the word is "motorcycle." One would have had great difficulty in discovering that the first example was the same word. So we see that the intelligibility of speech is carried more by high frequencies and therefore by consonants than by low frequencies and therefore by vowels. Hence, one could use a rather narrow band of frequencies to transmit speech if that band were judiciously chosen. Pierce and David (1958) observed that "a total band of 1500 cps, from, say, 400 to 1900 cps, provides reasonable conversational intelligibility in most instances."

Test Vocabulary Size. What else besides intensity and frequency can influence speech intelligibility? Earlier we suggested that one of the parameters of intelligibility is test vocabulary. An additional aspect of that parameter has to do with the *size* of the test vocabulary. If, for example, the listener knows that the test vocabulary consists of one and only one word, and if he knows what the word is, then his intelligibility score will always be 100 per cent, provided the intensity is above the threshold of detectability. That is to say, with a test vocabulary of one known word, the listener will always be correct if he simply hears anything. What if the test vocabulary consists of only two words, and similarly, four or eight of 16 or 256 or an infinity of words? This question was raised by Miller, Heise, and Lichten (1951) in a study having to do with the relation between the intelligibility score and the intensity of speech with reference to the magnitude of a background noise. Of course, this implies further that the presence of noise in varying amounts can also be a parameter of intelligibility (cf., Fig. 11–11). From their study, one may observe that if the test vocabulary consists of only two words and if the signal-to-noise ratio is −18 dB (that is, the noise exceeds the signal by 18 dB), then the intelligibility will be only 50 per cent. That is to say, when the choices are only two in number, and when the noise level is very high, the subject will do no better than chance. This holds also for larger test vocabularies, so that at a signal-to-noise ratio of −18 dB, a test containing only four words renders about 25 per cent correct, and so forth. On the other hand, if the test vocabulary is very small, intelligibility can be quite high indeed, even for very unfavorable signal-to-noise ratios. Again, for a test with only two words, 100 per cent intelligibility can be achieved at a ratio as poor as −9

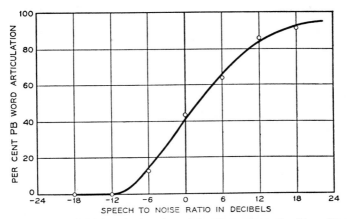

Figure 11–11 Intelligibility as a function of signal-to-noise ratio. (From Pierce, J. R., and David, E. E., Jr.: Man's World of Sound. Garden City, N.Y., Doubleday, 1958. Copyright 1958 by John R. Pierce and Edward E. David, Jr. Used by permission of Doubleday and Company, Inc.)

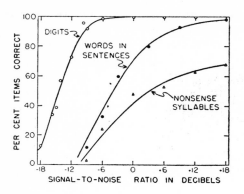

Figure 11–12 Intelligibility of three different types of speech material. (After Miller, Heise, and Lichten: J. Exp. Psychol., *41*:329–335, 1951.)

dB. On the other hand, if the test vocabulary is essentially unlimited (as it is potentially with a PB or CNC word list), then at −9 dB signal-to-noise ratio, the intelligibility is somewhat less than 10 per cent. So one can see that there is an exchange of noise level for test vocabulary size with certain limits. If the noise level is very high, then the test vocabulary size is not a relevant parameter. On the other hand, if the noise level is good, that is to say, if it is equal to or less than the signal level, then test vocabulary size becomes very important. At a signal-to-noise ratio of +3 dB (that is, an intensity level of signal double that of noise), the intelligibility of small test vocabularies is 100 per cent or very nearly so. For the essentially unlimited vocabulary at a signal-to-noise ratio of +3 dB, the intelligibility is

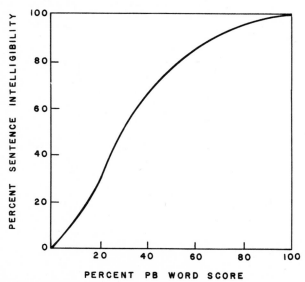

Figure 11–13 Conversion between word and sentence intelligibility. (From Egan: Laryngoscope, *58*:955–991, 1948.)

in the neighborhood of only 50 per cent. So again, it is apparent that test size becomes a parameter of intelligibility.

We mentioned earlier that the longer the utterance, the higher the intelligibility. This matter, too, was raised by Miller, Heise, and Lichten (1951), and their results are shown in Figure 11–12. That figure shows the effect of context upon word intelligibility. Again, if the noise level is high, there is no benefit from having words in context. But, even when the noise level is four times as great as the speech level (i.e., when the signal to noise ratio is −6dB), the benefit of context becomes apparent. The size of the benefit is about five per cent, but the intelligibility functions diverge. Therefore, one may observe that context renders an additional 30 per cent at 0 dB signal-to-noise ratio. Similarly, Egan (1948) measured the relation between word intelligibility and sentence intelligibility. Figure 11–13 shows Egan's conversion function. That curve shows the dependence of sentence intelligibility upon word intelligibility; 100 per cent for sentences requires very nearly 100 per cent for words; if words are unintelligible, sentences are also unintelligible. However, for values other than extremes, the higher intelligibility of sentences is apparent, so that fully half of the sentences may be understood when only about a quarter of the words are.

SUMMARY

All of the preceding suggests the limits of intelligibility to us. We have seen that intelligibility may be limited by the intensity of the signal. It may be limited by the relative intensity of the signal with respect to the intensity of a background noise. It may be limited by the frequency bandwidth through which it is to be transmitted, and we have a considerable amount of latitude in this parameter. We have seen further that a limit of intelligibility has to do with the nature and size of the test vocabulary which is to be intelligible. "High quality" means that the intensity was always more than adequate, that bandwidth always exceeded that of an ordinary telephone, that the vocabulary was familiar but unlimited.

REFERENCES

American Standards Association (1960): *American Standard Method for the Measurement of Monosyllabic Word Intelligibility, S 3.2.* New York, American Standards Association.

Buck, G. A. (1959): *The Conduct of Free Conversation Opinions Tests for Rating Speech Links.* Dollis Hill, Post Office Research Station.

Egan, J. P. (1944): *Articulation Testing Methods II.* OSRD Report No. 3802. Cambridge, Mass., Harvard University Psychoacoustic Laboratory.

Egan, J. P. (1948): Articulation testing methods. *Laryngoscope 58:*955–991.

Fairbanks, G. (1958): Test of phonemic differentiation: The rhyme test. *Journal of the Acoustical Society of America 30:*596–600.

Fletcher, H. (1953): *Speech and Hearing in Communication.* New York, D. van Nostrand Co.

Gerber, S. E. (1971): Perception of segmented diphthongs. Paper delivered to the 7th International Congress of Phonetic Sciences, Montreal.

Grinsted, W. H. (1937): The statistical assessment of standards of telephone transmission. *Siemens Magazine* (Engineering Supplement), No. 140.

Hanley, T. D., and Thurman, W. (1970): *Developing Vocal Skills.* (2nd Ed.) New York, Holt, Rinehart & Winston.

Hirsh, I. J. (1952): *The Measurement of Hearing.* New York, McGraw-Hill Book Co.

House, A. S., Williams, C., Hecker, M. H. L., and Kryter, K. D. (1963): *Psychoacoustic Speech Tests: A Modified Rhyme Test.* Cambridge, Bolt, Beranek & Newman.

Lehiste, I., and Peterson, G. E. (1959): Linguistic considerations in the study of speech intelligibility. *Journal of the Acoustical Society of America 31*:280–286.

Miller, G. A. (1951): *Language and Communication.* New York, McGraw-Hill Book Co.

Miller, G. A., Heise, G. A., and Lichten, W. (1951): The intelligibility of speech as a function of the context of the test materials. *Journal of Experimental Psychology 41*:329–335.

O'Neill, J. J., and Oyer, H. (1966): *Applied Audiometry.* New York, Dodd, Mead & Co.

Peterson, G. E., and Lehiste, I. (1962): Revised CNC lists for auditory tests. *Journal of Speech and Hearing Disorders 27*:62–70.

Pierce, J. R., and David, E. E., Jr. (1958): *Man's World of Sound.* New York, Doubleday & Co.

Sacia, C. F., and Beck, C. J. (1926): The power of the fundamental speech sounds. *Bell System Technical Journal 5*:393–403.

Verplanck, W. S. (1958): The control of the content of conversation: reinforcement of statements of opinion. *In* E. E. Maccoby, T. M. Newcomb, and E. I. Hartley (eds.): *Readings in Social Psychology.* New York, Holt, Rinehart & Winston.

Chapter Twelve

THE PERCEPTION
OF SPEECH

MARK P. HAGGARD

INTRODUCTION

Men have probably been listening to one another talk for hundreds of thousands of years, but this is not long enough for speech to have significantly influenced the evolution of the basic hearing mechanism. Non-linguistic requirements, such as spatial localization, have kept it essentially similar to the mechanism in other higher mammals. Apart from the link between speech perception and the cerebral localization of general language processes, we have as yet no physiological evidence of biological specialization for speech perception. Physiological and psychological acoustics contribute only indirectly to our picture of the way meaningful information is extracted from speech sounds. This account is at the psychological level. We have to know something about the *structure* of the information that is handled as the perceptual processes exploit that structure. Thus, we also require some acquaintance with phonetics and, to a certain extent, linguistics.

In this chapter we are concerned with essential concepts rather than

261

with the full range of empirical results on speech perception (for which the reader is referred to Studdert-Kennedy, 1972). A complete picture of speech perception would include the ways in which speech conveys emotional and attitudinal information. While this extra-linguistic, non-categorical information is very important, a scientific account of it is far off as the physical variables involved are just beginning to emerge.

DEFINITIONS

While this is not a treatise on phonetics, it is important that the reader be acquainted with some concepts of acoustic phonetics. A major treatise has been done on this subject, and the serious student is referred to Fant (1960).

In Chapter 10 we were introduced to the concept of "formant." A formant is a concentration of energy in a speech spectrum revealed as a peak in the spectral envelope or a dark concentration in the spectrogram. The formants are determined by the shape of the vocal tract above the glottis, and they are essentially independent of the glottal source. The term "glottal source" refers to the activity of the vocal cords which open and close quite rapidly, producing voiced speech. Later in this chapter we discuss the "voice onset time" which means the time when the vocal cords begin vibrating. For many speech sounds the vocal cords do not vibrate; they remain open, permitting the free passage of air. In such a case we speak of a voiceless sound (e.g., /s/) which gains its character by virtue of a constriction in the vocal tract above the glottis. These notions derive from a theory of speech production described as a *source-filter* theory which describes the activity of the vocal cords (or other constriction) as a source and the shape of the vocal tract as a filter (cf. Chapter 10) which modifies the source. This has been discussed recently by Lieberman (1972).

We may also refer to the acoustic properties of speech sounds (particularly consonants) by the nature of the noise caused by a constriction: fricatives, affricates, and stops. These sounds may be voiced or voiceless, that is, they may occur with or without a glottal source. A *fricative* consonant is one which is characterized by turbulent noise; a voiceless fricative, then, is one which consists only of such noise, while a voiced fricative is one which adds a glottal source to the turbulence. Examples of American English fricative pairs include /s/ (voiceless) and /z/ (voiced), /f/ and /v/, /Θ/ as in "*th*igh" and /Λ/ as in "*th*y." *Affricates*, like fricatives, are characterized by the presence of turbulence in addition to a momentary obstruction of the flow of air through the vocal tract. In a sense, affricates are a combination of stop and fricative. American English affricates are limited to the pair /tʃ/ as in "*ch*urch" and /Λ/ as in "*j*udge." Other affricates occur in some other languages. *Stops* (sometimes called plosives or stop-plosives) are characterized by a sudden rapid closing and opening of a constriction somewhere in the vocal tract. This results in a very brief stop of the airflow with an accompanying stop, often not quite complete, of acoustic energy followed by an abrupt resumption of airflow and energy. Again, this may or may not be accompanied by a glottal source, resulting in such pairs as /p/ and /b/ or /t/ and /d/. *Nasals* (/m/, /n/, /ŋ/) are made by admitting airflow to the nasal passages, resulting in voiced sounds of medium intensity, of relatively stable quality, for about 100 msec. The classes of sounds underlined so far differ in manner. Within each class there are differences of place of production that are reflected as differences of auditory quality, that is, of their formant frequency patterns (See Chapter 10 and also Figure 12–1.) *Vowels,* on the other hand, are always voiced and do not have complete constriction. Probably, the perception of vowels depends upon their steady-state (i.e., unchanging) properties, while consonant perception depends upon the dynamics (i.e., transitions) of their spectra.

CONTEXT

In connected speech the various sounds do not occur alone. They are found in association with other speech sounds with which they interact in such a way that it is hard to say where one ends and the next begins. Their representation is neither discrete in time nor absolute in the acoustical dimensions of intensity and frequency. However, meanings are conveyed in combinations of a set of discrete categorical units; this is a defining attribute of human language which creates a problem for perceptual processes since the parameters of the speech signal are essentially continuous. Most of this continuous information can be seen in the speech sound spectrogram (cf., Chapter 10). Formant movements reflect, in a fairly complicated way, the slow changes of articulator position as the articulators constrict the vocal tract at different places. If this were the whole story, then we could simply say that specified articulations produce specified acoustic patterns. However, an articulation is not the same as a phoneme — the linguistic unit that carries differences of meaning between words. The articulators are subject to situational modifications; for example, in the sound sequence /tr/ as in "try," spectrograms usually show no separate /t/ and /r/. Instead, the attempt to produce the two sounds often gives a two-part compromise sound similar to the initial or final sound of "church," /tʃ/. Furthermore, for most consonant sounds, only some articulator positions are critical. The ones which are not critical for a given phoneme are determined largely by the positions required for neighboring phonemes, both earlier and later in the sequence. This gives rise to a second context effect: the influences of neighboring phonemes contribute to the detailed vocal tract shape (coarticulation) and, hence, to the acoustic output (Fig. 12–1). As a further complication, in fast speech the

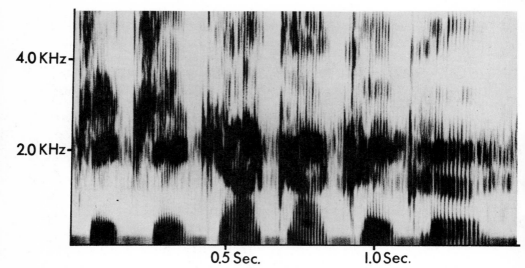

4.0 KHz

2.0 KHz

0.5 Sec.   1.0 Sec.

Figure 12–1 Coarticulation illustrated by changes in the formant transition and stop burst frequencies for /k/ in the utterance /kikikakakuku/. Note how the gradual lowering confirms that the tongue position and lip rounding parameters both before and after any particular /k/ have an effect upon it.

"target" position for a phoneme may not be reached by even the critical articulators. Phoneticians know these three types of context effects respectively as extrinsic allophones, coarticulation, and reduction. In speech perception we need to understand these effects because they produce the complicated relationships between acoustic patterns and phonemes. These context-dependent relationships are called *encoding* or *non-invariance*. Encoding is just as basic to spoken language as are grammatical transformations which affect meaning (Mattingly and Liberman, 1970).

These phonetic context effects require that our account of speech perception extend beyond psychoacoustics. In some sense, the perceptual mechanism must acount for encoding and must know about the factors which affect articulatory position. This is a complex task, executed very rapidly, and currently there is great interest in it. In this chapter, we are concerned with some of the ways in which the brain accomplishes the transformation from a continuous, context-dependent, acoustical representation to a discrete, categorical, *linguistic* representation.

PROSODY

There is yet another type of context which operates in speech perception. There are strong syntactic and semantic constraints upon words in sentences which are established directly by stress, pause, and intonation information derived from speech sounds and spread over the sentence. These influences, called *supra-segmentals* or *prosodic* factors are beginning to be understood. For example, the temporal pattern of fundamental frequency change and the relative durations of successive syllables are known to be important in the assignment of emphasis and in defining complex semantic and grammatical functions, such as interrogation and emphasis. Suprasegmental processing must take place simultaneously with the primary processing of speech. In addition, the identification of neighboring words can help to establish syntactic and semantic constraints; so, acoustical quality can be poor if context constraint is high, and vice versa. It has not been determined if global context information of this type affects the form or the accuracy of basic perceptual processing. Later we argue that it is economical for the basic processing to be passive, which implies that its form and accuracy cannot be changed even under extreme conditions.

VARIABLES IN SPEECH PERCEPTION

ACOUSTIC CUES

The chief acoustical variables which control the identification of sounds as members of one category or another are known for most languages. We also have some idea of the differences which the perceptual mechanism expects for different phonemes in different contexts. The results of Delattre (1965) on English and three other European languages show that the acoustical information below 4 kHz generally is most important. The critical acoustical variables for particular phoneme distinctions are known as *cues*. The cues for four important phonemic aspects of speech are as follows.

Vowel Quality. The main cues are the frequencies of the three (or even the first two) lowest formants during a short period between consonants. These values are taken relative to a particular speaker's average over several syllables.

Place of Consonant Articulation. The main cues are changes of the second and third formant frequencies adjacent to that part where output diminishes at the end of the articulation. For some consonants, the spectral structure of the sound produced by explosion or friction is also important. These values are also relative, this time relative to the vowel.

Manner of Consonant Articulation. The cues lie in the time structure of amplitude changes in various formant regions and in changes of excitation type (cf. Fig. 12–2). These cues give rise to identifications of the manners called stop, nasal, fricative, liquid, or semivowel.

Voicing of Consonants. The chief cue is the time structure of change of excitation type between glottal pulsing (for voiced sounds) and random noise due to supraglottal turbulence (for unvoiced sounds), as in stops and fricatives (cf. Fig. 12–3). But there are many cues. In prevocalic position minute differences in fundamental frequency can determine perceived

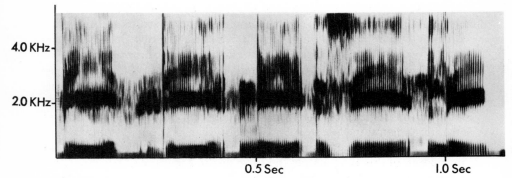

4.0 KHz

2.0 KHz

0.5 Sec   1.0 Sec

Figure 12–2 Spectrograms of /bi, di, ni, zi, li/. The /di/ differs from /bi/ in place of articulation and from /ni, zi, li/ in manner. The formant trajectories in the last four are similar because the vocal tract is constricted primarily in the same place, near the teeth ridge. Identification experiments have shown that the differences among the last four are carried by different aspects of the pattern. For the nasal /n/ a relatively steady state and relatively intense sound with characteristic frequencies is required, but the effects of nasalization also spill over into the vowel after the formant transitions in a way that is perceptually significant. Here effects may be seen in the F_1 region. For the voiced fricative, /z/, a low level voiced steady state must be accompanied or followed by a steady state of random excitation (fricative) with characteristic formant position. The liquid /l/ involves slower formant transitions, and, if there is not another consonant preceding it, a short steady state similar acoustically to a nasal in some respects.

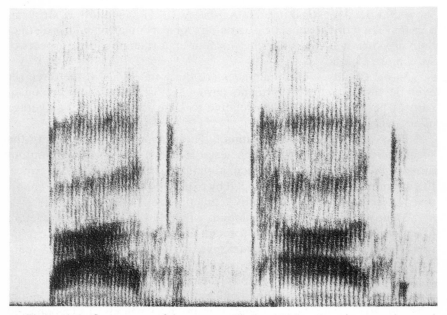

Figure 12–3 Spectrogram of the utterance "bad pad." Note the voice onset times and the formant transitions from stop to vowel and from vowel to stop.

voicing, and in final position the duration of the preceding vowel is important.

Most of the experimental work on acoustical cues has used the technique of speech synthesis (cf. Chapter 10) to give an approximate but controllable replica of the speech sound spectrogram. It has been found that the nearer the synthesizer output approximates a particular utterance from a real speaker, the better (i.e., more natural) it sounds. This is what we would expect; however, not all aspects of the spectrum are equally important for intelligibility. If we concentrate only on getting the major cues right, we can synthesize highly intelligible speech, although it will be in an unnatural, stilted style.

The cue concept is therefore a useful one; it allows us to describe the restricted aspects of the spectrogram on which the perceptual process *chiefly* depends and also to synthesize speech in an economical fashion. But we must be careful when talking about cues for a number of related reasons. We may discover that a certain physical variable makes a difference to people's perceptual responses but the way in which our measuring instruments lead us to express this variable does not guarantee the most exact, economical, and comprehensive specification of the cue. We find that it is often best to express cues as differences, ratios, or *changes* of the primary acoustic measurables; and there are both auditory and phonetic reasons for this. They more directly reflect the physical events being represented, and are more resistant to transmission disturbances. The "encoding problem" mentioned above may mean that a simple, yet general, acoustical expression of a cue is impossible, and phonetic context also has to be specified. Expressing a cue as a change goes part of the way toward expressing contextual influences, but there are still some cases where context may have to be specified more abstractly.

If we can sometimes contrive a perceptual difference by manipulating the phonetic context through certain acoustical changes in the vicinity of the acoustic cues rather than by changing the cues themselves, why then do we not call the context variable a cue also? If every variable were a cue, the description would be as complicated as the spectrogram itself, and the concept of cue would lose its power. We can avoid this by appealing to our knowledge of speech production: we can show that the context variable does not arise from the articulatory adjustments for a phonemic distinction, but from contextual aspects of articulatory performance. Therefore, a cue is established not solely by perceptual experiments, but also by insight into what information is being passed at each stage of the communication act.

Finally, adaptation techniques offer a way of distinguishing the effective cue extractors. After prolonged stimulation by a repeated stimulus pattern, perceptions change; that is, the feature extractors appear to become fatigued. Eimas and Corbit (1973) showed that the previous perception could be re-elicited by choosing extreme physical values, at least for the feature of voicing. Bailey (1972) showed the same effect for the place feature of stops. Because the adaptation in Bailey's experiments was restricted to individual formant transitions, we may conclude that adaptation takes place more at the level of acoustic cue extraction than at the level of linguistic feature decision.

PERCEPTUAL UNITS

The 24 consonants of spoken English can be specified as combinations of values of some eight articulatory features, such as stop/fricative or voiced/unvoiced. This mode of description appeals to the linguist who is concerned with characterizing a speaker's competence as well as to the psychologist concerned with accounting for how speech works. It is more economical to account for the perception of some eight consonant feature distinctions than for the perception of 24 individual consonant phonemes. This argument on its own does not give us any hint as to whether irreversible final decisions on linguistic units, such as features (or, for that matter, on phonemes, syllables, or words), actually occur in perception. Nor can considerations of economy alone determine which level of unit is the most psychologically important in any given situation. These are matters for experiment, but the problem of encoding must in general preclude a mechanism which makes a rigid series of perceptual decisions on features or phonemes which follow the acoustical structure of the utterance. But we can talk about "mapping" the input onto a phoneme string because apparently all that is retained (pending semantic analysis) is the critical information required to repeat an utterance. Nevertheless, a final decision about some feature of a particular phoneme may be suspended and then resolved only through a word identification or some other resolution of ambiguity.

Switching speech on and off or from ear to ear has been used to identify decision units. This process is most deleterious to intelligibility when it occurs at the average syllable rate (Huggins, 1964). This may be because chunks of this length in each ear lead to the switching action being interpreted as consonants because it sounds like a series of glottal stops. It does not mean that syllables are the only or even the important decision units. Indeed, it matters little exactly where in the syllable the switch acts, which rather suggests that syllables are *not* decision units. It is probably advisable to forget about units until we have some detailed models of how acoustical information in speech is processed. Then we may be able to say what the various levels of effective decision units are as each type of information gets processed under particular conditions.

FEATURES AND DIMENSIONS

The exact set of descriptive features to be used by linguists for distinguishing phonemes is open to argument. Therefore, efforts have been made to establish sets of feature dimensions by analyzing the pattern of confusions in identification tasks or in short-term memory tasks using nonsense syllables. Statistical procedures, such as factor analysis, have also been used to isolate the main dimensions which underlie confusions among items. Unfortunately, the results from these methods cannot always be given unambiguous interpretation. They may yield feature dimensions that totally conflict with the acoustical and articulatory facts, as Graham and House (1971) found with children's confusions. One problem is that confusion and identification arise at two levels: one reflects the arbitrary psychoacoustical similarities and differences between various sounds, and the other reflects linguistic feature dimensions. Factor-analytic methods have not yet cast any light upon the distinction between these two levels. In short-term memory tasks, however, confusions do appear to reflect those articulatory features which distinguish features in the listener's phonological system (Wickelgren, 1966). This is apparently because short-term memory relies upon an active rehearsal process using part of the speech *production* mechanism. The specifically *perceptual* role of features remains a relatively open question. Despite some claims, the adaptation techniques referred to above have not yet validated the feature (as opposed to the cue) perceptually.

MODELS OF PERCEPTION—AN ILLUSTRATION

It has been shown by Abramson and Lisker (1970) that, for English and diverse other languages, the chief acoustical differences between sets of unvoiced and voiced phonemes can be well summarized as "VOT"—the voice onset time (cf. Fig. 12–3). This time may be narrowly defined as the interval between the burst or release of a stop consonant articulation and the onset of periodic vibration of the vocal cords. In the articulatory realm, VOT corresponds to the time taken for the combination of muscular adjustment and restarting airflow to pull the vocal cords together into a position where they can vibrate and produce a regular train of pulses to excite the vocal tract. When a syllable beginning with a stop consonant is spoken repeatedly without change of rate or emphasis, the VOT is relatively constant. The VOT can be controlled by a prearranged setting of the degree of approximation of the vocal cords or by an actual command to close them at a certain time. These are the major adjustments used by speakers of English to make a difference between the voiced and unvoiced stops in initial position. The VOT is short (less than 20 to 30 msec) for voiced phonemes and long for unvoiced. In perceptual experiments, where the acoustical variables are fixed, the VOT can act as a cue to the voicing distinction in English. However, if we hold the VOT constant and vary other properties of the stimulus, subjects report differences in the number of times they hear /p/, /t/, or /k/ (unvoiced) versus /b/, /d/, or /g/ (voiced). Thus, there are other cues to voicing: for example, the number of /p/, /t/, or /k/ responses increases with the amplitude of the burst which occurs at the start of the stop articulation but decreases with first formant amplitude after onset of the glottal vibration (Delattre, 1965). Perception as unvoiced is also more frequent with falling pitch than with rising pitch at the onset of the glottal vibration (Haggard, Ambler, and Callow, 1970). This list of cues is slightly different when intervocalic and final positions are considered, and is slightly different again for voiced vs. unvoiced fricatives. The acoustical cues to voicing are multiple, even though the articulatory basis in any single speaker can be quite simple. But the situation is generally made more complicated, and communication consequently more reliable, by the use of more than one articulatory adjustment. Thus, the position of a stop consonant in a syllable determines which cues are most important. The problem for perception is giving appropriate weights and setting appropriate criteria for the cues in the position concerned. Other context factors which affect perception of voicing are the place of stop consonant articulation and the average rate of speech.

Thus, context effects in perception of voicing complicate the relationship between the critical articulator's position and the acoustical pattern produced, but the perceptual mechanism is able to solve the problem in each case. With slow, clear speech, context effects may not exert an important role as the cues take on distinct and unambiguous values; but many real speech situations are noisy, and people speak sloppily and in different ways. Thus, it is worthwhile for the perceptual mechanism to be able to retrieve individual feature distinctions such as voiced/unvoiced from minimal acoustical differences between sounds.

In the discussion of context effects, we have inevitably moved on from the barely psychological question, "What are the acoustic cues in speech?" to the highly psychological question, "How is the information in the cues processed?" This is a relatively new type of question, and not many of the answers are yet at hand. A model of speech perception, when that exists, may well be a family of block diagrams showing how the various cues are analyzed and mapped onto linguistic categories. This goal is still far off, but we can give some examples of limited block diagrams suggested by the study of context effects. Concentrating just on the effects of place of articulation, we found that perception in some way subtracts the effect of place when deciding voicing (see Fig. 12–4). Experiments show that this works in a rather specific way. Whatever the acoustical place information may be, the covert *decision* (right or wrong) about place appears to be what affects the voicing decision. We infer this because the distribution of voiced/unvoiced responses for stimuli of a given VOT is about the same within "wrong" /t/ and /d/ responses to stimuli normally giving identification as /p/ and /b/ as it is for "correct" /t/ and /d/ responses to /t/ and /d/ stimuli. Thus, the voicing response goes with the place *decision* and not necessarily with the acoustical place information, although the two are normally related. This dependence does not emerge in confusions of stimuli heard in white noise (Miller and

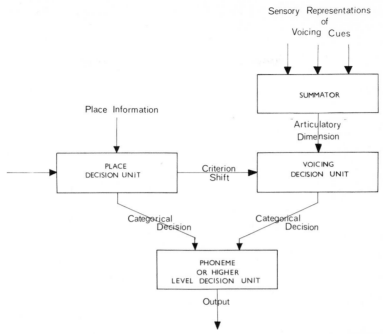

Figure 12–4 A block diagram model illustration of the operation of the place-context effect in voicing perception. Such diagrams serve to summarize our understanding of the process.

Nicely, 1955). Only with synthesized speech can one create the necessary condition of making *both* features ambiguous. With white noise the less distinct feature would become degraded first, making it unable to reflect a systematic relationship with the other feature. The finding of non-independence of the perceptual processing of the two features has been confirmed with a different technique. Inducing subjects to expect a single stimulus that is ambiguous on both features as a member of the /p, b/ set, results in a predominance of /p/ (i.e., unvoiced) responses; suggesting the /k, g/ set results in a predominance of /g/ (i.e., voiced) responses. The simplest pattern of internal information flow consistent with these results is that of Figure 12–4 with the place decision shifting the boundary value on the voicing dimension. It remains possible that the interdependence is partly at the peripheral level of the extraction of cues which contribute to both voicing and place, but that does not explain the induced expectation results.

Whatever final detailed model emerges from this research, it has been shown that there are ways of unraveling the processes underlying speech perception. We can ask again the old question, "What are the cues?" but with an orientation toward psychological processes rather than toward phonetic facts and linguistic generalizations. Inevitably this leads us to express perceptual mechanisms as block diagrams. One hesitates to call the diagrams "theories" because they are specific to a given distinction in a given language, and, possibly, parts of the diagram will be specific to an individual listener. Rather, they are detailed models around which a general theory might eventually be constructed.

UNIVERSALS AND BINARY FEATURES

The theoretical idea of binary distinctive features pervades discussion of both speech production and speech perception. This may result from asking more general — often biologically oriented — questions of the following type. How low in the perceptual system does the principle of categorical decision operate, and, specifically, decision between only two possible values of a feature? So far we have been talking as if the individual cues were extracted by lower psychoacoustical mechanisms as continuous variables which were then pooled onto some composite continuous dimension, best considered an articulatory dimension. This approach tends to emphasize the categorical processes that have arisen, presumably through learning, to deal with the arbitrary phonetics of one's own language. But a different emphasis is also possible.

Even if cues are multiple, they need not be registered as continuous dimensions, as we have assumed. They might be registered in a binary fashion as presence vs. absence of certain gross acoustical properties. As yet there is no very convincing evidence either for or against a "binary-properties" viewpoint, but it is a very interesting possibility for linguistic reasons. Some of the articulatory features of consonants are unquestionably binary — such as nasal/non-nasal — and it would be challenging to show that even those that were not binary in an articulatory description did initially affect the perceptual process in a binary fashion.

One intriguing experiment bears on this. Eimas et al. (1971), using selective habituation techniques, showed that very young infants can manifest a form of speech perception. When only two types of stop-vowel syllable appear in an experimental run, habituation of sucking following a stimulus syllable is more restricted to the syllable previously presented as the habituation stimulus. When the two syllables differ only in their values of VOT and associated lengths of voiced transition in the first formant, the habituation is most selective for pairs of syllables which straddle the normal English voiced/unvoiced category boundary. When an equivalent physical separation is arranged within a range of values that adult listeners would assign to a single category, habituation is not selective but spreads to the stimulus syllable not previously presented. The one-month-old infant thus exhibits a sort of categorical perception. Of course, we cannot conclude from this that either the category boundaries or the analyzers characteristic of the adult perceptual mechanism are innate. Several explanations are possible, among which the more likely should include: (a) while not yet linked to a linguistic system, analyzers registering the most frequent events in the auditory environment appear within a month or two of birth; (b) for psychoacoustical reasons, independent of language learning, certain ranges of temporal separation are more discriminable or there is a threshold value of extent of a formant transition that is detectable. This might explain why many (but not all) languages have evolved category boundaries at similar values on the VOT continuum. In summary, speech communication may employ discrete binary features because the production or sensory mechanisms (or both) are permanently set up to communicate via a restricted set of discrete states. Firm perceptual evidence on this point is lacking, but it has been convincingly argued that in production there are non-linear relationships between articulation and sound which constrain the variety of sounds that a speaker can easily produce into a set of categories, in some cases binary. Because encoding is such a great perceptual learning problem for the child, however, it is likely that the features used by language include a proportion with at least one salient acoustical correlate to which the auditory nervous system is especially responsive.

THEORETICAL VIEWS OF SPEECH PERCEPTION

MOTOR THEORY

Earlier we saw that the perceptual mechanism has to perform some quite sophisticated computation on the speech signal before decisions can be made, and that these computations appear to take some account of the mechanism that produces speech. One way of phrasing this idea has come to be called "the motor theory of speech perception" (Liberman et al., 1967). Actually, it is not a theory in the usual sense of that word. It is more an orientation designed to counter two less desirable orientations. One of these less desirable orientations was that of optimistic communications engineers of some 20 years ago who thought that speech could be automatically recognized by registering only direct cues to phonemic decisions from simple transformations on the raw waveform. The other orientation once prevailed among behavioristic psychologists: that the language code was exclusively a result of arbitrary cultural conditioning, categorical perception in speech being a general by-product of linguistic labeling and not indicating any special mode of processing peculiar to speech (Lane, 1965).

Contrary to the view that there is nothing "special" about speech perception, motor theory asserts that speech perception, in effect, is perception of events in *articulatory terms*. Let us call this a "weak" form of motor theory. We would not expect our internal representation of the speech mechanism to be perfect; by definition, categorical decision means a loss of information. We may infer that the perceiver's internal representation of the production mechanism need not be perfect to the extent of estimating precisely all articulatory parameters. It could use rules of thumb to enable economical shortcut processing. Such rules are called *heuristics,* and we may expect that further experiments will reveal many of the heuristics of speech perception. The idea of heuristics does not deny the existence of subtle constraints in speech, and the weak motor view can be held in this heuristic form without postulating an extremely detailed modeling of all the relevant articulatory constraints into the perceptual process.

Stronger versions of the motor point of view are possible. There are several arguments against the stronger forms of motor theory, of which two stem from its also implying an active, analysis-by-synthesis type of mechanism. The term *analysis-by-synthesis* refers to a process which synthesizes the signals to be analyzed, compares them with the signals for analysis, and generates an error measure. The process is repeated until the smallest possible error is achieved. There are basic logical difficulties with this idea. First, speech perception has to operate rapidly, especially as material may be allowed to accumulate to be decided upon in blocks longer than a phoneme. Any system involving even implicit production by the listener of a representation matching what the speaker is saying would be intrinsically slow. In a situation involving recognition of one of a large number of possible words, considerable delay would be needed to produce a set of possible matching representations before a successful match was reached. This is a conceptual disadvantage of any sort of analysis-by-synthesis theory, whether or not it advocates representations which are specifically motoric. Neisser (1967) and Stevens (1960) have presented arguments in favor of analysis-by-synthesis theories. There is some evidence bearing on this matter of delay in achieving a successful match. The element of active matching implies a selective mode of operation: a likely match from the list of possible words to be recognized is advanced first and compared with the input. The relevant feature analyzers have to be checked for presence or absence of the features which specify the phonemes of that word—in correct order. Insufficient correspondence will lead to no match being achieved, in which case another alternative will be advanced and a new set of analyzers checked. This means that we would have a *serial* searching model, and identification accuracy should be highest for first-matched alternatives. This should be so because storage of auditory information is imperfect, and during the period of unsuccessful matches it must become degraded. Thus, active analysis-by-synthesis models, whether or not the synthesized match is in a specifically articulatory form, imply greater accuracy for expected items; but this is not what the experimental data show. While a response bias is found toward the expected one of a small set of words (Haggard, 1968), no greater accuracy is found in distinguishing it from other words. Figures 12–5a and b give the general idea of models with active and with passive emphases. Note that a single over-all principle is probably not viable because of the many different levels of processing in the perception of speech.

Those who hold the motor view have suggested that an active ar-

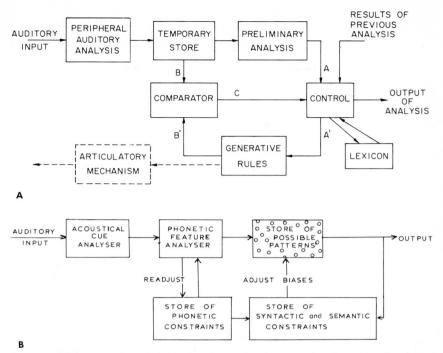

Figure 12–5 Two ways of thinking about speech perception, in terms of active or analysis-by-synthesis principle, after Stevens (1972), and a passive principle. It is not possible to say, in a way that is both precise and general, which of these models is preferable because they differ chiefly in how far up the scale of complexity of processing and in how far up the scale of unit size passive elements are involved. Another difficulty is that in a sufficiently complex network passive elements can contrive to simulate the function of active ones and vice versa. The active and passive principles are ways of meeting different types of constraints (memory space limitation and decision time limitation respectively) that must affect the perceptual process. In accordance with the respective general principles, adjustment of the analysis of phonetic features has been drawn in A as a function of higher level knowledge about what may have been said and in B as a function simply of consistencies at the same acoustic-phonetic level. In reality both factors appear to influence such adjustments. When we eventually have genuine models based on experimental data, they may turn out to have both active and passive components. (A, Reprinted from Language by Eye and Ear by Kavanagh and Mattingly by permission of The M.I.T. Press, Cambridge, Massachusetts. © Massachusetts Institute of Technology.)

ticulatory synthesis is economical by sharing certain processes between perception and production. The economy argument asserts that knowledge of articulation and knowledge of sound are the same, i.e., coded in the same nerve cells. But this economy is a real gain only if an extreme analysis-by-synthesis interpretation is already assumed. To economize on space (i.e., nerve cells) is to condemn the adult to a slow and painful recapitulation of childhood perplexity in every act of adult perception. Thus, the economy argument is a poor one for everyday speech perception.

Experiments show a lack of close relationships between perception and production in the individual. Denes (1967) found that practice in hearing one's own speech distorted did not specifically facilitate learning to hear correctly under the distortion. Bailey and Haggard (1973) showed that differences between individuals' productions of acoustical voicing cues did not correlate with corresponding individual differences in how the cues were perceived; this does not mean that correlations will not be found for some features, only that they may not be universal. Finally, there is no specific relationship between defects of articulation and defects of perception among children with developmental speech disorders. Children with /s/ defects are not relatively worse at discriminating /s/ than /r/ sounds (and vice versa), although /s/-defective children are generally more impaired perceptually (Haggard, Corrigall, and Legg, 1971). Thus, there is some support for the idea that an individual's processes of speech production are not *necessarily* relevant to his processes of speech perception, contrary to motor theory.

CATEGORICAL PERCEPTION

The motor theory was originally invoked to explain the phenomenon of *categorical perception*. While the acoustic cues for a distinction — such as that between /b/ and /d/ or between /b/ and /p/ — can easily be synthesized with a continuum of acoustical values between the extremes, perception of these classes of sounds is normally not continuous but categorical. Although we can produce continuously variable speech sounds, we normally perceive them discretely. That is to say, pairs of sounds differing by appropriate equal amounts on an acoustical continuum are well discriminated only if they happen to span the region (for that listener) which includes the boundary separating phoneme identifications. Physically equivalent, within-category differences tend to be poorly discriminated; this is also known as the "phoneme boundary" effect (cf. Fig. 12–6). There has been some controversy over the genuineness and interpretation of the categorical perception phenomenon. Lane (1965) has suggested that the effect is a general consequence of the trained availability of linguistic labels. This view underestimates the pervasive occurrence and compelling nature of categorical perception for the majority of naive subjects and its central role in our understanding of speech.

At one time it was thought that there might be a connection between the discreteness of articulatory gestures and the discreteness of perceptions, and that this might reflect the intervention of articulatory reference as a process for mapping sets of acoustic stimuli onto linguistic representations. But we have to divorce whatever we might like to say about subjective experiences of speaker's articulations, or about phoneticians' special judgments dependent on such experiences, from what we say about the process of identification by naive subjects. An empirical difficulty exists for the alleged link between categorical articulation and categorical perception. Unless very abbreviated and reduced, as in fast speech, vowels tend to be far less categorically perceived than stop consonants.

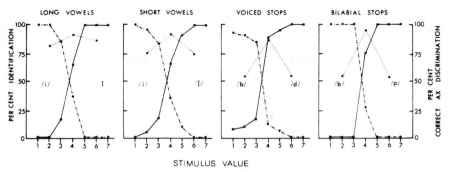

Figure 12–6 Typical data illustrating the phenomenon of categorical perception, from Pisoni (1973). For the vowels, the horizontal axis represents a physical continuum with equal steps in steady state frequencies of the second and third formants. For the place distinction /b/–/d/ the onset frequencies of these two formants at the start of the syllable provide the continuum; the frequencies are different but they co-vary. For the voicing distinction /b/–/p/, the continuum is provided by voice-onset-time. In each case the triangular-shaped dotted line curves, referring to the right vertical axis, represent the per cent correct discrimination of differences between syllables differing in small steps along the continuum. The pairs of crossed S-shaped functions represent the changes in the predominance of identification from one phenomenon to the other in the pair concerned. It can be seen that discrimination is better at the boundary than it is at the "within category" parts of the continuum where the predominance of one identification is very high. (After Pisoni: Perception and Psychophysics, *13*(2):256, 1973.)

This, along with data on brain asymmetries, suggests a special mode of processing for sounds which are "encoded." Motor theory handled this problem by excepting steady-state vowels on the grounds that they were more amenable to straightforward acoustical or musical processing; but one could equally argue the other way round. Vowels also have to carry information about speaker rate, identity, sex, and mood as well as contextual information needed for consonants. In contrast to this, consonants, especially the stops, employ rapid articulations giving brief, transient, encoded characteristics. These demand a rapid, passive, and heuristic treatment, oriented toward the most vital output—linguistic identification. This view is supported by studies of vowels and consonants in short-term memory and could explain the loss of information about all but the linguistically relevant aspects of the stimulus for consonants and the relatively good retention for vowels. We have come round to applying a type of motor hypothesis to vowels but not to consonants—the reverse of the original preference of the advocates of motor theory!

THE SPEECH MODE

There is strong subjective and objective evidence for a special mode of processing speech signals. This is the reason for saying that Lane's

(1965) view of categoricalness, while possibly correct in a limited way, is misleading in its assertion that there is nothing *especially* interesting about speech perception in general or about categoricalness in particular.

A compelling subjective instance of speech mode is the experience that accompanies faults in the parameter data controlling a speech synthesizer. If most of the data are correct, then the intended syllable is clearly heard. A small fault is heard separately as a "non-speech" residue—a buzz, hiss, click, or thump that quite detaches itself from the speech and is very difficult to locate objectively in time relative to the speech. That is, one hears a noise which is not speech, but one is quite unable to say precisely when in the utterance it occurred because a perceptual "filling-in" process renders the utterance itself clearly intelligible. If there are major faults, the whole utterance may not be heard as speech at all; whether it is or not depends both upon the listener's expectations and the gross naturalness of the utterance. Sometimes the listener's perceiving system suddenly switches into speech mode, and a confusing cacophony then becomes intelligible speech.

Turning to more objective data, we find that quite different patterns of performance can be obtained in speech and non-speech mode. Mattingly et al. (1971) compared discrimination for formant transition patterns corresponding to initial and final stop consonants at different places of articulation, and also employed an equivalent non-speech series ("chirps") consisting of the same stimuli but with the first formant missing. The speech series gave higher discrimination and also gave phoneme boundary peaks in discrimination that were lacking in the non-speech series. Furthermore, for speech the initial transitions were discriminated better than the final, while for non-speech the opposite was true. This suggests completely different sets of analyzers are activated by speech and non-speech stimuli, possibly related to different hemispheres of the brain.

Activating the speech mode is the major requirement we must fulfill before extending the results obtained with artificial stimulus patterns to perception of real speech. This satisfied, we have no reason to believe that the mechanism will rewire itself into a new configuration for the duration of our experiments just because our stimuli are not totally natural. We have to be careful on the response side as well. Unless we ask the subject simply to repeat what was said, we may be giving him an unnatural task, and an elaborate pattern of predictions may be required to relate the laboratory results to real life.

THE NEUROPSYCHOLOGICAL BASIS

At present we can say virtually nothing about the neural processes underlying speech perception, but introduction of more precise techniques in clinic and laboratory offers some hope of being able to say something worthwhile about the gross localization of perceptual functions. Occasionally, a brain-damaged patient is seen who has a virtually total incomprehension of speech but a relatively good audiogram. In one such patient seen by the author, there was no general language deficit as written communication with him was relatively easy, nor was it connected with acoustical perception in general as he professed still to be able to hear bird song and traffic noise and performed relatively well on pitch discriminations. Pathologies so specific in both modality and level are rare, however, and they will probably only contribute to gross anatomical localizations rather than make any contribution to the understanding of the neurophysiological processes of speech perception. This is because sufficiently large numbers of patients are unlikely to be given the same sets of tests over several decades to enable comparison of homogeneous subgroups.

A more promising approach involves investigation of evoked electroencephalographic potentials in the temporal lobe in controlled experimental situations. A difference has been observed in the averaged evoked left hemisphere potential for the same stimulus between conditions where the judgment required was a non-linguistic one (high/low) and one where subjects had to identify a stop consonant (Wood, Goff, and Day, 1971). Thus, electrophysiological techniques may well be able to assist our exploration of perceptual processes as well as to corroborate brain asymmetries, but few studies to date have incorporated the elaborate electrophysiological controls necessary for unambiguous interpretations.

We know that structured auditory perception demands intact temporal lobes. The left hemisphere (for normal right-handed people), dominant for other aspects of language, is dominant also for perception at the level of phonetic features; while the right is dominant for music, environmental sounds, and for non-linguistic information carried on a speech signal such as the emotional tone of an utterance. Demonstrations of asymmetry in neurologically intact subjects depend upon a psychological technique involving synchronized dichotic stimulation (cf. Chapter 9) and also on the anatomical fact that most ascending fibers from a given ear go to the contralateral cortex, tending to inhibit the ipsilateral pathways. Thus, for most linguistic tasks, we get a right-ear advantage (REA) in the normal, right-handed listener. REA appears to depend upon several factors, one of which is a predisposition toward linguistic processing. Another factor is the presence in the stimuli of acoustical features that normally bear an encoded relationship to phoneme categories.

In discussing speech perception, it is worth placing some importance on these results because they appear to be quite separate from another cause of REA. In language tasks, functional specialization of the left cerebral hemisphere is most clearly revealed by language tasks involving temporal structuring, and hence memory for strings of sufficient length to enable decoding of the temporal structure. Thus, if a string of words has to be processed or remembered, and the emphasis is put on word *order* as a syntactic cue, or if there is a stipulation to get the order correct in recall, asymmetries can be revealed with stimulation of one ear only.

The results at the level of speech-sound structure are functionally somewhat different. A dichotic presentation is normally required to show REA with nonsense syllables. Too much should not be made of the fact that many encoded cues, such as VOT and formant transitions, involve a fine temporal structuring. Vowel identification depends upon some sort of vocal tract estimation when there is more than one alternative speaker, and this condition is one which encourages REA. The functional asymmetry appears to characterize phonetic processing without a truly linguistic task; Doehring and Bartholomeus (1971) have shown REA for recognition of the speaker. In addition, Papçun, Krashen, and Terbeek (1971) have shown REA for Morse code; that is, linguistic structure without a speech stimulus. These last two experiments give a double dissociation between processing of lengths of linguistically structured material and processing of phonetic context; each can give REA in the absence of the other. Therefore, we have good reason to believe that there is cerebral asymmetry for the specific decoding processes underlying speech perception as well as for language processing in general. Why hemispheric specialization should extend to this level of performance can only be a subject of speculation at present. Possibly, the speech decoding processes are asymmetrically organized in the brain because they are activated on the same occasions as the higher-level operations on word sequences are activated.

Earlier we suggested that the rapid-transition information underlying place, manner, and voicing of consonants appeared responsible for the most robust of categorical perception effects. It also appears to be responsible for the most robust right-ear advantages, as especially difficult tasks have to be devised to make vowels show right-ear advantages. There is no evidence that this difference is due to phonological class per se: one possible underlying factor is the different contributions to acoustical storage by consonants and vowels. Vowels are acoustically distinctive and of long duration in stressed syllables; hence, a more resistant acoustical representation exists. This can be used as a basis for making the non-linguistic judgments of a discrimination task. It may also be available longer in the right hemisphere for transmission to the left hemisphere under dichotic stimulation conditions than is transient or degraded information, thus alleviating the competition for left-hemisphere categorical processing and reducing the apparent right-ear advantage.

This involvement of acoustical storage is consistent with the basic picture of the speech perception process given by the phenomena of categorical perception and REA. It now becomes virtually impossible to dissociate the role of encoded stimulus-response relationships from the role of poor acoustical storage because their physical correlates are so similar. However, we should not think of acoustical storage as a memory with fixed properties. Different survival times of different types of information in it will reflect the usefulness of those types of information to the perceptual system. Vowels provide a context for consonants as well as categorical information of their own. It is necessary to provide context for decoding some parameters of consonants, as well as extracting prosodic information that assists with syntactic and semantic analysis plus determination of the speaker's mood, style, and identity. It is only economical that speech production should have developed in a way that makes vowels long enough for precise auditory analysis. Preserving the results of this analysis in sensory storage for relatively long periods (up to about two seconds) is possible because of the relatively small amount of change involved in the acoustical pattern for vowels (and also for some consonants having steady states). In this light, acoustical storage (not to be confused with memory for categorically identified material) is seen as a necessary component of efficient perception. Information will persist and appear to endure in store in proportion to its usefulness in processing over protracted periods and also in proportion to its distinctiveness and acoustical simplicity.

CONCLUSIONS

From this discussion, speech perception emerges as a set of related automatic heuristic processes for transforming a continuous, variable, multidimensional, acoustical code into a discrete context-free string of linguistic units. These processes must be determined by the structure of speech signals possible with a human vocal tract constricted by a limited set of articulators, and also by the intrinsic limitations of the auditory system, although at present the former influence appears to be the more important and interesting. The perceptual processes are also constrained by the need to provide discrete categorical information for higher-level linguistic analyses. Information is lost in transforming to a phonemic string or equivalent, but such a representation appears to be held in short-term memory for repeating or for further linguistic analysis. There is a well-substantiated functional and neural separation between speech perception and non-speech perception or non-linguistic judgments about speech. Despite some possible analogies between levels, there is a separation between the phonemic level of perceptual functioning and those levels that segment the phonemes into words in syntactical relation or those that use the total linguistic message to revise an internal model of the state of the world.

REFERENCES

Abramson, A. S., and Lisker, L. (1970): Discriminability along the voicing continuum. *Proceedings of the Sixth International Congress of Phonetic Sciences.* Prague, Academia.

Bailey, P. J. (1972): Personal communication.

Bailey, P. J., and Haggard, M. P. (1973): Perception and production: Some correlations on voicing of an initial stop. *Language and Speech, 16*:189–195.

Delattre, P. (1965): *Comparing the Phonetic Features of English, French, German, and Spanish.* Heidelberg, Julius Groos Verlag.

Denes, P. (1967): On the motor theory of speech perception. *In* W. Wathen-Dunn (ed.): *Models for Perception of Speech and Visual Form.* Cambridge, Mass., The M.I.T. Press.

Doehring, D. G., and Bartholomeus, B. N. (1971): Laterality effects in voice recognition. *Neuropsychologia, 9:*425–430.

Eimas, P. D., and Corbit, J. D. (1973): Selective adaptation of linguistic feature detectors. *Cognitive Psychology, 4:*99–109.

Eimas, P. D., Siqueland, E. R., Jusczyk, P., and Vigorito, J. (1971): Speech perception in infants. *Science, 171:*303–306.

Fant, G. (1960): *Acoustic Theory of Speech Production.* The Hague, Mouton & Co.

Graham, L. W., and House, A. S. (1971): Phonological oppositions in children's speech. *Journal of the Acoustical Society of America, 49:*559–566.

Haggard, M. P. (1968): Selectivity in speech perception models. *Zeitschrift für Phonetik, 21:*70–73.

Haggard, M. P., Ambler, S., and Callow, M. (1970): Pitch as a voicing cue. *Journal of the Acoustical Society of America, 47:*613–617.

Haggard, M. P., Corrigall, J. M., and Legg, A. G. (1971): Perceptual factors in articulatory defects. *Folia Phoniatrica, 23:*33–40.

Huggins, A. W. F. (1964): Distortion of the temporal pattern of speech: interruption and alternation. *Journal of the Acoustical Society of America, 36:*1055–1064.

Lane, H. L. (1965): The motor theory of speech perception: a critical review. *Psychological Review, 72:*275–309.

Liberman, A. N., Cooper, F. S., Shankweiler, D. P., and Studdert-Kennedy, M. (1967): Perception of the speech code. *Psychological Review, 74:*431–461.

Lieberman, P. (1972): *Speech Acoustics and Perception.* Indianapolis, Bobbs-Merrill Co.

Mattingly, I. G., and Liberman, A. M. (1969): The speech code and the physiology of language. *In* K. N. Leibovic (ed.): *Information Processing in the Nervous System.* New York, Springer Verlag.

Mattingly, I. G., Liberman, A. M., Syrdal, A. K., and Halwes, T. (1971): Discrimination in speech and non-speech modes. *Cognitive Psychology, 2:*131–157.

Miller, G. A., and Nicely, P. (1955): An analysis of perceptual confusions among some English consonants. *Journal of the Acoustical Society of America, 27:*338–352.

Neisser, U. (1967): *Cognitive Psychology.* New York. Appleton-Century-Crofts.

Papçun, G., Krashen, S., and Terbeek, D. (1971): Is the left hemisphere specialized for speech, language, or something else? *UCLA Working Papers in Phonetics, 19:*69–77.

Stevens, K. N. (1960): Toward a model for speech recognition. *Journal of the Acoustical Society of America, 32:*47–51.

Stevens, K. N. (1972): Segments, features, and analysis by synthesis. *In* J. F. Kavanagh and I. G. Mattingly (eds.): *Language by Ear and by Eye.* Cambridge, MIT Press.

Studdert-Kennedy, M.: (1972): The perception of speech. *In* T. A. Sebeok (ed.): *Current Trends in Linguistics, No. 12.* The Hague, Mouton & Co.

Wickelgren, W. (1966): Distinctive features and errors in short-term memory for English consonants. *Journal of the Acoustical Society of America, 39:*388–398.

Wood, C. C., Goff, W. R., and Day, R. S. (1971): Auditory evoked potentials during speech perception. *Science, 173:*1248–1251.

GLOSSARY

Acoustic: designating things which have the physical properties of sound waves (e.g., acoustic energy).

Acoustical: designating things which deal with, but do not have, the properties of sound waves (e.g., acoustical measurement).

Acoustics: that branch of physics dealing with sound in all its aspects.

Amplifier: a device to increase signal amplitude.

Amplitude: the vertical dimension at a given point on a graph of a sound wave scaled in power, intensity, or pressure.

Aperiodic: describing a wave with amplitude changes which occur irregularly in time.

Audiology: the science of hearing in all its aspects.

Audiometer: a device for the measurement of hearing.

Audiometry: the science and technology associated with the measurement of hearing.

Auditory flutter: perception of the discontinuity of any interrupted sound.

Auditory flutter fusion: loss of the perception of discontinuity due to increased rapidity of interruption.

Basilar membrane: in the cochlea, the membrane which supports the end organs of hearing and which separates the scala media from the scala tympani.

Bel: a dimensionless unit (named for Alexander Graham Bell) expressing the logarithm to the base 10 of the ratio between two powers; hence, *decibel*: 10 times said logarithm, or one-tenth of a bel.

Binaural: designating *any* arrangement in which signals are heard with both ears.

Binaural fusion: designating the fact that one percept may be derived in spite of differences between signals arriving at each ear.

Binaural summation: designating the fact that the threshold of hearing for two ears is normally better than for the better one of those same two ears.

Categorical perception: the hypothesis that speech communication may function via a restricted set of discrete states.

Click pitch: perception of a click which seems to have some tonality.

Complex wave: designating a sound wave produced by combination of any number of simple sinusoidal components of different frequencies.

Compression amplification: a form of output-limiting modifying the shape of high-amplitude waves.

Critical band: designating the range of frequencies beyond which noise will not further decrease the audibility of a particular sinusoid.

Cycle: designating each completed repetition of a waveform; the number of such repetitions occurring in one second is the *frequency* (q.v.) of the signal and its unit of measurement is the *Hertz* (q.v.).

Dichotic: designating an arrangement in which each ear receives a different signal.

Difference limen: the just-noticeable difference of stimulus change observed in a specified number of trials.

Diffraction: designates the bending of waves around obstacles.

Diotic: designating an arrangement in which each ear receives the same signal.

Directivity: designating that some sound sources radiate more efficiently in some directions than in others.

Directivity factor: the ratio of the amplitude in a given direction to the amplitude averaged over all directions at a certain distance.

Distortion: designating a waveform change which is not desired.

Electroacoustic: designating relations and conversions of energy between electrical and acoustical forms.

Envelope: the overall output signal of an acoustic or electroacoustic device.

Filter: designating any acoustic or electroacoustic device which permits some frequencies to pass and discriminates against all others; hence, *low-pass filter:* one which passes all frequencies less than some value; *high-pass filter:* one which passes all frequencies greater than some value; *band-pass filter:* one which passes all frequencies between two selected values.

Field: the area over which a sound wave may be distributed; hence, *sound field:* designating one which is limited by reflections and boundaries; and *free field:* designating one free of boundaries, as in an anechoic (i.e., without reflections) chamber or space.

Formant: designating concentrations of energy in a sound spectrum, especially of speech.

Fourier analysis: designating that a complex wave may be decomposed into a finite set of sinusoids; after Jean Baptiste Joseph Fourier (1768–1830), French mathematician whose discovery this was.

Fourier synthesis: the composition of a complex wave from a set of sinusoids.

Frequency: the number of complete repetitions of a wave occurring per unit time.

Frequency response: the range of frequencies over which an acoustic or an electroacoustic device operates.

Fundamental frequency: in a complex wave, designating the basic waveform which repeats itself within a *period* (q.v.).

Gain: designating the amount by which the output amplitude of an acoustic or an electroacoustic device exceeds the input amplitude.

Harmonic: designating a component of a complex wave which is an integral multiple of the fundamental frequency.

Hertz: the unit of measurement of frequency named for Heinrich Rudolph Hertz (1857–1894), German physicist.

Impedance: indicating, in harmonic systems, a ratio between force and particle velocity important for *transducers* (q.v.); its unit is the Ohm.

Intensity: designating *power* (q.v.) in watts per unit area in square centimeters; therfore, the unit of intensity is the watt/cm^2.

Intensity level: in decibels, 10 times the logarithm to the base 10 of the ratio between a given intensity and a reference intensity; the reference intensity in acoustics is usually taken as 10^{-16} watt/centimeter^2.

Just-noticeable difference: usually called simply "jnd," is a name for what is now called the *difference limen* (q.v.).

Line spectrum: designating a spectrum with components which occur at a number of discrete frequencies.

Longitudinal wave: designates one in which the direction of displacement is perpendicular to the wavefront.

Loudness: refers to the intensive attribute of auditory sensations by which one may report sounds as being loud or soft, louder or softer; its unit is the sone.

Loudness level: or equal loudness, refers to the comparative intensive attributes of signals of different spectra; its unit is the *phon* (q.v.).

Mel: the unit of measurement of *pitch* (q.v.)

Microphone: an electroacoustic *transducer* (q.v.) which responds to sound waves and delivers essentially equivalent electric waves.

Monaural: refers to listening with one ear.

Monophonic: designates *diotic* (q.v.) listening to only one source of sound.

Monotic: designates an arrangement where signals are provided to one ear only.

Newton: designates the unit of force after the great philosopher and mathematician, Sir Isaac Newton (1642–1727).

Ossicles: the smallest bones of the body, the malleus, incus, and stapes, found in the middle ear.

Period: designates the reciprocal of frequency; hence, the period of frequency f is l/f in time.

Periodic: designates a wave with amplitude changes which occur regularly in time.

Phase: refers to any particular point of a cycle.

Phase difference: describes the relative locations of two waves at a point in time.

Phon: the unit of measurement of *loudness level* (q.v.).

Piezoelectricity: from the Greek *piesoein,* meaning to squeeze; designates a property of some materials to develop an electrical potential when strained; such materials are useful as electroacoustic transducers.

Pink noise: in contrast to white noise (q.v.), designates one with equal energy per octave.

Pitch: refers to that attribute of auditory sensations by which one may report sounds as being high or low, higher or lower; its unit is the *mel* (q.v.).

Power: designates the amount of energy transferred per unit time; its unit is the *watt* (q.v.).

Power level: in decibels, 10 times the logarithm to the base 10 of the ratio between a given power and a reference power; the reference power in acoustics is usually taken as 10^{-13} watt.

Prosody: designates the stress and intonation patterns of speech.

Recruitment: refers to the abnormal growth of loudness.

Resonance: refers to that property of mechanical or electrical systems which prolongs sounds due to reflection or reverberation.

Reverberation: designates the persistence of sound due to reflections in an enclosed space after the sound source has stopped.

Sensation level: refers to the level in decibels above the threshold of hearing for a particular ear, individual, or group.

Sensitivity level: refers to the response of a transducer being the ratio of its amplitude sensitivity to a reference sensitivity.

Sine wave: designates a periodic oscillation or simple harmonic motion.

Sinusoid: any waveform having the same shape as a sine wave.

Sound pressure: refers to the variation of air pressure due to a disturbance in the acoustic range; its unit may be the dyne per square centimeter (d/cm^2), the Newton per square meter (N/m^2), or the microbar (μbar).

Sound pressure level: in decibels, 20 times the logarithm to the base 10 of the ratio between a given sound pressure and a reference sound pressure; in acoustics, the reference sound pressure is usually taken as 2×10^{-5} N/m^2 or 2×10^{-4} μbar but sometimes as 1 μbar.

Spectrograph: a device which displays a sound spectrum from instant to instant.

Spectrum: refers to the array of entities arranged according to frequency; hence, the spectrum of a sound is its frequency content.

Stereophonic: designates an arrangement of signals differently in two transducers and heard diotically.

Temporal numerosity: refers to an observer's accuracy in reporting the number of signals presented.

Threshold: in psychophysics, the physical value of a stimulus to which an observer will respond a specified number of times, usually 50 per cent.

Threshold of audibility: designates the sound pressure level which will evoke a response on a specified fraction of trials by one or some listeners.

Timbre: usually designates the quality of sound whereby a listener may distinguish between two sounds of equal pitch and loudness.

Transducer: a device capable of converting one form of energy to another (e.g., electroacoustic transducer).

Watt: the unit of measurement of power named for James Watt (1736–1819), Scottish inventor.

Wavelength: designates the distance between any two analogous points on a wave.

White noise: refers to a random noise with equal energy per cycle.

GENERAL REFERENCES

It has become evident that there are certain books and journals pervaded by the kinds of information we have discussed. This list is not a bibliography of the whole text; it is a list of the most important, most general works. A serious student should be familiar with them all.

Beranek, L. L. (1954): *Acoustics*. New York, McGraw-Hill Book Co., Inc.
Beranek, L. L. (ed.) (1971): *Noise and Vibration Control*. New York, McGraw-Hill Book Co., Inc.
Davis, H., and Silverman, S. R. (1970): *Hearing and Deafness* (3rd ed.). New York, Holt, Rinehart and Winston, Inc.
Fant, G. (1960): *Acoustic Theory of Speech Production*. The Hague, Mouton and Co.
Fletcher, H. (1953): *Speech and Hearing in Communication*. New York, D. van Nostrand Co.
Green, D. M., and Swets, J. A. (1966): *Signal Detection Theory and Psychophysics*. New York, John Wiley and Sons, Inc.
Hirsh, I. J. (1952): *The Measurement of Hearing*. New York, McGraw-Hill Book Co., Inc.
Jerger, J. F. (1973): *Modern Developments in Audiology* (2nd ed.). New York, Academic Press.
Katz, J. (ed.) (1972): *Handbook of Clinical Audiology*. Baltimore, Williams and Wilkins Co.
Littler, T. S. (1965): *The Physics of the Ear*. Elmsford, N.Y., Pergamon.
Pierce, J. R., and David, E. E., Jr. (1958): *Man's World of Sound*. Garden City, N.Y., Doubleday and Co., Inc.
Plomp, R., and Smoorenberg, G. F. (eds.) (1970): *Frequency Analysis and Periodicity Detection in Hearing*. Leiden, Netherlands, A. W. Sijthoff.
Stevens, S. S. (ed.) (1951): *Handbook of Experimental Psychology*. New York, John Wiley and Sons, Inc.
Stevens, S. S., and Davis, H. (1938): *Hearing: Its Psychology and Physiology*. New York, John Wiley and Sons, Inc.
Tobias, J. V. (ed.) (1970): *Foundations of Modern Auditory Theory*, Vol. I. New York, Academic Press.
Tobias, J. V. (ed.) (1972): *Foundations of Modern Auditory Theory*, Vol. II. New York, Academic Press.
van Bergeijk, W. A., Pierce, J. R., and David, E. E., Jr. (1960): *Waves and the Ear*. Garden City, N.Y., Doubleday and Co., Inc.
von Békésy, G. (1960): *Experiments in Hearing*. New York, McGraw-Hill Book Co., Inc.
Wever, E. G., and Lawrence, M. (1954): *Physiological Acoustics*. Princeton, N. J., Princeton University Press.

Similarly, a few journals carry the bulk of the publications in the field. These include:

IEEE Transactions on Audio and Electroacoustics
Journal of the Acoustical Society of America
Journal of the Audio Engineering Society
Journal of Auditory Research
Journal of Experimental Psychology
Journal of Speech and Hearing Disorders
Journal of Speech and Hearing Research
Perception and Psychophysics
Psychonomic Science
Quarterly Journal of Experimental Psychology

INDEX

Note: Page references to illustrations are set in *italics*; page references to tables include the designation (t).

291